# Orofacial Pain Case Histories with Literature Reviews

*Editors*

DAVID A. KEITH
RONALD J. KULICH
MICHAEL E. SCHATMAN
STEVEN J. SCRIVANI

# DENTAL CLINICS OF NORTH AMERICA

www.dental.theclinics.com

January 2023 • Volume 67 • Number 1

# ELSEVIER

1600 John F. Kennedy Boulevard • Suite 1800 • Philadelphia, Pennsylvania, 19103-2899

http://www.dental.theclinics.com

**DENTAL CLINICS OF NORTH AMERICA Volume 67, Number 1**
**January 2023 ISSN 0011-8532, ISBN: 978-0-323-97290-1**

Editor: John Vassallo; j.vassallo@elsevier.com
Developmental Editor: Ann Gielou M. Posedio

*Dental Clinics of North America* (ISSN 0011-8532) is published quarterly by Elsevier Inc., 360 Park Avenue South, New York, NY 10010-1710. Months of issue are January, April, July, and October. Business and Editorial Offices: 1600 John F. Kennedy Boulevard, Suite 1800, Philadelphia, PA 19103-2899. Periodicals postage paid at New York, NY and additional mailing offices. Subscription prices are $333.00 per year (domestic individuals), $692.00 per year (domestic institutions), $100.00 per year (domestic students/residents), $388.00 per year (Canadian individuals), $897.00 per year (Canadian institutions), $100.00 per year (Canadian students/residents) $454.00 per year (international individuals), $897.00 per year (international institutions), and $200.00 per year (international students/residents). International air speed delivery is included in all *Clinics* subscription prices. All prices are subject to change without notice. **POSTMASTER:** Send address changes to *Dental Clinics of North America*, Elsevier Health Sciences Division, Subscription Customer Service, 3251 Riverport Lane, Maryland Heights, MO 63043. **Customer Service (orders, claims, online, change of address): Elsevier Health Sciences Division, Subscription Customer Service, 3251 Riverport Lane, Maryland Heights, MO 63043. Tel: 1-800-654-2452 (U.S. and Canada). Fax: 314-447-8029. E-mail: journalscustomerservice-usa@elsevier.com (for print support); journalsonlinesupport-usa@elsevier.com (for online support).**

*Reprints.* For copies of 100 or more, of articles in this publication, please contact the Commercial Reprints Department, Elsevier Inc., 360 Park Avenue South, New York, NY 10010-1710. Tel.: 212-633-3874; Fax: 212-633-3820; E-mail: reprints@elsevier.com.

*The Dental Clinics of North America* is covered in *MEDLINE/PubMed (Index Medicus), Current Contents/Clinical Medicine, ISI/BIOMED* and *Clinahl.*

# Contributors

## EDITORS

**DAVID A. KEITH, BDS, FDSRCS, DMD**
Professor, Department of Oral and Maxillofacial Surgery, Massachusetts General Hospital, Harvard School of Dental Medicine, Boston, Massachusetts, USA

**RONALD J. KULICH, PhD**
Professor, Department of Diagnostic Sciences, Tufts University School of Dental Medicine, Departments of Anesthesia, Critical Care and Pain Medicine, and Psychiatry, Massachusetts General Hospital/Harvard Medical School, Boston, Massachusetts, USA

**MICHAEL E. SCHATMAN, PhD**
Clinical Instructor, Department of Anesthesiology, Perioperative Care, and Pain Medicine, Department of Population Health–Division of Medical Ethics, NYU Grossman School of Medicine, New York, New York, USA; School of Social Work, North Carolina State University, Raleigh, North Carolina, USA

**STEVEN J. SCRIVANI, DDS, DMedSc**
Adjunct Lecturer, Formerly Adjunct Professor, Craniofacial Pain Center, Department of Diagnostic Sciences, Tufts University School of Dental Medicine, Boston, Massachusetts, USA

## AUTHORS

**OMAR F. ALASWAITI, DDS**
Resident, Orofacial Pain Program, Tufts University School of Dental Medicine, Boston, Massachusetts, USA

**SHURUQ A. ALTURKI, DDS**
Former Orofacial Pain Resident, Craniofacial Pain Center, Department of Diagnostics Sciences, Tufts University School of Dental Medicine, Boston, Massachusetts, USA

**SOWMYA ANANTHAN, BDS, DMD, MSD**
Department of Diagnostic Sciences, Associate Professor, Center for Temporomandibular Disorders and Orofacial Pain, Rutgers School of Dental Medicine, Newark, New Jersey, USA

**ROXANNE BAVARIAN, DMD, DMSC**
Department of Oral and Maxillofacial Surgery, Massachusetts General Hospital, Department of Oral and Maxillofacial Surgery, Harvard School of Dental Medicine, Boston, Massachusetts, USA

**TORE BJORNLAND, DDS, PhD**
Professor, Department of Oral Surgery and Oral Medicine, Institute of Clinical Dentistry, Faculty of Dentistry, University of Oslo, Oslo, Norway

**BRIANA J. BURRIS, DDS**
Department of Oral and Maxillofacial Surgery, Massachusetts General Hospital,
Department of Oral and Maxillofacial Surgery, Harvard School of Dental Medicine,
Boston, Massachusetts, USA

**CONRAD CHRABOL, MD**
Department of Biologic and Materials Sciences and Prosthodontics, University of
Michigan School of Dentistry, Michigan Neuroscience Institute (MNI), Headache &
Orofacial Pain Effort (H.O.P.E.) Laboratory, Ann Arbor, Michigan, USA

**ALEXANDRE F. DASILVA, DDS, DMEDSC**
Department of Biologic and Materials Sciences and Prosthodontics, University of
Michigan School of Dentistry, Michigan Neuroscience Institute (MNI), Headache &
Orofacial Pain Effort (H.O.P.E.) Laboratory, Ann Arbor, Michigan, USA

**RENY DE LEEUW, DDS, PhD, MPHA**
Professor, Division Orofacial Pain, University of Kentucky College of Dentistry, Lexington,
Kentucky, USA

**DIEGO FERNANDEZ-VIAL, DDS**
Division Orofacial Pain, University of Kentucky College of Dentistry, Lexington, Kentucky,
USA

**PATRICIA GUERRERO, DDS**
Assistant Professor, Craniofacial Pain Center, Department of Diagnostics Sciences, Tufts
University School of Dental Medicine, Boston, Massachusetts, USA

**SHRUTI HANDA, BDS, DMD**
Division of Orofacial Pain, Oral and Maxillofacial Surgery, Department of Surgery,
Massachusetts General Hospital, Harvard School of Dental Medicine, Boston,
Massachusetts, USA

**RACHEL HARRIS, DMD**
Harvard School of Dental Medicine, Boston, Massachusetts, USA

**GARY M. HEIR, DMD**
Department of Diagnostic Sciences, Professor and Program Director, Robert and Susan
Carmel Chair in Algesiology, Professor, Program and Clinical Director, Center for
Temporomandibular Disorders and Orofacial Pain, Rutgers School of Dental Medicine,
Newark, New Jersey, USA

**ESPEN HELGELAND, DDS, PhD**
Department of Clinical Dentistry, Faculty of Medicine, University of Bergen, Department of
Oral and Maxillofacial Surgery, Haukeland University Hospital, Bergen, Norway

**MARÍA F. HERNÁNDEZ-NUÑO DE LA ROSA, DDS, MS**
Assistant Professor and Director of Clinical Research, Department of Oral and
Maxillofacial Surgery, Tufts University School of Dental Medicine, Boston,
Massachusetts, USA

**NICOLE HOLLAND, DDS, MS**
Tufts University School of Dental Medicine, Boston, Massachusetts, USA

**XIAO-SU HU, PhD**
Department of Biologic and Materials Sciences and Prosthodontics, University of
Michigan School of Dentistry, Michigan Neuroscience Institute (MNI), Headache &
Orofacial Pain Effort (H.O.P.E.) Laboratory, Ann Arbor, Michigan, USA

**MYTHILI KALLADKA, GDS, MSD**
Institute for Oral Health, University of Rochester, Rochester, New York, USA

**SHEHRYAR NASIR KHAWAJA, BDS, MSc**
Consultant, Orofacial Pain Medicine, Department of Internal Medicine, Shaukat Khanum Memorial Cancer Hospital and Research Centers, Lahore, Pakistan

**DAJUNG J. KIM, PhD**
Department of Biologic and Materials Sciences and Prosthodontics, University of Michigan School of Dentistry, Michigan Neuroscience Institute (MNI), Headache & Orofacial Pain Effort (H.O.P.E.) Laboratory, Ann Arbor, Michigan, USA

**MANVITHA KUCHUKULLA, BDS, MDS**
Private Practice, Vermont, USA

**RONALD J. KULICH, PhD**
Professor, Department of Diagnostic Sciences, Tufts University School of Dental Medicine, Departments of Anesthesia, Critical Care and Pain Medicine, and Psychiatry, Massachusetts General Hospital/Harvard Medical School, Boston, Massachusetts, USA

**MANYOEL LIM, PhD**
Department of Biologic and Materials Sciences and Prosthodontics, University of Michigan School of Dentistry, Michigan Neuroscience Institute (MNI), Headache & Orofacial Pain Effort (H.O.P.E.) Laboratory, Ann Arbor, Michigan, USA

**PEER MORK-KNUTSEN, DDS**
Senior Resident, Department of Oral Surgery and Oral Medicine, Institute of Clinical Dentistry, Faculty of Dentistry, University of Oslo, Oslo, Norway

**THIAGO D. NASCIMENTO, DDS, MMEDSC, MS**
Department of Biologic and Materials Sciences and Prosthodontics, University of Michigan School of Dentistry, Michigan Neuroscience Institute (MNI), Headache & Orofacial Pain Effort (H.O.P.E.) Laboratory, Ann Arbor, Michigan, USA

**TORBJØRN Ø. PEDERSEN, DDS, PhD**
Associate Professor, Department of Clinical Dentistry, Faculty of Medicine, University of Bergen, Department of Oral and Maxillofacial Surgery, Haukeland University Hospital, Bergen, Norway

**TARA RENTON, BDS, MDSc, PhD**
Department of Oral Surgery, King's College London Dental Institute, London, United Kingdom

**ANNIKA ROSÈN, DDS, Dr Med Sci**
Professor, Department of Clinical Dentistry, Faculty of Medicine, University of Bergen, Department of Oral and Maxillofacial Surgery, Haukeland University Hospital, Bergen, Norway

**SHAIBA SANDHU, BDS, DDS**
Division of Orofacial Pain, Oral and Maxillofacial Surgery, Department of Surgery, Massachusetts General Hospital, Harvard School of Dental Medicine, Boston, Massachusetts, USA

**MICHAEL E. SCHATMAN, PhD**
Clinical Instructor, Department of Anesthesiology, Perioperative Care, and Pain Medicine, Department of Population Health–Division of Medical Ethics, NYU Grossman School of Medicine, New York, New York, USA; School of Social Work, North Carolina State University, Raleigh, North Carolina, USA

**STEVEN J. SCRIVANI, DDS, DMedSc**
Adjunct Lecturer, Formerly Adjunct Professor, Craniofacial Pain Center, Department of Diagnostic Sciences, Tufts University School of Dental Medicine, Boston, Massachusetts, USA

**JEFFRY R. SHAEFER, DDS, MS, MPH**
Department of Oral and Maxillofacial Surgery, Massachusetts General Hospital, Department of Oral and Maxillofacial Surgery, Harvard School of Dental Medicine, Boston, Massachusetts, USA

**FRÉDERIC VAN DER CRUYSSEN, MD, DDS, MHPM**
Department of Oral and Maxillofacial Surgery, University Hospitals Leuven, Department of Imaging and Pathology, OMFS-IMPATH Research Group, Faculty of Medicine, University Leuven, Leuven, Belgium

# Contents

> Masticatory myofascial pain disorders (MMPD) are a common group of orofacial pain conditions affecting the muscles of mastication, with headache and cervical disorders as well as chronic widespread pain and psychosocial disorders being common comorbid conditions. As their pathophysiology is multifactorial in nature, a multimodal and interdisciplinary approach should be considered. Overall treatment goals include decreasing pain and disability, increasing mandibular range of motion, and improving quality of life. This article describes a complex case exhibiting common characteristics of MMPD while additionally reviewing the literature on classification, pathophysiology, and evidence-based treatment planning.

> The improvement in diagnostic accuracy, improvement of the endoscopic equipment, better selection of patients for open TMJ surgery, and increased focus on research and education are promising for the treatment of the group of patients with TMJ derangements. In the future, prospective randomized clinical trials need to be performed to give the clinician guidelines as to which type of intervention should be chosen in a particular patient base on accepted criteria for diagnosis and treatment of TMJ derangement.

> Temporomandibular joint (TMJ) arthropathy is an umbrella term that may be applied to mechanical dysfunction or disease of one or both TMJs. This article presents a case of a 24-year-old woman who presented with symptoms of TMJ pain and jaw locking as an example to provide evidence-based recommendations for conducting a patient evaluation, initiating a diagnostic workup, formulating an assessment, and instituting various non-surgical modalities for the treatment of TMJ arthropathies.

Trigeminal neuralgia (TN) is a rare neuropathic pain disorder characterized by recurrent, paroxysmal episodes of short-lasting severe electric shock-like pain along the sensory distribution of the trigeminal nerve. Recent classification systems group TN into 3 main categories depending on the underlying pathophysiology. This article will present a case history and review the epidemiology, diagnostic criteria, classification, clinical features, diagnostic investigations, pathophysiology, and management of TN.

A case of a 64-year-old woman is reported, who developed new-onset pain over a preexisting area of right mandibular fullness. Clinical examination, MRI, and fine-needle aspiration cytology confirmed the diagnosis of a benign parotid gland tumor-pleomorphic adenoma, which was treated by total parotidectomy with complete removal of the tumor. When evaluating a patient with orofacial pain, oral health care providers should be cognizant of all potential differential diagnoses, especially in the setting of red flags such as persistent or enlarging facial swelling/fullness.

Pain is a common and most debilitating symptom of head and neck cancers (HNC). The prevalence of pain in HNC is nearly 70%. There are no universally accepted classification or diagnostic criteria for HNC-related pain, and currently, HNC-related pain is classified based on the underlying pathophysiological mechanism, the location of the tumor, and the protagonist of pain. The clinical presentation of HNC-related pain varies and can be similar to primary pain disorders. The management of HNC-related pain primarily consists of pharmacotherapy. However, in some cases, interventions may be needed. This article will present a case study and review the epidemiology, diagnostic criteria and classification, clinical features, pathophysiology, and HNC-related pain management.

This article presents the case of a patient with persistent right-sided jaw pain with a history of multiple temporomandibular joint surgeries in the setting of persistent widespread body pain, the causes of which were fibromyalgia and osteoarthritis with multiple joint replacements, as well as psychological diagnoses of PTSD and depression. Despite extensive treatment from her orofacial pain team in combination with neurology and neurosurgery, her severe pain persisted, likely due to the consequences of untreated PTSD and depression, which led to avoidance of activities that would exacerbate her pain and thus to further disability and emotional deterioration.

Migraine is a highly prevalent neurovascular disorder that affects approximately 15% of the global population. Migraine attacks are a complex cascade of neurologic events that lead to debilitating symptoms and are often associated with inhibitory behavior. The constellation of severe signs and symptoms during the ictal phase (headache attack) makes migraine the third most common cause of disability globally in both sexes under the age of 50. Misuse of pharmaceuticals, such as opiates, can lead to devastating outcomes and exacerbation of pain and headache attacks. A safe and well-tolerated non-pharmacological research approach is high-definition transcranial direct current stimulation over the M1.

This presentation describes a patient's extensive and expensive search for relief of pain in the orofacial area. The journey includes many diagnostic errors and failed and likely unnecessary treatments. A systematic approach to problem definition and rule-out reasoning for the differential diagnoses based on the International Classification of Orofacial Pain is described. Conservative treatment was implemented with satisfactory results. Common pitfalls in the management and treatment of complex pain patients are discussed.

Clear and effective communication is vital to quality patient care. More than 66 million Americans (21.5%) speak a language other than English at home, with more than 25 million (8.2%) speaking English "less than very well." Addressing language differences in the orofacial pain setting is of utmost importance to care quality, treatment outcomes, and overall health equity. In the case presented, language-related communication challenges affect the diagnosis and management of a patient with orofacial pain. This case highlights the significance of language discordance in the clinical setting and demonstrates the need for greater language access in the orofacial pain field.

# DENTAL CLINICS OF NORTH AMERICA

**FORTHCOMING ISSUES**

*April 2023*
**Temporomandibular Disorders: The Current Perspective**
Davis C. Thomas and Steven R. Singer, *Editors*

*July 2023*
**Clinical Decisions in Medically Complex Dental Patients, Part I**
Mel Mupparapu and Andres Pinto, *Editors*

*October 2023*
**Clinical Decisions in Medically Complex Dental Patients, Part II**
Mel Mupparapu and Andres Pinto, *Editors*

**RECENT ISSUES**

*October 2022*
**Dental Biomaterials**
Jack L. Ferracane, Luiz E. Bertassoni, and Carmem S. Pfeifer, *Editors*

*July 2022*
**Smile Design**
Behnam Bohluli, Shahrokh C. Bagheri, and Omid Keyhan, *Editors*

*April 2022*
**Special Care Dentistry**
Stephanie M. Munz, *Editor*

**SERIES OF RELATED INTEREST**

*Atlas of the Oral and Maxillofacial Surgery Clinics*

*Oral and Maxillofacial Surgery Clinics*

**THE CLINICS ARE AVAILABLE ONLINE!**
Access your subscription at:
www.theclinics.com

# Preface

# Orofacial Pain Case Histories with Literature Reviews

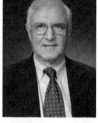
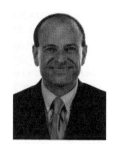

David A. Keith, BDS, FDSRCS, DMD      Ronald J. Kulich, PhD      Michael E. Schatman, PhD

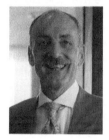

Steven J. Scrivani, DDS, DMedSc

*Editors*

Patients with orofacial pain (OFP) present to dental practices for treatment on a regular basis. In the United States, temporomandibular disorders (TMD) and OFP affect up to 15% of the adult population[1] with the prevalence of temporomandibular joint and muscle disorders ranging from 5% to 12%[2] and other OFP disorders reported in 10% to 25% of the general population.[3] While dentists receive excellent education regarding caries, periodontal disease, and other common dental disorders, their education in the broader area of pain and OFP, specifically, is frequently inadequate.

The field of OFP has been in existence for several decades[4] and has recently been recognized as a Specialty of Dentistry by the American Dental Association Committee of Dental Accreditation (CODA).[5] Currently, there are 12 CODA-approved OFP training programs in the United States,[6] although the number of specialists is small and unevenly distributed ("Language Access and Orofacial Pain"). Worldwide, several professional organizations exist[7]; however, OFP is poorly represented in certain countries.

In our work as educators, researchers, and authors, we have encountered a dearth of resources for the general dental practitioner seeking to advance their knowledge in this field. Textbooks tend to be out of date, and journal articles generally provide little

Dent Clin N Am 67 (2023) xiii–xvi
https://doi.org/10.1016/j.cden.2022.08.001
0011-8532/23/© 2022 Published by Elsevier Inc.

dental.theclinics.com

practical information. Continuing education courses exist but are frequently biased toward commercial products or procedures. These resources may provide valuable content but lack actual case histories with follow-up and current evidence-based literature reviews. The case-based teaching method has become popular in professional education, and OFP lends itself to this approach, as dentists can learn how to formulate a differential diagnosis, develop a treatment plan, and follow the patient's response, thus providing information they can use on a daily basis. The literature reviews have allowed the authors to expand on the case in a more traditional didactic style and cover the topic in a comprehensive manner. This approach is consistent with new curriculum standards for dental school education.[8]

In this issue, we have brought together authors from the clinical world, education, and research to present case histories of patients suffering from a wide variety of OFP conditions and headaches. The histories are comprehensive and represent real-life situations commonly encountered by clinicians. The authors offer differential diagnoses for each case and justify their choices and treatment plans. In many instances, as in real life, the diagnoses may be revised, and the treatment plan changed over time. The results are not always ideal. In addition to the case histories, each article contains an up-to-date, evidence-based review of the available literature on the subject that allows the practitioner to gain a broader view of the field.

The *Dental Clinics of North America* has been published for many years, with issues in 2007, 2013, and 2018 having concentrated on OFP, as well as an issue covering controlled substance risk and pain.[9] All have been authored by experts in the field and have covered the topic comprehensively. The approach of the editors of those issues was based on the common format of the *Dental Clinics of North America* and on our understanding of the field at that time. In recent years, much has changed. Hence, there is a need to update practicing dentists in new development in the field.

The OPPERA study (a 5-year study of 4000 patients funded by the National Institute of Dental and Craniofacial Research) has provided scientific evidence regarding TMD and accurately describes them as multifactorial, overlapping, and chronic pain conditions[10] ("Masticatory Muscle Pain," "Surgical Treatment of Temporomandibular Joint Derangement: 30-year Follow-Up of TMJ Discectomy, A Case Report and Literature Review," and "Temporomandibular Joint Arthropathy—Nonsurgical Management"). The International Classification of Orofacial Pain[11] has furthered our understanding of the numerous neuralgic pain conditions we see in the mouth and face; however, the definitions are by no means definitive ("Burning Mouth Disorder," "Chronic Facial Pain," "Persistent Idiopathic Dentoalveolar Pain Disorder," "Posttraumatic Trigeminal Neuropathic Pain Disorder," and "Trigeminal Neuralgia"). Research is shedding light on the nature of headaches such as migraines, which will determine innovative treatments in the future ("Headache and Orofacial Pain"). A common theme throughout these articles is the emphasis on Axis II diagnoses, that is, the diagnostic category in OFP practice that classifies comorbid psychological factors. It is well recognized that the psychological comorbidities of pain in general and OFP specifically are central to our understanding of patients' pain behaviors and the treatment outcomes. The article entitled, "Psychosocial Issues in Chronic Facial Pain," explores that connection in detail.

While cancer pain is ideally managed by specialists within the field of cancer care, such as palliative medicine, the lessons learned by our colleagues who do see these patients ("Cancer Pain") can be used in other chronic OFP conditions. The OFP patient brings many clinical and administrative challenges to dental practices, and these are considered in the articles "Pathology Mimicking Orofacial Pain" and "Challenges for the Dentist in Managing Orofacial Pain." By the very nature of the conditions with which they present, pain patients can be disruptive to the smooth running of a dental office, and special efforts may need to be taken to accommodate them. Overcoming racial, language, socioeconomic, and literacy barriers is a high priority in dentistry, as is becoming the case in medicine, generally, and the article, "Language Access and Orofacial Pain," addresses aspects of this problem.

The Editors thank John Vassallo and his talented team at Elsevier for guiding us through this process and for allowing us to step outside of the normal format of the *Dental Clinics of North America* to present this issue in an innovative fashion. They were "intrigued by the idea of having case studies along with the literature review—almost like a hybrid model of publishing," agreeing that "there is a new paradigm in dental education using case-based formats." We thank our colleagues, the article authors, for their commitment to this developing field and for the insights they have provided on the many challenging issues with which our patients present. Their dedication to clinical care, research, and education will ensure that the specialty of OFP will continue to make a significant impact on patient care in the future.

David A. Keith, BDS, FDSRCS, DMD
Department of Oral and Maxillofacial Surgery
Massachusetts General Hospital
Harvard School of Dental Medicine, Fruit St.
Boston, MA 02114, USA

Ronald J. Kulich, PhD
Department of Diagnostic Sciences
Tufts University School of Dental Medicine, 1, Kneeland St
Boston, MA 02111, USA

Department of Anesthesia
Critical Care and Pain Medicine
Massachusetts General Hospital/Harvard Medical School, 1, Kneeland St
Boston, MA 02111, USA

Michael E. Schatman, PhD
Department of Anesthesiology
Perioperative Care, & Pain Medicine
NYU Grossman School of Medicine, 550 1st Ave
New York, NY 10016, USA

Department of Population Health–Division of Medical Ethics
NYU Grossman School of Medicine, 550 1st Ave
New York, NY 10016, USA

Steven J. Scrivani, DDS, DMedSc
Formerly Craniofacial Pain Center
Department of Diagnostic Sciences
Tufts University School of Dental Medicine, 1, Kneeland St.
Boston, MA 02111, USA

*E-mail addresses:*
dkeith@mgh.harvard.edu (D.A. Keith)
RKulich@mgh.harvard.edu (R.J. Kulich)
Michael.Schatman@nyulangone.org (M.E. Schatman)
sjscrivani1@gmail.com (S.J. Scrivani)

**REFERENCES**

1. List T, Jensen RH. Temporomandibular disorders: old ideas and new concepts. Cephalalgia 2017;37(7):692–704.
2. National Institute of Dental and Craniofacial Research. Prevalence of TMJD and its signs and symptoms. https://www.nidcr.nih.gov/research/data-statistics/facial-pain/prevalence. [Accessed 16 March 2022].
3. Macfarlane TV, Glenny AM, Worthington HV. Systematic review of population-based epidemiological studies of oro-facial pain. J Dent 2001;29(7):451–67.
4. American Academy of Orofacial Pain. Home page. https://aaop.clubexpress.com/. [Accessed 16 March 2022].
5. Heir GM. Guest editorial. Orofacial pain, the 12th specialty: the necessity. J Am Dent Assoc 2020;151(7):469–71.
6. https://aaop.org/orofacial-pain-programs/. [Accessed 16 March 2022].
7. https://aaop.org/sister-academy/. [Accessed 16 March 2022].
8. Fricton J, Chen H, Shaefer JR, et al. New curriculum standards for teaching temporomandibular disorders in dental schools: a commentary. J Am Dent Assoc 2022;153(5):395–8. https://doi.org/10.1016/j.adaj.2021.11.013. PMID: 35184865.
9. Kulich RJ, Keith DA, Schatman ME. Controlled substance risk mitigation in the dental setting. Dent Clin NA 2020;64:3.
10. Slade GD, Ohrbach R, Greenspan JD, et al. Painful temporomandibular disorder: decade of discovery from OPPERA studies. J Dent Res 2016;95(10):1084–92.
11. International Classification of Orofacial Pain, 1st issue (ICOP). Cephalalgia 2020; 40(2):129–221.

# Masticatory Myofascial Pain Disorders

María F. Hernández-Nuño de la Rosa, DDS, MS[a],*, Patricia Guerrero, DDS[b], Shuruq A. Alturki, DDS[b], Steven J. Scrivani, DDS, DMedSc[b]

## KEYWORDS

- Temporomandibular disorders • Masticatory myofascial pain disorders
- Orofacial pain • Masticatory muscle pain • Interdisciplinary treatment

## KEY POINTS

- Temporomandibular disorders (TMD) are a heterogeneous group of musculoskeletal conditions affecting the orofacial region. Masticatory myofascial pain disorders (MMPD) are the most common subtype.
- The pathophysiology of MMPD is complex and multifactorial. Given that psychological comorbidities and sleep disturbances are considered contributing factors, the use of validated tools for behavioral and sleep screening is recommended.
- Proper management of MMPD will require a multimodal and interdisciplinary approach, including home care programs, pharmacotherapy, physical therapy, oral orthotic devices, behavioral therapy, and injection therapy.
- The prognosis of MMPD will be determined by the complexity of the case and patient compliance with the treatment plan.

## CASE PRESENTATION

A 28-year-old woman presents to the authors' clinic for a consultation at the request of her primary care physician. Her chief complaint is bilateral jaw pain, neck pain, and headaches ("this pain is killing me").

The patient states that she initially sought consultation with her general dentist shortly after her symptoms began, where she was evaluated and instructed to perform jaw stretching exercises daily at home. She was also recommended to use heat therapy consisting of hot compresses applied periodically to the affected areas. She reports that her symptoms "slightly improved" with this regimen but adds that she continued experiencing pain. She then had an oral orthotic appliance fabricated

[a] Department of Oral and Maxillofacial Surgery, Tufts University School of Dental Medicine, 1 Kneeland Street, Boston, MA 02111, USA; [b] Department of Diagnostics Sciences, Craniofacial Pain Center, Tufts University School of Dental Medicine, 1 Kneeland Street, Boston, MA 02111, USA
* Corresponding author.
*E-mail address:* maria.hernandez@tufts.edu

Dent Clin N Am 67 (2023) 1–11
https://doi.org/10.1016/j.cden.2022.07.001
0011-8532/23/© 2022 Elsevier Inc. All rights reserved.

that only had contacts on her front teeth. She had to stop using this device after a short period of time as she felt it was not helping at all to alleviate her symptoms and was causing much more pain and discomfort because of the excessive pressure on her front teeth. Subsequently, she sought consultation for her symptoms with her primary care physician, who prescribed an over-the-counter nonsteroidal anti-inflammatory drug (NSAID) and a low dose of a muscle relaxant to be taken as needed along with a course of physical therapy. She reports that this treatment was "somewhat helpful" in controlling her symptoms but states that they continued being troublesome for her. She was finally referred to the authors' clinic by her primary physician for further evaluation and management of her symptoms.

The patient states that her symptoms began abruptly around 4 years ago with no specific etiology and points to the preauricular, masseter, and temple areas bilaterally as well as to the cervical area. She does not report any history of trauma of any sort that might be associated with the onset of her symptoms. The pain is present every day, and she describes it as being continuous in duration, dull/pressure-like in quality, and moderate in intensity (Visual Analogue Scale or VAS = 6), but she adds that it fluctuates during the day, being usually more severe (VAS = 8) and throbbing in nature in the morning upon awakening. She reports having difficulty opening her mouth but denies having experienced or experiencing any bite changes, temporo-mandibular joint sounds, or episodes of jaw locking. Functional mandibular activities such as yawning or chewing hard foods, and several neck movements including side-bending and rotation exacerbate her pain. Daily life stressors also make her symptoms worse. She reiterated that prior treatments of a combination of neck and jaw stretching exercises, heat therapy with hot compresses, and relaxation techniques such as mindfulness along with over-the-counter ibuprofen and tizanidine 2 mg to be taken as needed seem to alleviate her symptoms (VAS = 2) but just temporarily.

Regarding the headaches, she states that they began shortly after her facial pain and adds that they seemed to be triggered by stressful events. She points to the fronto-temporal area bilaterally and describes them as pulsating in quality, and moderate (VAS = 6) in intensity. They occur once or twice a week, usually toward the end of the day, and last no longer than 2 to 3 hours or until she takes ibuprofen or acetaminophen. They are aggravated by routine physical activity. She reports sensitivity to light and sounds and mild nausea associated with her headaches but denies experiencing any visual, motor, or sensory disturbances or vomiting. She also denies experiencing autonomic symptoms such as upper eyelid ptosis, lacrimation, rhinorrhea, or conjunctival injection.

Her medical history is positive for seasonal allergies. She is otherwise healthy and denies having any other medical condition. However, she reports significant fatigue associated with her pain. She has not undergone any surgical procedure nor has she been hospitalized for this or any other medical condition. She reports being allergic to penicillin. Her family history is noncontributory. She uses an over-the-counter antihistamine as needed for her seasonal allergies and denies currently being on any other medication or medical treatment.

She is single and works full-time as a mental health counselor. She feels this occupation is stressful and the main source of her anxiety. She drinks 16 ounces of coffee and 24 ounces of water on average daily. She consumes one glass of alcohol 2 to 3 times a week, mostly wine and beer, but never alone. She currently smokes marijuana about once a month but denies using any other illegal substances. She has never smoked cigarettes. She states that she catches herself clenching her teeth often during the day and feels that she also does it at nighttime while asleep. She

**Table 1**
**Commonly used questionnaires for behavioral and sleep disturbances screening**

| Domain | Questionnaire | Case Patient's Score | Interpretation |
|---|---|---|---|
| Substance use | Tobacco, Alcohol, Prescription medications, and other Substance use (TAPS) tool | 0 | No use in the past 12 months |
| Anxiety | General Anxiety Disorder-7 (GAD-7) | 10 | Moderate anxiety |
| Depression | Patient Health Questionnaire (PHQ-9) | 0 | No depression |
| Sleep quality | Pittsburgh Sleep Quality Index (PSQI) | 7 | Poor sleep quality |
| Daytime sleepiness | Epworth Sleepiness Scale (ESS) | 12 | Mild sleepiness |
| Obstructive sleep apnea | Snoring, Tiredness, Observed apnea, high blood Pressure, Body mass index, Age, Neck circumference, and Male gender (STOP-BANG) questionnaire | 1 | Low risk |

cracks her neck on a regular basis as it provides temporary relief for her neck pain (**Table 1**).

She feels that she has a relatively high level of stress, mostly because of work. She defines herself as an anxious person with some significant generalized worry. She is being seen regularly by a therapist and feels that this approach has been beneficial for her (see **Table 1**).

She reports occasional inability to fall asleep and adds that she sometimes wakes up tired in the morning. She denies snoring or experiencing episodes of apnea during sleep. As stated previously, she feels that she might clench and grind her teeth while asleep (see **Table 1**).

Her vital signs were within normal limits (Pulse = 65, BP = 129/78, relative risk (RR) = 12, Temperature = 99.0°F). The patient had a coordinated and smooth gait. She was alert and oriented with a full range of affect. She answered all the questions appropriately but reported feeling anxious, worried, and fatigued.

Upon visual inspection of the head and neck, no gross atrophy or asymmetry was observed. Her skin was warm, dry, and intact with no lesions, rashes, areas of discoloration, or masses. A forward head and neck posture with rotation and side bending to the right was observed.

Upon further examination, there was moderate pain bilaterally (VAS = 6) upon palpation of the masseter and temporalis muscles. There was also mild pain bilaterally (VAS = 3) upon palpation of the sternocleidomastoid muscles, the suboccipital area, the posterior cervical paraspinal muscles, and the upper shoulder area. There was no pain or discomfort upon palpation of the lateral and posterior aspects of the temporomandibular joints. The cervical range of motion was within normal limits. The unassisted opening was 32 mm without pain, and the examiner-assisted opening was 38 mm with moderate pain (VAS = 6) in the masseter and temporalis muscles bilaterally. The path of opening/closing was straight. The range of motion in the horizontal axis was within normal limits bilaterally. There was no palpable or audible clicking, popping, or crepitus during the mandibular range of motion. There was no temporomandibular joint locking or subluxation during the examination. The clench and stretch tests were positive for pain in the masticatory muscles bilaterally and replicated the patient's chief complaint.

The dentition was sound and well restored. The oral mucosa and gingival tissues were pink and normal in appearance. The floor of the mouth was soft and nontender. The tongue appeared normal with no surface lesions, masses, or areas of discoloration. The tongue movements were normal. The hard and soft palate appeared normal, and there were no masses, lesions, or discoloration. The uvula was in the midline, and the palate had symmetric movement. The oral cavity was moist. The salivary flow was adequate upon palpation and stimulation of the glands. A Mallampati classification type I was observed. There was moderate pain bilaterally (VAS = 6) upon lateral resistance of lateral pterygoid muscle and palpation of the temporalis tendon, with referral toward the masseter and temporalis muscles. The occlusion was stable with posterior bilateral contacts. Signs of attrition were observed in the upper and lower molars.

The cranial nerve examination was normal.

The anterior area of the neck was soft and nontender. There were no palpable masses or lymphadenopathy. The thyroid did not present any masses and was mobile. The carotid pulsations were full and equal bilaterally, and no carotid bruit was heard upon auscultation.

A panoramic radiograph was taken (**Fig. 1**). The maxillary sinuses were symmetric and well aerated with no masses. The mandibular condyles were seated within the glenoid fossa. There appeared to be a distinct and intact cortical margin on both condylar heads with slight overlap superimposition of the glenoid fossa on the left. There were no signs of significant degenerative remodeling. The full dentition was present with erupted third molars in occlusion and minimal dental restorations. There were no signs of any gross dental or periodontal pathology. No bony lesions were observed in the maxilla or the mandible. The cortical margin of the mandibular bone was intact. No areas of calcification in the carotid artery system were observed.

Based on the history, clinical examination, and imaging study, this patient was diagnosed with masticatory myofascial pain disorder with referral, cervical myofascial pain disorder, and episodic migraine without aura. The awake and sleep bruxism and the anxiety, stress and sleep impairment were likely contributing to her symptoms.

As a treatment, a home care program was established. This program comprised patient education and reassurance, parafunctional behavior awareness and modification, a set of jaw and neck self-stretching exercises to be performed daily along

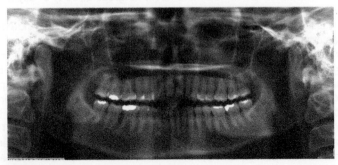

**Fig. 1.** Panoramic radiograph - Initial evaluation

with a gentle massage, and heat therapy with moist hot compresses. In addition, a course of pharmacotherapy consisting of meloxicam 15 mg to be taken once a day in the morning for 10 days along with cyclobenzaprine 10 mg to be taken at bedtime for 3 weeks was prescribed. A trial of magnesium 600 mg/d in divided doses to be used as a preventive medication for her migraine headaches was also suggested. An oral orthotic hard stabilization appliance to be used at nighttime consistently and during the day as needed was recommended. Lastly, the patient was referred for behavioral therapy evaluation and was advised to return to our clinic periodically for follow-up. She agreed to this treatment plan, and the oral orthotic appliance was made and inserted at this initial visit.

A few weeks later, at the first follow-up visit, the patient stated that she was following the self-management plan diligently. She was also using the oral orthotic hard stabilization appliance along with the prescribed medications and felt that this approach was being somewhat helpful to control her symptoms (VAS = 3) with her headaches presenting less frequently (3 episodes/month on average). She was also sleeping better. The patient reported that she preferred to hold off on consulting with a behavioral therapist but added that she decided to resign from her current job and pursue other professional opportunities. She stated that this decision had a positive impact on her life, as her level of stress and anxiety as well as her pain symptoms significantly decreased since then.

At the second follow-up office visit, the patient stated that she noticed a worsening in her symptoms and in her sleep quality shortly after completing the pharmacotherapy. She reported an increase in her bruxism, jaw pain/stiffness, and migraine headaches. She was using the oral orthotic hard stabilization appliance and following the home care program as she thought they were helpful in controlling her symptoms, but she discontinued the magnesium as it was not providing significant relief. The patient was prescribed nortriptyline 10 mg to be taken at bedtime and a course of physical therapy. Again, the benefits of behavioral medicine for the management of her pain and sleep symptoms were emphasized.

At the third follow-up office visit, the patient reported a significant improvement in her symptoms with occasional mild jaw pain (VAS = 1) and no headaches. She had been evaluated by a behavioral pain psychologist and was undergoing cognitive-behavioral therapy as well as practicing meditation regularly, which she reported as being helpful. Overall, she was doing well and felt that her symptoms had significantly improved since her initial evaluation. The patient was pleased with the outcome of the treatment plan. She was advised to continue with the home care program, the oral orthotic hard stabilization appliance, and the nortriptyline as prescribed along with the behavioral therapy treatment. At this point, she was asked to follow up as needed.

## CLINICS CARE POINTS

- Pre-existing psychological variables are etiologic risk factors for the development of temporomandibular disorders (TMD).[1] Thus, it is advised that a battery of standardized and validated tools for behavioral screening such as the GAD-7, the PHQ-9, and the TAPS tool be routinely completed by the patient with suspected TMD at the initial evaluation.

- Given the bidirectional relationship that exists between pain and sleep,[2] it is recommended that orofacial pain patients are screened for comorbid sleep disturbances at the initial evaluation via questionnaires such as the PSQI, ESS, and the STOP-BANG questionnaire. A multidisciplinary approach, including a potential referral to a sleep physician, will be required to properly manage these patients.

- Bruxism can occur during wakefulness (awake bruxism) and during sleep (sleep bruxism). The available evidence suggests that biologic, psychological, and exogenous factors might play a more important role than morphologic factors in the etiology of this clinical entity. A multimodal approach involving reversible treatments such as patient education, oral orthotic devices, pharmacotherapy, physiotherapy, and behavioral therapy is recommended for the management of bruxism.[3] In some cases, botulinum toxin injections might also be needed.[4]

- Low levels of magnesium have been linked to several neurologic diseases, including migraine headaches.[5] National and international guidelines suggest the use of several nutraceuticals, including oral magnesium, for the prophylaxis of this primary headache disorder.[6,7]

- Tricyclic antidepressants (TCAs) are commonly used in migraine prevention. Amitriptyline has the best evidence and is recommended as first-line therapy when comorbid sleep impartment is present.[8] Nortriptyline represents a good alternative because of its more favorable tolerability profile. TCAs, particularly nortriptyline, are also effective in the management of chronic masticatory muscle pain.[9]

## LITERATURE REVIEW
### Introduction

TMD are a broad group of musculoskeletal conditions that affect the masticatory muscles, temporomandibular joints, and associated structures.[10] Their pathophysiology is complex and multifactorial in nature. TMD are fairly common clinical entities with an estimated prevalence of 3% to 15% in western populations and a female-to-male ratio of approximately 2:1.[11] Around 50% of TMD patients are diagnosed with some type of masticatory myofascial pain disorder. TMD can manifest at any age, being the highest prevalence in young and middle-aged subjects (20 and 40 years of age) compared with the child and the elderly populations.[12] It is worth mentioning that this prevalence may differ for certain TMD conditions such as disc displacements and inflammatory-degenerative joint disorders, which are more predominant in subjects over the age of 30 and 50 years, respectively.[13]

The Diagnostic Criteria for Temporomandibular Disorders (DC/TMD), a validated screening and diagnostic tool published in 2014, describes the 12 most common types of TMD: myalgia, local myalgia, myofascial pain, myofascial pain with referral, arthralgia, headache attributed to TMD, 4 disc-related disorders, degenerative joint disease, and subluxation.[14] The classification released by the American Academy of Orofacial Pain in 2018 presents an expanded TMD taxonomy that also includes less common temporomandibular joint conditions such as movement disorders and muscle/joint neoplasms.[15] The International Classification of Headache Disorders (ICHD) 3rd edition, also published in 2018, classifies TMD as a subtype of secondary headaches, whereas the recently released International Classification of Orofacial Pain (ICOP) 1st edition categorizes them in two separated clusters of conditions, myofascial orofacial pain and temporomandibular joint pain.[16,17]

Masticatory myofascial pain disorders (MMPD) are considered a subtype of TMD. They affect the muscles of mastication, but often coexist with other conditions including headache and cervical disorders, as well as chronic widespread pain and psychosocial disorders such anxiety and depression. They might also present with masticatory muscle hypertrophy and parafunctional-related occlusal wear.[15] Proper history taking, evaluation, and diagnosis are essential to effectively treat patients with MMPD.

## Classification

The DC/TMD further divides myalgia (pain of muscle origin) into more specific sub-classes known as local myalgia, myofascial pain, and myofascial pain with referral, which can all be differentiated by provocation testing with palpation. In general, all these conditions can be modified by jaw movement, function, or parafunction. Local myalgia is defined as pain of muscle origin localized only to the site of palpation. Meanwhile, myofascial pain is similar to local myalgia with the difference being pain spreading beyond the site of palpation but within the boarder of the muscle. Lastly, myofascial pain with referral is described as local myalgia; however, the pain spreads beyond the boundary of the muscle, often to other portions of the head and face. The DC/TMD proposes a dual-axis criteria comprised of an Axis I for the physical assessment and an Axis II which focuses on the pain-related disability and on the psychosocial status of the patient, being both essential to achieve a proper diagnosis and subsequent management of TMD.[14]

The International Classification of Orofacial Pain Disorders (ICOP) 1st edition subcategorizes pain of muscle origin differently than the DC/TMD. This new classification adds a temporal distinction between conditions, with the aim of possibly improving therapeutic outcomes after further studies. The ICOP builds its diagnostic subcategories on whether the pain is primary or secondary. Under the umbrella of "primary myofascial orofacial pain," the terms "acute," "chronic," and "chronic infrequent/chronic frequent/chronic highly frequent" are used along with the description of "with/without referral." Within the subtype of secondary myofascial orofacial pain, the diagnostic terms of myositis, tendonitis, and muscle spasm are used.[17]

## Pathophysiology

The pathophysiology of MMPD is complex and controversial, with little evidence available on the presence of gross pathologic change in the muscle tissues in those patients suffering from these conditions.[18] Current literature supports the involvement of intrinsic and extrinsic variables such as environmental, emotional, behavioral, genetic, and physical factors in the initiation and maintenance of chronic muscle pain and dysfunction.[19]

Peripheral and central sensitization are believed to play an important role in the pathophysiology of MMPD. After muscle nociceptors become sensitized, neuropeptides are released peripherally increasing the response, and surpassing the normal threshold. This can translate to long-term changes in the central nervous system, known as central sensitization, which plays a role in the maintenance of chronic pain.[20] These neuroplastic changes have much in common with other comorbid conditions such as tension-type headache (TTH) and fibromyalgia.[18]

Sleep disturbances and psychological comorbidities such as anxiety and depression are considered strong contributing factors for MMPD with the potential to enhance the perception of pain. Thus, patients should be screened for any of these conditions and referred to the appropriate specialist. There are other elements such as genetics, gender, and lifestyle habits that can influence the perfection of pain. Certain genes (e.g., catechol-O-methyltransferase or COMT gene) code for different pain sensitivities making some individuals naturally more sensitive to pain than others.[21] Women are also more likely to suffer from these pain conditions.[11] Lastly, lifestyle habits such as nutrition, exercise, and smoking are also thought to contribute to MMPD, but further studies are needed.

### Treatment

Treatment options available for the management of MMPD are numerous and include various noninvasive modalities such as home care programs, pharmacotherapy, physical therapy, oral orthotic appliance therapy, behavioral therapy, and injection therapy. Given the complex and multifactorial nature of the pathophysiology of MMPD, an interdisciplinary approach including multiple modalities of treatment will be required. The treatment goals will be to decrease pain, increase mandibular range of motion and decrease disability, improving the overall quality of life of the patient.[19]

A comprehensive home care program is an essential component of any musculoskeletal pain management plan. This program should comprise a set of jaw and neck self-stretching exercises along with gentle massage and heat therapy with moist hot compresses over the affected areas. For some patients, the use of cold compresses might also provide pain relief. However, if the case is too complex or the patient does not comply with the recommended program, he or she should be referred to physical therapy for further management. Patient education and reassurance as well as awareness and modification of mandibular parafunctional habits will also play an important role in the management of MMPD.[15]

Various forms of pharmacotherapy are indicated in the management of MMPD. NSAIDs and steroids have been widely used for their analgesic and anti-inflammatory properties in these patients. However, their administration should be limited to the short term for the management of acute symptoms because of their adverse effect profile.[22] Skeletal muscle relaxants such as cyclobenzaprine can be beneficial and are commonly used for muscle pain, although there is insufficient evidence to strongly conclude their effectiveness.[23] TCAs are also used in the management of chronic pain conditions, including MMPD, because of their analgesic effect. Aside from sedation, which might be beneficial for these patients, common adverse effects are dizziness, dry mouth, palpitations, nausea, increased appetite, and constipation. Nortriptyline is preferred over amitriptyline because of its more favorable tolerability profile.[9] Of note, cyclobenzaprine is structurally similar to TCAs, which is important to consider when prescribing.[24] TCAs and selective serotonin reuptake inhibitors (SSRIs) and serotonin norepinephrine reuptake inhibitors (SNRIs) should be prescribed with caution in the elderly population and when managing polypharmacy. The clinician should also limit the prescription of benzodiazepines to the short term because of risk for addiction and screen the patient for potential substance use disorders before initiating therapy.[22,25] The patient's Prescription Drug Monitoring Program (PDMP) should be consulted periodically and the primary care physician should be kept informed when prescribing controlled substances.[25]

Oral orthotic appliances are commonly used in the management of TMD. Well-adjusted hard stabilization appliances have moderate quality evidence supporting their use, in particular for the management of myogenic TMD, when compared with other types of appliances and no treatment. Interestingly, they are equally effective when compared with other treatment modalities such as pharmacotherapy and physical and behavioral therapies. However, better-designed randomized control trials with larger samples sizes remain needed. Although still unclear, the hypothesized function of these devices includes a more even load distribution along with a reduction in the activity of masticatory muscles and an increase in the parafunctional habits awareness. Oral appliances can also serve to protect the teeth from the forces of attrition. Appliance therapy should always be considered as part of a broader rehabilitation treatment program.[26,27]

Behavioral therapy has shown to be successful in treating habit and lifestyle variables that contribute to chronic pain including myogenic conditions. After a thorough evaluation, psychologists will manage comorbid anxiety, depression, poor sleep, and sometimes, catastrophizing. Extreme focus on pain is known as catastrophizing, which has been suggested to increase pain severity, and sometimes disable patients.[28] Behavioral therapy treatment modalities focus on education, coping strategies, encouragement to engage in physical activity, sleep hygiene, stress reduction and habit changes.[29] Motivation to comply with treatment plans and ultimately improve quality of life are fundamental goals for the patient.

For those refractory patients, injection therapy with trigger point and/or botulinum toxin type A (BoT-A) injections might be good alternative. Trigger point injections (TPIs) using local anesthesia (LA) have shown to combine the antinociceptive effects of the LA along with the mechanical disruption of needling muscle fibers, resulting in pain relief. Although LA has not been demonstrated to improve MMPD, it has been shown to reduce muscle soreness and discomfort at the time of the procedure.[30] Lidocaine 0.25% without vasoconstrictor is recommended because of its low muscle toxicity.[31] TPIs are more invasive than other treatment modalities for MMPD; however, if pain reduction is not easily achieved, TPIs should be considered, because they have a low side-effect profile and are cost-effective for the patient.[32] Botulinum toxin type A (BoT-A) has shown to reduce pain in about one-third of patients with refractory MMPD. The presence of muscle hypertrophy was found to be a positive predictor for BoT-A therapy in these patients.[33] Interestingly, muscle hypertrophy is not considered to be a diagnostic criterion for identification of masticatory myalgia or myofascial pain disorders, as per the guidelines of the American Academy of Orofacial Pain and the DC/TMD.[14,15] BoT-A therapy can provide significant relief for up to 10 weeks, the reduction in size of the masticatory muscles being the most common adverse effect reported by these patients.[33] It is also an effective and well-tolerated preventive treatment for chronic headache disorders, in particular chronic migraine headache.[34]

## SUMMARY

MMPD are a common subtype of TMD affecting the muscles of mastication. Headache and cervical disorders as well as chronic widespread pain and psychosocial disorders are common comorbid conditions. Replication of the pain complaints along with a comprehensive history taking and clinical examination are the gold standard for diagnosis. MMPD present a complex and multifactorial pathophysiology. Their proper management will require a multimodal and interdisciplinary approach including various alternatives such as home care programs, pharmacotherapy, physical therapy, oral orthotic appliance therapy, behavioral therapy, and injection therapy. The treatment goals encompass the improvement of the patient's quality of life by decreasing pain, increasing mandibular range of motion, and decreasing disability. The prognosis will depend on the complexity of the case and on patient compliance with the treatment plan.

## REFERENCES

1. Fillingim RB, Ohrbach R, Greenspan JD, et al. Psychological factors associated with development of TMD: the OPPERA prospective cohort study. J Pain 2013; 14(12):T75–90.

2. Klasser GD, Almoznino G, Fortuna G. Sleep and orofacial pain. Dent Clin North Am 2018;62(4):629–56.

3. Lobbezoo F, Ahlberg J, Glaros AG, et al. Bruxism defined and graded: an international consensus. J Oral Rehabil 2013;40(1):2–4.
4. Fernandez-Nunez T, Amghar-Maach S, Gay-Escoda C. Efficacy of botulinum toxin in the treatment of bruxism: systematic review. Med Oral Patol Oral Cir Bucal 2019;24(4):e416–24.
5. Kirkland AE, Sarlo GL, Holton KF. The role of magnesium in neurological disorders. Nutrients 2018;10(6):730.
6. Holland S, Silberstein SD, Freitag F, et al. Evidence-based guideline update: NSAIDs and other complementary treatments for episodic migraine prevention in adults: report of the Quality Standards Subcommittee of the American Academy of Neurology and the American Headache Society. Neurology 2012; 78(17):1346–53.
7. Evers S, Afra J, Frese A, et al. EFNS guideline on the drug treatment of migraine–revised report of an EFNS task force. Eur J Neurol 2009;16(9):968–81.
8. Burch R. Migraine and tension-type headache: diagnosis and treatment. Med Clin North Am 2019;103(2):215–33.
9. Haviv Y, Zini A, Sharav Y, et al. Nortriptyline compared to amitriptyline for the treatment of persistent masticatory myofascial pain. J Oral Facial Pain Headache 2019;33(1):7–13.
10. Scrivani SJ, Keith DA, Kaban LB. Medical progress: temporomandibular disorders. N Engl J Med 2008;359(25):2693–705.
11. LeResche L. Epidemiology of temporomandibular disorders: implications for the investigation of etiologic factors. Crit Rev Oral Biol Med 1997;8(3):291–305.
12. Leresche L, Drangsholt M. Epidemiology of orofacial pain: prevalence, incidence, and risk factors. In: Sessle BJ, Lavigne GJ, Lund JP, et al, editors. Orofacial pain: from basic science to clinical management. 2nd edition. Chicago: Quintessence Publishing; 2008. p. 13–8.
13. Manfredini D, Piccotti F, Ferronato G, et al. Age peaks of different RDC/TMD diagnoses in a patient population. J Dent 2010;38(5):392–9.
14. Schiffman E, Ohrbach R, Truelove E, et al. Diagnostic criteria for temporomandibular disorders (DC/TMD) for clinical and research applications: recommendations of the International RDC/TMD consortium network* and orofacial pain special interest groupdagger. J Oral Facial Pain Headache 2014;28(1):6–27.
15.. de Leeuw R, Klasser G. Orofacial pain: guidelines for assessment, diagnosis and management. 6th edition. Hanover Park, IL: Quintessence Publishing Co, Inc; 2018. p. 143–207.
16. Headache classification committee of the international headache society (IHS) the international classification of headache disorders, 3rd edition. Cephalalgia 2018;38(1):1–211.
17. International classification of orofacial pain, 1st edition (ICOP). Cephalalgia 2020; 40(2):129–221.
18. Lorduy KM, Liegey-Dougall A, Haggard R, et al. The prevalence of comorbid symptoms of central sensitization syndrome among three different groups of temporomandibular disorder patients. Pain Pract 2013;13(8):604–13.
19. Svensson P, Sharav Y, Benoliel R. Myalgia, myofascial pain, tension-type headaches, and fibromyalgia. In: Sharav Y, Benoliel R, editors. Orofacial pain and headache. 2nd edition. Chicago: Quintessence Publishing Co, Inc.; 2015. p. 195–256.
20. Mense S. The pathogenesis of muscle pain. Curr Pain Headache Rep 2003;7(6): 419–25.

21. Slade GD, Ohrbach R, Greenspan JD, et al. Painful temporomandibular disorder: decade of discovery from OPPERA studies. J Dent Res 2016;95(10):1084–92.
22. Kalladka M, Young A, Khan J. Myofascial pain in temporomandibular disorders: Updates on etiopathogenesis and management. J Bodyw Mov Ther 2021;28: 104–13.
23. Leite FM, Atallah AN, El Dib R, et al. Cyclobenzaprine for the treatment of myofascial pain in adults. Cochrane Database Syst Rev 2009;CD006830.
24. Honda M, Nishida T, Ono H. Tricyclic analogs cyclobenzaprine, amitriptyline and cyproheptadine inhibit the spinal reflex transmission through 5-HT2 receptors. Eur J Pharmacol 2003;458(1–2):91–9.
25. Keith DA, Hernández-Nuño de la Rosa MF. Special screening resources: strategies to identify substance use disorders, including opioid misuse and abuse. Dental Clin 2020;64(3):513–24.
26. Fricton J, Look JO, Wright E, et al. Systematic review and meta-analysis of randomized controlled trials evaluating intraoral orthopedic appliances for temporomandibular disorders. J Orofac Pain 2010;24(3):237–54.
27. Al-Moraissi EA, Farea R, Qasem KA, et al. Effectiveness of occlusal splint therapy in the management of temporomandibular disorders: network meta-analysis of randomized controlled trials. Int J Oral Maxillofac Surg 2020;49(8):1042–56.
28. Reiter S, Eli I, Mahameed M, et al. Pain catastrophizing and pain persistence in temporomandibular disorder patients. J Oral Facial Pain Headache 2018;32(3): 309–20.
29. Williams ACC, Fisher E, Hearn L, et al. Psychological therapies for the management of chronic pain (excluding headache) in adults. Cochrane Database Syst Rev 2020;8(8):CD007407.
30. Walker JW, Shah BJ. Trigger point injections: a systematic, narrative review of the current literature. SN Compr Clin Med 2020;2(6):746–52.
31. Iwama H, Akama Y. The superiority of water-diluted 0.25% to neat 1% lidocaine for trigger-point injections in myofascial pain syndrome: a prospective, randomized, double-blinded trial. Anesth Analg 2000;91(2):408–9.
32. Borg-Stein J, Iaccarino MA. Myofascial pain syndrome treatments. Phys Med Rehabil Clin N Am 2014;25(2):357–74.
33. Khawaja SN, Scrivani SJ, Holland N, et al. Effectiveness, safety, and predictors of response to botulinum toxin type a in refractory masticatory myalgia: a retrospective study. J Oral Maxillofac Surg 2017;75(11):2307–15.
34. Herd CP, Tomlinson CL, Rick C, et al. Cochrane systematic review and meta-analysis of botulinum toxin for the prevention of migraine. BMJ Open 2019;9(7): e027953.

# Surgical Treatment of Temporomandibular Joint Derangement

## 30-Year Follow-Up of Temporomandibular Joint Discectomy, a Case Report and Literature Review

Tore Bjornland, DDS, PhD*, Peer Mork-Knutsen, DDS

### KEYWORDS

- Temporomandibular joint derangement • Surgical treatment • Arthroscopy
- Discectomy • Disc repair

### KEY POINTS

- The diagnosis and treatment of temporomandibular joint (TMJ) derangement has evolved during the past 4 decades. Surgical interventions have evolved simultaneously, but different treatment modalities have been used without clear descriptions of the surgical procedure used for the different diagnoses. Numerous reports have been published, but there have been few long-term follow-up studies. Some procedures (eg, discectomy with replacement with Teflon-Proplast implants) have resulted in destruction of the TMJ by heavy foreign body reactions. This has resulted in skepticism among some providers regarding the advisability of TMJ surgery for this condition. .

- It is important that patients with TMJ derangement undergo the appropriate surgical treatment after examination, imaging, and as indicated, conservative treatment, which should not continue for more than 6 months if unsuccessful. In this presentation, the different surgical treatment modalities are discussed, and the authors present a case with a 30-year follow-up after bilateral discectomy without replacement of the disc.

- The wide range of functional changes and pathologic conditions represented by the term TMD (temporomandibular disorders) may be more confusing than clarifying in the decision-making process. When dealing with patients with complex TMJ symptomatology one should consider a multidisciplinary approach in both diagnosis and treatment.

- With appropriate decision making and use of the appropriate surgical techniques, treatment of TMJ derangement can be successful in the long term with few complications.

---

Department of Oral Surgery and Oral Medicine, Institute of Clinical Dentistry, Faculty of Dentistry, University of Oslo, Box 1109 Blindern, Oslo N-0371, Norway
* Corresponding author.
*E-mail address:* tore.bjornland@odont.uio.no

Dent Clin N Am 67 (2023) 13–25
https://doi.org/10.1016/j.cden.2022.07.002
0011-8532/23/© 2022 Elsevier Inc. All rights reserved.

## INTRODUCTION

During the past few decades, diagnosis and treatment of temporomandibular joint (TMJ) derangement have evolved tremendously. In a short communication with 2 case reports, Annandale[1] was the first to describe open TMJ surgery with repositioning of the disc for this condition. Up until the 1970s, the diagnosis of joint disease was mainly based on the osseous changes, but with the introduction of arthrography, many studies described internal derangement of the TMJ disc.[2–8] Wilkes[3] is credited with the first classification system. Since then, other efforts have been made to standardize the diagnostic criteria, and one is the Diagnostic Criteria for Temporomandibular Disorders (DC/TMD).[9] Another focused on the surgical classification,[10] and a third one used the Delphi process aiming to produce recommendations for a standardized evaluation in relation to TMJ dysfunction.[11]

As technology evolved, arthrographic examination was combined with computerized tomography (CT),[12] and now evaluation of the osseous changes are performed with CT, while MRI studies are used to evaluate soft tissue changes, joint effusions, osteoarthritis, and the different stages of disk displacement. Ultrasound may also be used in the examination of the TMJ, but the interpretation is difficult (**Fig. 1**). Despite the development of these newer imaging techniques and the effort to make accurate classifications, it has been difficult to apply strict diagnostic criteria in order to determine the correct treatment option, as the signs and symptoms that can occur among patients with the same diagnosis may vary substantially.

Indeed, the definition of TMJ derangement has been debated, and there is common agreement that it includes different stages of disc displacement. For many years, the classification of internal derangement by Wilkes[13] has been looked upon as a standard and has been used in the diagnosis of TMJ derangement and in describing the indications for different surgical approaches. One of the questions raised is whether the diagnosis and treatment decisions should be based solely on the position of the disc, or if deterioration of the TMJ, such as osteoarthritis, remodeling, and ankylosis, should be included in the definition, and if so should additional types of disease focused classification be used.[9–11]

Positive treatment outcomes for derangement of the TMJ will vary considerably depending on diagnostic accuracy, the patient's symptoms, and the treatment modalities offered by the providers, among other factors.

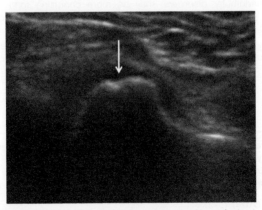

**Fig. 1.** Ultrasound of left TMJ in a 56-year old woman. An irregularity is seen on the top of the condyle (*arrow*) indicating remodeling and osteoarthritis.

Surgical intervention for TMJ derangement may include a wide range of procedures from injections, arthrocentesis, arthroscopy, eminectomy, condylotomy, disc repair and discectomy, to total joint prosthesis.[14–36] The various diagnoses with types of suggested surgical procedures are listed in **Table 1**. Most of the publications are not randomized controlled studies, and some have only short-term follow-up periods. There are, however, some exceptions with long-term follow-up of discectomies,[17,26,37–39] and some important systematic reviews have recently been published[40,41]. Liapaki and colleagues[41] performed a systematic review of randomized clinical trials (RCT) on different intra-articular drugs for TMJ osteoarthritis, and they found that all injectables in conjunction with arthrocentesis were effective in alleviating pain and improving mandibular function. In a meta-analysis of RCTs, Al-Moraissi and colleagues[40] concluded that minimally invasive TMJ procedures, both on a short- and intermediate-term basis, showed superiority in the treatment of arthrogenous TMJ conditions.

**Table 1**
**Account of symptom and pathology based conditions and their possible surgical treatment options**

| Diagnosis | Putative Treatment Alternatives |
|---|---|
| Disc displacement with reduction (mild or no pain) | Nonsurgical treatment |
| Disc displacement with reduction (moderate-to-severe pain) | 1. Nonsurgical treatment<br>2. Surgical treatment<br>• Discectomy with or without replacement<br>• Modified condylotomy<br>• Disc repositioning<br>• Arthroscopy<br>• Arthrocentesis |
| Disc displacement without reduction | 1. Nonsurgical treatment<br>2. Surgical treatment<br>• Arthrocentesis<br>• Arthroscopy<br>• Discectomy with or without replacement |
| Osteoarthritis | 1. Nonsurgical treatment<br>2. Surgical treatment<br>• Arthrocentesis<br>• Arthroscopy<br>• Cortisone injection<br>• Hyaluronic acid injection<br>• Open surgery may be indicated |
| Arthritis | 1. Nonsurgical treatment<br>2. Surgical treatment<br>• Cortisone injection<br>• Arthrocentesis<br>• Arthroscopy<br>• Open surgery may be indicated |
| Ankylosis | Surgical treatment<br>• Gap-osteotomy<br>• Gap-osteotomy with interpositioning of muscle/fascia or fat<br>• Total joint replacement (prosthesis)<br>• Costochondral graft<br>• Distraction osteogenesis |

*Data from* Lund B, Ulmner M, Bjørnland T, et al. A disease-focused view on the temporomandibular joint using a Delphi-guided process. J Oral Sci 2020; 62: 1-8.

Open surgery for TMJ disc displacement with or without reduction and the associated deterioration of the joint may be indicated.[10,11] Some long-term studies have been published, but without reference to control groups.[17,37,39] To the best of the authors' knowledge, no reports of sham operations have been published for TMJ surgery as has been done for shoulder surgery,[42] which have shown that sham operations may give the same results compared with labial repair or biceps tenodesis.

Treatment of any type of TMD should always be based on subjective measures of functional disability and screening for psychosocial factors, which may need to be dealt with before treatment. Surgical interventions should be as minimally invasive as possible, and it is important that the interventions used have been documented with long-term follow-up studies.

For this case presentation, the authors have chosen discectomy as the surgical treatment of TMJ derangement.

## CASE PRESENTATION

A 22-year-old man was referred to the Department of Oral Surgery and Oral Medicine, Faculty of Dentistry, University of Oslo, because of pain in both TMJ areas. He had a history of blunt trauma to the face 4 to 5 years previously (car accident), and had since experienced TMJ pain and reduced opening of the mouth, which had amplified after a forced mouth opening during a regular dental checkup. The pain was mainly referred to the right TMJ, was of constant character and exacerbated during eating, and increased in the afternoon. In addition, he reported headache that was diagnosed as tension type headache that was described as 7 on a Visual Analogue Scale (0–10 cm). He had previously been treated with physical therapy and a hard acrylic orthotic appliance, without improvement. There was no previous history of illness or allergy, and he had not had any need of psychological or neurologic consultations. There was no history of sleep disturbances, bruxism, or other pain syndromes. The patient used naproxen 250 mg 3 times daily for pain relief.

On examination, the patient presented with a maximal interincisal opening of 42 mm. The dentition showed a stable occlusion without signs of excessive wear or parafunctional habits. On opening the mouth, a click was noted after 30 mm, with deviation of the mandible toward the left. There were normal lateral movements, and pain was elicited from the muscles of mastication when palpated. At the time that this case was being treated, tomograms and arthrography in addition to panoramic radiographs were the only available radiographic images of the TMJ. The patient was referred for a panoramic radiograph and transcranial TMJ images (**Fig. 2**), and adjustment to the previously made acrylic appliance was done. A preliminary diagnosis of disc displacement with reduction was established, and a follow-up appointment was scheduled for 3 months.

On returning, the patient described little to no reduction in pain relief after using the acrylic appliance. He was then referred for arthrography (available at the time) that confirmed the suspected diagnosis of an anterior disc displacement with a late reduction in both TMJs, with no hard tissue changes observed in the articular fossa or mandibular condyle and normal translational movements of both condyles (**Fig. 3**). Before the arthrography, local anesthesia of the right TMJ joint was performed with 1.8 mL lidocaine 20 mg/mL with adrenaline 12.5 μg/mL. The anesthesia served 2 purposes: to minimize pain during the arthrographic procedure and to examine if this could influence on the present joint pain. The patient could immediately report on a good effect on the TMJ pain. Another adjustment to the orthotic appliance was done, and the patient was instructed to try physical therapy.

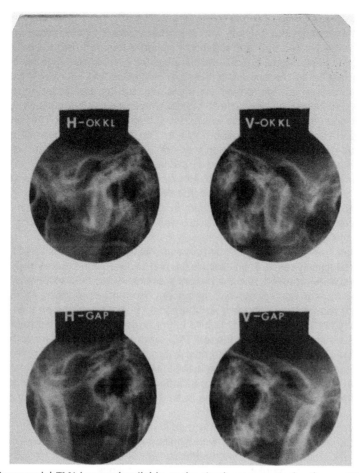

**Fig. 2.** Transcranial TMJ images (available at the time) preoperatively of case, 22-year old man. H means right side, V means left side. Upper images in centric occlusion, lower two in maximal mouth opening.

Twenty-one months after the initial consultation, the patient had not experienced reduction in pain after use of an acrylic appliance or physical therapy. Discectomy of the right TMJ seemed indicated, because his symptoms had not been relieved by conservative measures. Discectomy had achieved much acceptance in the

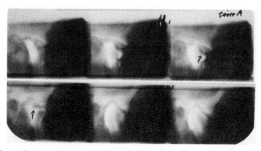

**Fig. 3.** Arthrography taken preoperatively of right TMJ in a 22-year old man. Arrows indicate inferior part of the displaced disc.

Scandinavian countries with long-term observations,[17,37] and therefore this surgical procedure was offered to patients with disc displacement where conservative treatment had not alleviated pain and reduced function. After informing the patient about the possibility of a surgical option, and the possible complications of this treatment, the patient accepted discectomy of the right TMJ based on informed consent. The surgical procedure was performed via a preauricular incision under general anesthesia. After injecting 5 mL lidocaine 10 mg/mL with adrenaline 5 μg/mL, a skin incision was made, and the temporal fascia was exposed by blunt dissection. The joint capsule was exposed via an inverted L-shaped incision. The radiologic diagnosis of an anterior disc displacement with late reduction was confirmed by surgical observations. The disc was excised, and the wound was closed in layers. The patient had normal motor and sensory function postoperatively. He was given a prescription for cephalexin 500 mg 2 times daily for 7 days and paracetamol 500 mg with codeine 30 mg and given instructions to eat only soft foods for the next 2 weeks before gradually starting with jaw exercises. A scheduled check-up was arranged 7 days later. There was no change in the occlusion postoperatively.

A week later, he described a red rash covering his whole body, which was thought to be a hypersensitivity reaction on cephalexin, and this was immediately discontinued. The sutures were removed, and the patient was scheduled for a follow-up 3 months later. Three months postoperatively, the patient had a mouth opening of 45 mm and a significant reduction in TMJ pain and the tension type headache on the right side. Tomography showed satisfactory results in the right TMJ (**Fig. 4**). However, he had developed similar symptoms in the left TMJ, and he was referred for arthrography of the left TMJ, with follow-up in 6 months. Arthrography of the left TMJ revealed anterior disc displacement with adhesions in the lower joint compartment. The same procedure with local anesthesia was also performed on the left side prior to arthrography, with good effect on the TMJ pain. The patient was offered a discectomy of the left TMJ, which he accepted.

Discectomy of the left TMJ was performed in the same manner as on the right side, and an anterior disc displacement with significant adhesions in the lower compartment with the mandibular condyle was observed. The wound was closed in layers, and the surgery was completed without any complications.

After 1 week, the patient had a mouth opening of 32 mm. He was instructed in jaw exercises and use of the acrylic appliance. A follow-up 3 months postoperatively was scheduled. At this time, the patient presented with no pain but experienced muscle fatigue after longstanding jaw activity. He had an interincisal opening of 44 mm, and crepitation from the left TMJ. The patient was scheduled for a follow-up after 12 months.

One year after discectomy of the left TMJ, the patient had an interincisal opening of 45 mm but reduced lateral movements measuring 3 mm bilaterally. There was some crepitation from the left TMJ, and mild myalgia. The patient was scheduled for follow-up in another year.

Three-years postoperatively, the patient experienced no pain from the TMJs. He had crepitation sounds in the left TMJ, maximal interincisal opening of 45 mm, and laterotrusive movements of 3 mm bilaterally. Transcranial images revealed bony changes in the left TMJ, with insignificant reduced translational movement (**Fig. 5**).

The patient was followed annually for the first 5 years and at 10 years and 30 years after the operations, with clinical and radiologic examinations. The initial preoperative visual analog scale (VAS)-score was 7 out of 10, and on the 10-year follow-up 0 out of 10. Ten years postoperatively, crepitation on the left TMJ was observed, and he had a

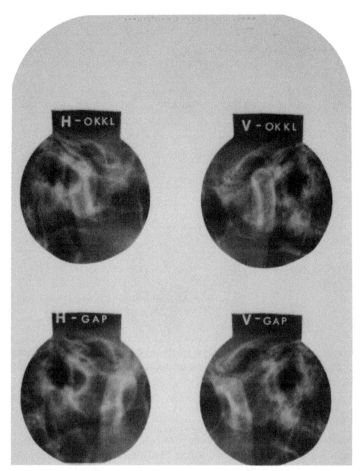

**Fig. 4.** Transcranial TMJ images (available at the time) 3 months postoperatively after right discectomy, in case, 22-year old man. H means right side, V means left side. Upper images in centric occlusion lower 2 images in maximal mouth opening.

maximum interincisal opening of 50 mm. The laterotrusive movements were 12 mm to the right and 10 mm to the left, which was a significant improvement compared with the results of the 3-year follow-up. Tomographic radiographs (available at the time) showed close to normal intra-articular findings in the right TMJ, and osteoarthritis and remodeling in the left TMJ. There were satisfactory translational movements in the right joint, and slightly reduced translational movements in the left joint.

Thirty years postoperatively, the patient had no pain in the TMJs. Crepitation sounds from both TMJs were noted. The patient had a maximum interincisal opening of 47 mm, and 10 mm laterotrusive movements bilaterally. He had not experienced any temporomandibular or myofascial pain since the last follow-up. Tomographic radiographs showed normal intra-articular findings in the right TMJ, which was comparable with preoperative findings, with normal translational movements. The left TMJ showed comparable results with radiographs taken 20 years earlier, with slightly reduced condylar translation, but without obvious changes indicating osteoarthritis. Panoramic radiograph (**Fig. 6**) indicated no abnormal attrition of teeth.

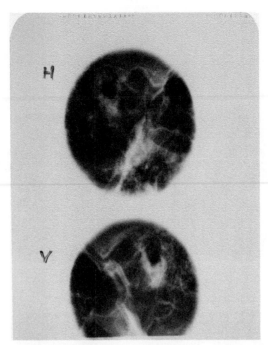

**Fig. 5.** Transcranial TMJ images (available at the time) 3 years postoperatively after bilateral discectomies in case, 22-year old man. H means right side, V means left side. Both images taken during maximal mouth opening.

## DISCUSSION

Surgical treatment of TMJ derangement is controversial and sometimes contradictory. Despite long traditions with different surgical TMJ interventions, surprisingly, few systematic reviews and RCTs dealing with surgical TMJ intervention have been performed.[40,41] Even with the focus on establishing diagnostic criteria for TMJ disease and treatment options,[9–11] the results may have included too many diagnoses under the TMD umbrella. The wide range of functional changes and pathologic conditions represented by the term TMD may be more confusing than clarifying in the treatment decision-making process. Should the conditions be treated conservatively with

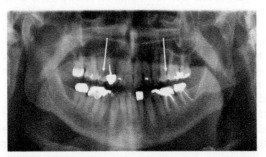

**Fig. 6.** Panoramic radiograph of case, 30 years after bilateral discectomies indicating no abnormal attrition of teeth (*arrows*).

counseling, medication, or splints, or with surgical interventions? Moreover, how long should conservative treatment be performed prior to surgical interventions? These questions are still to be answered. The ultimate decision as to which surgical technique one should chose depends on patient and surgeon preference but should be guided by long-term evidence based on studies and not anecdotal information.[17,37,39]

Furthermore, the providers' preferences and their skills may influence the different treatment options. Scrutinizing review articles, it seems obvious that the treatment of TMJ/TMD should start with less invasive procedures,[40,41,43] mainly because of the fear of possible surgical complications. Laskin[44] stated that one should focus on specific diagnostic entities instead of including too many symptoms under 1 diagnostic umbrella. There might be situations where the optimal treatment for the patient is delayed, because the whole treatment panorama from conservative to surgical interventions is being employed. It is of great importance that the provider establish a disease-focused view of the TMJ[11] and that the surgical methods should be based on well-defined and well-characterized patient populations. In the absence of a clear diagnostic classification, studies on surgical procedures may give the unfortunate impression of a technique in search of a disease. In dealing with patients with complex TMJ symptoms, the provider should consider a multidisciplinary approach in diagnosis and treatment. There are now more centers dealing with diagnosis, treatment, education of health providers, and research in oro-facial pain.

Symptoms from the TMJ are frequently reported with some differences between men and women, with an overall prevalence of 16% to 52%.[45] How many are in need of the different treatments is not clear, and may depend on the availability of health providers working with TMJ-related problems. Recent publications emphasize the importance of using the right diagnostic criteria and prospective randomized controlled studies.[25,36,46–49] Furthermore, long-term observations of the results are of high importance[17,37,39] to determine the success rate of the different procedures. Likewise, complications during the surgical procedures may be serious for the patient and may also negate the results of the procedures.[50]

In their case, the authors performed open surgery with discectomy without replacement with either alloplastic or autogenous materials. Disc repositioning has been a successful treatment with the use of arthroscope,[51] but long-term follow-up has indicated that even with favorable results regarding function and pain, the disc may persist in an abnormal anterior position.[52] In this present case, the authors performed discectomy on the left side 6 months after discectomy on the right side. During that period, the patient had self-exercise as prescribed after surgery, but no other treatment. It was an assumption that because the first surgery was successful, the other side would be similar successful. This may not always be the case, but it worked in this case after the evaluation of the clinical and radiological findings. Pain from the TMJ and the surrounding musculature may also make a decision for surgery difficult, but in previous studies, the authors have shown that TMJ surgery may also have positive effect on pain from the masticatory muscles, not only TMJ pain.[39,53]

Discectomy and replacement with an alloplast was used with promising results in open TMJ surgery, but later it was shown that some of these materials created foreign body reactions.[54] The use of temporalis myofascial flap or different autografts such as auricular cartilage graft and abdominal dermis-fat graft has been used, and favorable results have been reported. In a meta-analysis, discectomy without or with different autogenous grafts showed comparable success rates, and the conclusion was that interpositional autogenic grafts were not superior to discectomy alone. Comparisons between alloplastic materials and discectomy alone were in favor of discectomy without replacement.[55]

In discectomy without replacement, as in this case, one may see changes such as flattening of the condyle and osteophytes and reduced joint space that may resemble osteoarthrosis. These changes may also be seen in nontreated joints[47] observed on CT, indicating that these changes may by adaptive rather than pathologic changes. Before the 1990s, arthrography was widely used, as in this case, and could be compared with the observations made on MRI.[56] MRI has great advantages in that it is not necessary with interventions in the TMJ with injection of contrast material, it is not radiation, and the diagnostic accuracy now is superior to arthrotomography concerning all soft tissue changes in the TMJ.

## SUMMARY

The improvement in diagnostic accuracy, improvement of the endoscopic equipment, better selection of patients for open TMJ surgery, and increased focus on research and education are promising for the treatment of the group of patients with TMJ derangements. In the future, prospective randomized clinical trials need to be performed to give the clinician guidelines as to which type of intervention should be chosen in a particular patient base on accepted criteria for diagnosis and treatment of TMJ derangement.

## CLINICS CARE POINTS

- TMJ surgery should be performed after a period with conservative treatment/counseling.
- Clinical and radiological evaluation should be performed according to international guidelines.
- Minimal invasive TMJ surgery should be performed if possible.
- TMJ surgical procedures should be based on long-term evidence based studies.
- Physical therapy and self exercise should be performed after TMJ surgery in order to achieve good function.

## ACKNOWLEDGMENTS

The authors thank Dr Caroline Hol, University of Oslo for providing the radiographic images.

## DISCLOSURE

No disclosure or funding.

## CONFLICT OF INTEREST

None.

## REFERENCES

1. Annandale T. On displacement of the inter-articular cartilage of the lower jaw, and its treatment by operation. Lancet 1887;1:411.
2. Farrar WB. Diagnosis and treatment of anterior dislocation of the articular disc. NYJ Dent 1971;41:348–51.
3. Wilkes CH. Arthrography of the temporomandibular joint in patients with the TMJ pain-dysfunction syndrome. Minn Med 1978;61:645–52.

4.  Katzberg RW, Dolwick MF, Bales DJ, et al. Arthrotomography of the temporomandibular joint: new technique and preliminary observations. Am J Roentgenol 1979;132:949–55.

5.  Farrar WB, McCarty WL Jr. Inferior joint space arthrography and characteristics of condylar paths in internal derangements of the TMJ. J Prosthet Dent 1979;41: 548–55.

6.  Westesson P-L. Double-contrast arthrography and internal derangement of the temporomandibular joint. Swed Dent J (Suppl) 1982;13:1–57.

7.  Isacsson G, Isberg A, Johansson A-S, et al. Internal derangement of the temporomandibular joint: radiographic and histologic changes associated with severe pain. J Oral Maxillofac Surg 1986;44:771–8.

8.  Isberg A, Isacsson G, Johansson A-S, et al. Hyperplastic soft-tissue formation in the temporomandibular joint associated with internal derangement. A radiographic and histologic study. Oral Surg Oral Med Oral Pathol 1986;61:32–8.

9.  Schiffman E, Ohrbach R, Truelove E, et al. Diagnostic criteria for temporomandibular disorders (DC/TMD) for clinical and research applications: recommendations of the international RDC/TMD consortium network and orofacial pain special interest group. J Oral Facial Pain Headache 2014;28:6–27.

10. Dimitroulis G. A new surgical classification for temporomandibular joint disorders. Int J Oral Maxillofac Surg 2013;42:218–22.

11. Lund B, Ulmner M, Bjørnland T, et al. A disease-focused view on the temporomandibular joint using a Delphi-guided process. J Oral Sci 2020;62:1–8.

12. Helms CA, Katzberg RW, Morrish R, et al. Computed tomography of the temporomandibular joint meniscus. J Oral Maxillofac Surg 1983;41:512–7.

13. Wilkes CH. Internal derangements of the temporomandibular joint. Pathological variations. Arch Otolaryngol Head Neck Surg 1989;115:469–77.

14. Courtemanche AD, Son-Hing QR. Eminectomy for chronic recurring subluxation of the temporomandibular joint. Ann Plast Surg 1979;3:22–5.

15. Dunn MJ, Benza R, Moan D, et al. Temporomandibular joint condylectomy: a technique and postoperative follow-up. Oral Surg Oral Med Oral Pathol 1981; 51:363–74.

16. Dolwick MF, Riggs RR. Diagnosis and treatment of internal derangements of the temporomandibular joint. Dent Clin North Am 1983;27:561–72.

17. Eriksson L, Westesson PL. Long-term evaluation of meniscectomy of the temporomandibular joint. J Oral Maxillofac Surg 1985;43:263–9.

18. Nitzan DW, Dolwick MF, Martinez GA. Temporomandibular joint arthrocentesis: a simplified treatment for severe, limited mouth opening. J Oral Maxillofac Surg 1991;49:1163–7.

19. Lundh H, Westesson PL, Eriksson L, et al. Temporomandibular joint disk displacement without reduction. Treatment with flat occlusal splint versus no treatment. Oral Surg Oral Med Oral Pathol 1992;73:655–8.

20. Feinberg SE. Use of local tissues for temporomandibular joint surgery disc replacement. Atlas Oral Maxillofac Surg Clin North Am 1996;4:51–74.

21. Gynther GW, Holmlund AB. Efficacy of arthroscopic lysis and lavage in patients with temporomandibular joint symptoms associated with generalized osteoarthritis or rheumatoid arthritis. J Oral Maxillofac Surg 1998;56:147–51.

22. Hall HD, Navarro EZ, Gibbs SJ. Prospective study of modified condylotomy for treatment of nonreducing disk displacement. Oral Surg Oral Med Oral Pathol Oral Radiol Endod 2000;89:147–58.

23. Saeed N, Hensher R, McLeod N, et al. Reconstruction of the temporomandibular joint autogenous compared with alloplastic. Br J Oral Maxillofac Surg 2002;40: 296–9.

24. Bartlett SP, Reid RR, Losee JE, et al. Severe proliferative congenital temporomandibular joint ankylosis: a proposed treatment protocol utilizing distraction osteogenesis. J Craniofac Surg 2006;17:605–10.

25. Bjørnland T, Gjærum AA, Møystad A. Osteoarthritis of the temporomandibular joint: an evaluation of the effects and complications of corticosteroid injection compared with injection with sodium hyaluronate. J Oral Rehabil 2007;34:583–9.

26. Abramowicz S, Dolwick MF. 20-year follow-up study of disc repositioning surgery for temporomandibular joint internal derangement. J Oral Maxillofac Surg 2010; 68:239–42.

27. Loveless TP, Bjornland T, Dodson TB, et al. Efficacy of temporomandibular joint ankylosis surgical treatment. J Oral Maxillofac Surg 2010;68:1276–82.

28. Miloro M, Henriksen B. Discectomy as the primary surgical option for internal derangement of the temporomandibular joint. J Oral Maxillofac Surg 2010;68: 782–9.

29. Dimitroulis G. A critical review of interpositional grafts following temporomandibular joint discectomy with an overview of the dermis-fat graft. Int J Oral Maxillofac Surg 2011;40:561–8.

30. Granquist EJ, Quinn PD. Total reconstruction of the temporomandibular joint with a stock prosthesis. Atlas Oral Maxillofac Surg Clin North Am 2011;19:221–32.

31. Khadka A, Hu J. Autogenous grafts for condylar reconstruction in treatment of TMJ ankylosis: current concepts and considerations for the future. Int J Oral Maxillofac Surg 2012;41:94–102.

32. Holmlund A, Lund B, Weiner CK. Mandibular condylectomy with osteoarthrectomy with and without transfer of the temporalis muscle. Br J Oral Maxillofac Surg 2013;51:206–10.

33. Leandro LF, Ono HY, Loureiro CC, et al. A ten-year experience and follow-up of three hundred patients fitted with the Biomet/Lorenz microfixation TMJ replacement system. Int J Oral Maxillofac Surg 2013;42:1007–13.

34. Forshaw RJ. Reduction of temporomandibular joint dislocation: an ancient technique that has stood the test of time. Br Dent J 2015;218:691–3.

35. Ulmner M, Kruger-Weiner C, Lund B. Patient-specific factors predicting outcome of temporomandibular joint arthroscopy: a 6-year retrospective study. J Oral Maxillofac Surg 2017;75:e1641–3.

36. Bergstrand S, Ingstad HK, Møystad A, et al. Long-term effectiveness of arthrocentesis with and without hyaluronic acid injection for treatment of temporomandibular joint osteoarthritis. J Oral Sci 2019;61:82–8.

37. Eriksson L, Westesson P-L. Results of temporomandibular joint discectomies in Sweden 1965-85. Swed Dent J 1987;11:1–9.

38. Eriksson L, Westesson P-L. Temporomandibular joint diskectomy. No positive effect of temporary silicone implant in a 5-year follow-up. Oral Surg Oral Med Oral Pathol 1992;74:259–72.

39. Bjørnland T, Larheim TA. Discectomy of the temporomandibular joint: 3-year follow-as a predictor of the 10-year outcome. J Oral Maxillofac Surg 2003;61: 55–60.

40. Al-Moraissi EA, Wolford LM, Ellis E III, et al. The hierarchy of different treatments for arthrogenous temporomandibular disorders: a network meta-analysis of randomized clinical trials. J Cranio Maxillo Fac Surg 2020;48:9–23.

41. Liapaki A, Thamm JR, Ha S, et al. Is there a difference in treatment effect of different intra-articular drugs for temporomandibular joint osteoarthritis? A systematic review of randomized controlled trials. Int J Oral Maxillofac Surg 2021;50:1233–43.
42. Schrøder CP, Skare Ø, Reikerås O, et al. Sham surgery versus labial repair or biceps tenodesis for type II SLAP lesions of the shoulder: a three-armed randomized clinical trial. Br J Sports Med 2017;51:1759–66.
43. Eliassen M, Hjortsjö C, Olsen-Bergem HG, et al. Self-exercise programmes and occlusal splints in the treatment of TMD-related myalgia – evidence based medicine? J Oral Rehab 2019;46:1088–94.
44. Laskin DM. Temporomandibular disorders: a term past its time? J Am Dent Assoc 2008;139:124–8.
45. Bueno CH, Pereira DD, Pattussi MP, et al. Gender differences in temporomandibular disorders in adult populational studies: a systematic review and meta-analysis. J Oral Rehabil 2018;45:720–9.
46. Møystad A, Mork-Knutsen BB, Bjørnland T. Injection of sodium hyaluronate compared to a corticosteroid in the treatment of patients with temporomandibular joint osteoarthritis: a CT evaluation. Oral Surg Oral Med Oral Pathol Endod 2008;105:e53–60.
47. Møystad A, Bjørnland T, Mork-Knutsen BB, et al. Injection of sodium hyaluronate compared to a corticosteroid in the treatment of patients with temporomandibular joint osteoarthritis: clinical effects and CT evaluation of osseous changes. Oral Surg 2008;1:88–95.
48. Malekzadeh BÖ, Cahlin BJ, Widmark G. Conservative therapy versus arthrocentesis for the treatment of symptomatic disk displacement without reduction: a prospective randomized controlled study. Oral Surg Oral Med Oral Pathol Oral Radiol 2019;128:18–24.
49. Rao JKD, Sharma A, Kashyap R, et al. Comparison of efficacy of sodium hyaluronate and normal saline arthrocentesis in the management of internal derangement of temporomandibular joints – a prospective study. Natl J Maxillofac Surg 2019;10:217–22.
50. Keith DA. Success, failure, and complications of temporomandibular joint surgery. In: Keith DA, editor. Surgery of the temporomandibular joint. Boston: Blackwell Scientific Publications; 1992. p. 298–315.
51. McCain JP, Hossameldin RH, Srouji S, et al. Arthroscopic discoplexy is effective in managing temporomandibular joint internal derangement in patients with Wilkes stage II and III. J Oral Maxillofac Surg 2015;73:391–401.
52. Montgomery MT, Gordon SM, Van Sickels JE, et al. Changes in signs and symptoms following temporomandibular joint disc repositioning surgery. J Oral Maxillofac Surg 1992;50:320–8.
53. Bjørnland T, Larheim TA. Synovectomy and diskectomy of the temporomandibular joint in patients with chronic arthritic disease compared with diskectomies in patients with internal derangement. A 3-year follow-up study. Eur J Oral Sci 1995;103:2–7.
54. Dolwick MF, Aufdemorte TB. Silicone-induced foreign body reaction and lymphadenopathy after temporomandibular joint arthroplasty. Oral Surg Oral Med Oral Pathol 1985;59:449–52.
55. Kramer A, Lee L, Beirne O. Meta-analysis of TMJ discectomy with or without autogenous/alloplastic interpositional materials: comparative analysis of function outcome. J Oral Maxillofac Surg 2004;62:49–50.
56. Larheim TA, Bjørnland T, Smith H-J, et al. Imaging temporomandibular joints in patients with rheumatic disease. Comparison with surgical observations. Oral Surg Oral Med Oral Pathol 1992;73:494–501.

# Nonsurgical Management of Temporomandibular Joint Arthropathy

Briana J. Burris, DDS[a,b,c], Roxanne Bavarian, DMD, DMSc[a,b,*],
Jeffry R. Shaefer, DDS, MS, MPH[a,b]

KEYWORDS

• TMJ • TMD • Arthopathy • Orofacial pain • Arthritis • Diagnosis • Management

KEY POINTS

- The management of a TMJ arthropathy is dependent on an accurate diagnosis that helps understand the etiology of the condition.
- There are many non-surgical treatment options available with proven efficacy, which can be initiated while patients complete the diagnostic work up of their TMJ arthropathies.
- The majority of patients with a TMJ arthropathy will have symptomatic relief with non-surgical treatment modalities, which often include a combination of patient education, occlusal appliance therapy, pharmacotherapy, physical therapy, and behavioral therapy.
- For patients with persistent symptoms of TMJ arthralgia or limited range of motion after completing conservative, non-surgical treatment, a surgical consultation is recommended for further evaluation and possible intervention.

## CASE REPORT

A 24-year-old woman presented to the orofacial pain clinic with the chief complaint of jaw locking and pain. She stated that her symptoms began about 4 months prior during a visit with her primary care physician when she opened her mouth wide during evaluation of a sore throat and her jaw became locked in an open position. The open lock persisted for approximately 2 hours before she was seen by her dentist, who helped manually reposition her jaw. Following this initial locking episode, she developed a persistent, dull ache of her jaw, localized to her bilateral masseter and preauricular areas. The symptoms were constant but fluctuated in severity, with

[a] Department of Oral and Maxillofacial Surgery, Massachusetts General Hospital, 55 Fruit St, Boston, MA 02114, USA; [b] Department of Oral and Maxillofacial Surgery, Harvard School of Dental Medicine, 188 Longwood Ave, Boston, MA 02115, USA; [c] Department of Oral and Maxillofacial Surgery, Harvard Medical School, 25 Shattuck St, Boston, MA 02115, USA
* Corresponding author. Department of Oral and Maxillofacial Surgery, Harvard School of Dental Medicine, 188 Longwood Ave, Boston, MA, 02115.
*E-mail address:* roxanne_bavarian@hsdm.harvard.edu

Dent Clin N Am 67 (2023) 27–47
https://doi.org/10.1016/j.cden.2022.07.003
0011-8532/23/© 2022 Elsevier Inc. All rights reserved.

intensity ranging from 2 to 6 on a visual analog scale (VAS) of 10 points, and typically worsened throughout the day. She reported aggravating activities including chewing, yawning, and clenching. The patient is aware of a daytime clenching habit as well as nighttime bruxism, both exacerbated by stress. When her pain is severe, it radiates to her temples as well as to her neck and shoulders. The patient tearfully stated that she recently experienced a second episode of open locking, 1 week before her initial visit at the authors' clinic, which required an emergency visit to an outside oral surgeon for intravenous sedation and manual reduction of her jaw. The patient was not aware of a history of jaw clicking or pain before her first locking episode 4 months previously. She had not noticed any symptoms of swelling, erythema, numbness, or tingling of the face.

Review of her medical records revealed a history of psoriatic arthritis, migraines, anxiety, polycystic ovarian syndrome, and type 2 diabetes. Upon discussion, the patient reported receiving a diagnosis of psoriatic arthritis during childhood, at which time she experienced oligoarticular symptoms at her bilateral hips, knees, and hands. Her generalized symptoms are now quiescent without the use of medication, and she denies pain in other joints. Her family history was negative for rheumatoid arthritis or other connective tissue diseases. She also has a 10-year history of migraines and will take sumatriptan 25 mg as needed, on average once a week. Her migraines are sometimes triggered by her jaw and neck pain. Her polycystic ovarian syndrome is medically managed with hormonal treatment. Her type 2 diabetes mellitus is well controlled with oral metformin. She reported that her anxiety is well controlled with citalopram 20 mg once daily. She is in graduate school for nursing. She does not drink alcohol and has never used tobacco. She has no history of illicit drug use or substance misuse.

Her initial clinical examination revealed no facial asymmetry or swelling. Her mandibular range of motion was limited to 22 mm without pain, although she was able to stretch to 40 mm with symptoms of pressure and stiffness reported in the bilateral masseter muscles. Her lateral excursions were 10 mm bilaterally, and her protrusive excursion was 8 mm. She had no palpable clicking or popping sounds during mandibular movements. Pain was elicited on palpation of her bilateral temporomandibular joint (TMJs), bilateral deep and superficial masseters, and bilateral temporalis muscles. She also had tenderness on palpation of her sternocleidomastoid, splenius capitis, and posterior digastric muscles, with her right side generally being more

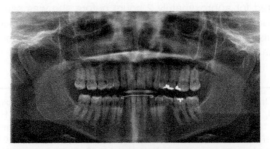

**Fig. 1.** Panoramic radiograph reveals no obvious osseous pathology and no significant condylar remodeling bilaterally. Her dentition is grossly intact with a minimally restored dentition, with all 4 third molars and left mandibular second premolar missing. She has a mandibular lingual fixed retainer from teeth # 22 to 27. She also has retained primary left second molar, with evidence of distal decay as well as mesial decay on the adjacent left first permanent molar.

sensitive than the left. Her occlusion was evaluated with shimstock and demonstrated a stable and repeatable bite with bilateral posterior occlusion. An initial panoramic radiograph was obtained and was negative for degenerative condylar changes, odontogenic lesions, and bony pathology (**Fig. 1**).

Her initial diagnoses included bilateral TMJ arthropathy with associated arthralgia and myofascial pain of the masticatory and cervical muscles. The cause of these conditions was thought to be secondary to parafunctional bruxism and anxiety as well as possibly related to her history of psoriatic arthritis.

Given her history of open locking, an MRI of her TMJs was ordered. Further diagnostic testing and nonsurgical treatment were initiated simultaneously. The patient was recommended for conservative, nonsurgical treatment, including patient education, physical therapy modalities, oral appliance therapy, and pharmacotherapy. Physical therapy modalities included instruction in jaw stretching exercises to be held for 30 to 60 seconds, 6 times daily, as well as a referral to physical therapy. The patient had an occlusal appliance (maxillary anterior bite plane) previously fabricated by her local dentist, which fit well and subjectively reduced her pain, and she was advised to continue wearing this nightly. The patient was also prescribed a 2-week course of naproxen 500 mg twice daily to treat her TMJ arthralgia as well as metaxalone 800 mg, which could be used nightly as needed for masticatory muscle spasms and pain. A follow-up clinic visit was scheduled.

The patient returned for reassessment 2 months after the initial consultation. At that time, she reported improvement of her symptoms, with her jaw pain decreasing from a 6 to an average intensity of 2 on a 10-point VAS. Her migraine frequency also reduced from 3 migraines weekly to 1 migraine weekly. Her pain-free range of motion increased from 22 to 34 mm, with a maximum opening of 40 mm with pain felt in the bilateral masseters. She had not experienced further episodes of open locking of her jaw and was experiencing less discomfort during mastication and speaking. The diagnostics were subsequently reviewed, and the MRI of her TMJs demonstrated appropriate disk-condyle relationship, without effusion, although minimal translation of the condyles was appreciated in the open-mouth series (**Figs. 2** and **3**). Her diagnoses remained bilateral TMJ arthropathy, with significant reduction of the intensity and frequency of her TMJ arthralgia and myofascial pain of the masticatory and cervical muscles. A plan was reiterated for continued nonsurgical treatment, including continued

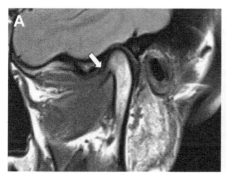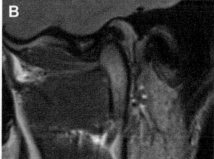

**Fig. 2.** (*A*) Right mandibular condyle and articular disk as seen in proton density-weighted closed-mouth position. Articular disk (*white arrow*) appears deformed, flattended, and is not well visualized in the closed-mouth position. (*B*) Right mandibular condyle and articular disk as seen in proton density-weighted open-mouth position. Despite normal disk-condyle relationship, minimal translation is noted.

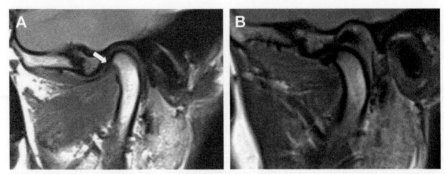

**Fig. 3.** (A) Left mandibular condyle and articular disk as seen in proton density-weighted closed-mouth position. Articular disk (*white arrow*) appears deformed, flattened, and is not well visualized in the closed-mouth position. (B) Left mandibular condyle and articular disk as seen in proton density-weighted open-mouth position. Despite normal disk-condyle relationship, minimal translation is noted.

physical therapy. A referral to rheumatology was ordered to evaluate for psoriatic arthritis as the cause of her symmetric TMJ pain. During the rheumatology consultation, a detailed history, serology, and imaging of the TMJs were reviewed. The rheumatologist provided the diagnosis of quiescent childhood psoriatic arthritis, with low suspicion for inflammatory arthritis of her bilateral TMJ, given imaging, negative serology, and positive response to nonsurgical treatment (see **Fig. 3**).

## LITERATURE REVIEW: NONSURGICAL MANAGEMENT OF TEMPOROMANDIBULAR JOINT ARTHROPATHIES

The aforementioned case report represents the initial evaluation and management of a patient presenting with the chief complaint of bilateral TMJ pain and intermittent open locking of her jaw. Arthropathy is a broad diagnostic term for any pathologic condition afflicting one or more joints of the body. TMJ arthropathy is an umbrella term that may be applied to mechanical dysfunction or disease of one or both TMJs. The most common subtypes of TMJ arthropathies are listed in **Fig. 4**. The remainder of this article provides evidence-based recommendations for conducting a patient evaluation, initiating a diagnostic workup, formulating an assessment, and instituting various nonsurgical modalities for the treatment of TMJ arthropathies.

## EXAMINATION OF A PATIENT WITH TEMPOROMANDIBULAR DISORDER AND DIAGNOSTIC MODALITIES
### Patient Interview with History

In the evaluation and diagnosis of TMJ arthropathies, a comprehensive approach to both history and physical examination is recommended. Developing an algorithm to review pertinent aspects of a patient's history and key clinical examination findings will allow for the establishment of appropriate working diagnoses and initial treatment recommendations. Use of the *Diagnostic Criteria for Temporomandibular Disorders* is recommended when a patient presents with clinical signs and/or symptoms of pain or dysfunction affecting their TMJ.[1] Identifying intra-articular and extra-articular signs and a suspected cause is the first clinical challenge. One must determine if the patient's chief complaint is *predominantly* a sequelae of an intra-articular problem (ie,

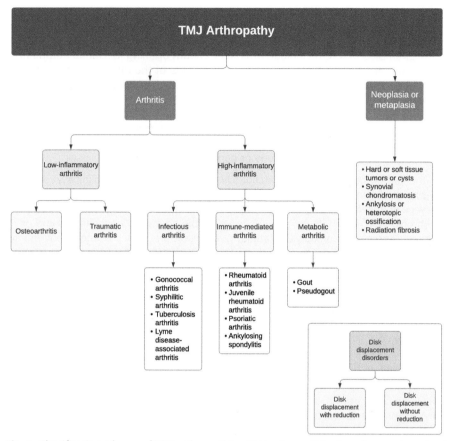

**Fig. 4.** Classification scheme of TMJ arthropathies. TMJ arthropathies have been categorized as low inflammatory or high inflammatory.[2] Of note disk displacement disorders are featured in a separate box, because disk displacement is being recognized as a clinical and radiographic finding that may or may not be present in combination with various TMJ arthropathies.

arthropathy) or an extra-articular problem, such as myogenous pain or a centrally mediated pain process.

Obtain a history of presenting illness with particular focus on
- Specific chief complaint (in the patient's own words)
  - Is there a clear duration of the complaint?
  - Does the patient recall a specific inciting event?
  - Is the patient able to localize the complaint to 1 area?
- Quality and intensity of the chief complaint
- Alleviating or exacerbating factors
- Known and witnessed parafunctional habits
- Known history and/or symptoms of dentofacial anomalies with a malocclusion
  - History of orthodontic correction
  - History of orthognathic surgery recommendations or consultations

- Treatment to date, including pharmacotherapy, physical therapy, occlusal appliance therapy, injection-based interventions, or TMJ surgery
- History of traumatic events and/or cervical sprain (whiplash) injuries:
  - Examples of trauma include prolonged mouth opening for dental treatments, traumatic bite of food, direct blow to the side of the face while playing with children or during sports activities, direct blow to chin due to a ground-level fall.
- Prior medical history with attention to previous psychological diagnoses
- Known history and/or symptoms of multiple joint involvement
  - Previous orthopedic or rheumatologic treatment
  - Familial history of autoimmune or connective tissue diseases

In the author's case study, the patient's history was detailed and clinically relevant, and provided information about comorbidities. The history raised suspicion for the presence of an inflammatory TMJ arthropathy and highlighted the presence of comorbid chronic pain disorders (migraines) and possible contribution of one or more psychological domains (anxiety). Chronic pain disorders are the most commonly associated comorbidities for patients presenting with symptoms of temporomandibular disorder (TMD).[2–4] Anxiety, whether in response to personal stress or related to catastrophizing, can increase nociceptor response to a stimulus and predispose one to and/or perpetuate chronic pain. Patients with reports of chronic pain, history of psychological and psychosocial diagnoses, or positive responses to psychological screening tools, require a multidisciplinary approach for their differential diagnosis and assessment.[5]

### Physical Examination

Perform a complete head and neck examination with focused attention on
- Gross facial asymmetries, deviation of chin point, skeletal malocclusion
- Maximum unassisted incisal opening
  - Hypomobility is considered less than 35 mm
- Lateral excursive and protrusive range of motion
  - Limited lateral excursive movements greater than or equal to 7 mm
  - Limited protrusion greater than or equal to 6 mm
- Deviation on opening
  - Anterior disk displacement may result in deviation toward the affected side during early opening, because contraction of the lateral pterygoid muscle is unable to overcome the internal derangement and produce contralateral motion
- Reproducible clicking on palpation of the TMJ during 2 of 3 trials of vertical range of motion
  - Note whether clicking occurs during opening or closing movements
- Joint loading test
  - Instruct patient to localize provoked pain with 1 finger
  - Positive direct pressure loading: Biting force between maxillary canine and mandibular canine (or premolar) elicits pain in the contralateral TMJ
  - Positive indirect pressure loading: Biting force between maxillary canine and mandibular canine (or premolar) elicits pain in the ipsilateral TMJ
- Palpation of lateral condylar poles, masticatory muscles
  - Recommended force of palpation of 0.5 kg to the TMJ
  - Recommended force of palpation of 1.0 kg to the masticatory muscles

The totality of the clinical examination findings may cumulatively suggest a specific diagnosis, although signs frequently provide evidence of one or more possible

TMJ arthropathies. Physical examination findings should be taken into account with findings from the patient history, imaging, serology, and clinical judgment to arrive at a diagnosis.[6] For example, joint loading tests may provide clinical signs of intra-articular pathology, because the application of biting force will transmit localized pain to the contralateral joint.[6] The test involves the placement of a tongue depressor over the unilateral canine-premolar region, instructing the patient to bite and hold the tongue depressor, and point with one finger to where they feel pain. Specificity in localization helps identify whether the patient is pointing directly to the TMJ or to a masticatory muscle (masseter). Deviation toward the affected TMJ in early mouth opening clinically represents restricted condylar translation and possibly an abnormality in ipsilateral lateral pterygoid muscle function, which physiologically provides contralateral movement during normal translation.[6] Patients with limited mouth opening due to coronoid hyperplasia will retain the ability to protrude within normal excursive limits, despite a notable hard-end feel during maximum opening. The ability to manually stretch the patient to a maximum opening that falls within normal limits is suggestive of a significant concomitant or predominant masticatory myalgia.[6] Tenderness to palpation of the lateral condyle poles is thought to be sensitive for intra-articular pathology, although not specific to one particular type of TMJ arthropathy.[2,3]

The clinical examination in our case was notable for limited mouth opening, with the ability to manually stretch the patient to a range of motion within normal limits. The absence of clicking, popping, deviation, or limited excursions lowers suspicions for an internal derangement as the primary cause of this patient's TMJ arthropathy, despite her history of locking episodes. Nonspecific signs (ie, unilateral tenderness of the lateral pole) or mixed clinical signs were noted, but no significant emphasis is placed on these findings. Evidence of masticatory myalgia and cervical myofascial pain were significant, as indicated by familiar tenderness to palpation of masticatory muscles and cervical muscles bilaterally.

## Imaging

### Panoramic
A panoramic radiograph provides an overall 2-dimensional view of the mandibular condyles, mandibular bodies and rami, maxilla, and odontogenic structures. Panoramic radiographs are recommended for all patients presenting with symptoms of TMJ pain or dysfunction as a screening to assess for the presence of an odontogenic source of symptoms, presence of osseous abnormalities in the alveolar bone or either of the bilateral TMJs, such as condylar fracture, osseous lesions, or condylar asymmetries.[6-8] Panoramic radiographs are a convenient first-line diagnostic images to obtain given the clinical ease and minimal radiation exposure. However, cautious interpretation of TMJ arthropathies is necessary due to low diagnostic reliability beyond gross osseous changes.[8,9]

### MRI
MRI of the TMJs offers the clearest view of the joint's anatomy and is recognized as the most sensitive imaging tool for evaluating the TMJ and diagnosing pathologic processes of intra-articular soft tissues.[4] The standard protocol for an MRI of the TMJ includes 3 scanning sequences: proton density (PD), T1-weighted, and T2-weighted sequences. Typically, the PD or T1-weighted scanning sequences are taken in both open and closed-mouth positions. The aforementioned sequences allow for assessment of anatomy at rest and with mouth opening, in an effort to capture anatomy during function. Although MRIs are regarded as the gold standard for diagnosis of an

internal derangement, the disk-condylar relationship is only one piece of information gathered from an MRI. An MRI of the TMJ also allows for assessment of disk shape and/or deformity suggesting compromised disk quality, intra-articular pathology such as a joint effusion or synovial chondromatosis, condylar anatomy and/or the presence of hard tissue pathology such as osteomyelitis, or soft tissue lesions in close relationship, such as a synovial cyst. The standard protocol for MRI diagnosis of anterior disk displacement uses the most superior surface (12-o'clock position) of the condyle as a reference point for normal position of the posterior band. Greater than 10° (11-o'clock or 1-o'clock) of displacement relative to the 12-o'clock position is considered disk displacement.[10] Alternative methods of MRI interpretation have been explored. Shaefer and colleagues[11] found a closer relationship between TMJ disk displacement and arthralgia when a line perpendicular to the posterior slope of the eminence is used to determine disk displacement rather than the 12-o'clock position. Classification of internal derangement applied to MRI findings depend on the presence of disk displacement, with or without disk reduction in the open-mouth view, and more advanced classification is assigned based on the presence or absence of degenerative changes of the mandibular condyle and fossa component.[6] **Table 1** reviews the most commonly used classification schemes in articular disk disorders: the diagnostic criteria (Diagnostic Criteria for Temporomandibular Disorder [DC/TMD]) and Wilkes classifications. The DC/TMD classification is a validated, research-based classification system for the diagnosis of articular disk disorders. The Wilkes classification is a descriptive classification that is not a validated diagnostic classification but is widely used among oral and maxillofacial surgeons to describe the symptoms and clinical and radiographic findings associated with the

**Table 1**
**Comparison between the diagnostic criteria for temporomandibular disorder and the Wilkes classification of TMJ internal derangement**

| DC/TMD[1] | Wilkes Classification[12,13] |
| --- | --- |
| *Disc displacement with reduction (ICD-10 M26.63):* reproducible clicking/popping with jaw movement | *Stage 1:* early reducing disk displacement: clicking without pain or limitation |
| *Disc displacement with reduction with intermittent locking (ICD-10 M26.63):* clicking/popping with history of transient catching/locking in the past 30 d | *Stage 2:* late reducing disk displacement: one or more episodes of pain, mid to late opening click, transient catching and locking |
| *Disc displacement without reduction with limited opening (ICD-10 M26.63):* limited range of motion on opening < 40 mm | *Stage 3:* nonreducing disk displacement: multiple painful episodes, locking, restricted mobility |
| *Disc displacement without reduction without limited opening (ICD-10 M26.63):* history of limited range of motion but now with ≥ 40 mm mouth opening | *Stage 4:* nonreducing disk displacement: chronic increasing functional disturbance |
| *Degenerative joint disease (ICD-10 19.91):* crepitus with jaw movement | *Stage 5:* nonreducing disk displacement: chronic with osteoarthritis, crepitus, pain, restricted motion and difficulty functioning |

Notably, the Wilkes classification includes pain in its staging system, whereas the The Diagnostic Criteria for Temporomandibular Disorders considers TMJ arthralgia (ICD-10 M26.62) as a separate diagnosis that can accompany any stage of arthropathy.
*Abbreviations:* ICD, International Classification of Diseases.

diagnosis of an articular disk disorder. Both the DC/TMD and Wilkes classifications are included in **Table 1** for comparison.

### Computed tomography/cone beam computed tomography
Computed tomography (CT) is the imaging modality regarded for superior visualization of hard tissue anatomy and further has the ability to render 3-dimensional reconstructions.[7] Although the T1-weighted image or PD MRI scanning protocols are typically used to assess hard tissue anatomy of the TMJ, CT or cone beam CT (CBCT) may also be obtained to allow for assessment of hard tissues in 3 dimensions. CT scans are frequently used for assessment of structural relationships and are routinely obtained for pathology, after trauma, or before total joint replacement. CBCT or CT imaging should be pursued if suspicions of hard tissues abnormalities are evident in panoramic radiograph, and/or inadequately described in an MRI report.[6,8] It is not uncommon to obtain both an MRI and CT, with the goal of accurately assessing both the hard and soft tissues.

### Serology

In the case presented, the patient presented with a history of psoriatic arthritis. A history of symptoms in other joints or a familial history of immune-mediated or inflammatory arthritis may raise suspicion for an immune-mediated arthropathy and is a reasonable rationale for serologic screening tests.[6] By obtaining a rheumatoid factor and anti-cyclic citrullinated peptide (anti-CCP), most patients with rheumatoid arthritis may be identified.[2] Less-specific screening tests like the anti-nuclear antibody and HLA-B27 may suggest the presence of an immune-mediated arthritis, psoriatic arthritis, ankylosing spondylitis, or mixed connective tissue disease.[2,14] Patients should be informed that obtaining serology is a screening tool, and that no formal diagnosis will be made from these results alone. Referral to a rheumatologist may be appropriate for a definitive diagnosis and subsequent medical management. In the case presented, the suspicion for an immune-mediated arthropathy was low, given her negative serology, negative family history, and no evidence of degenerative arthritis apparent on imaging; however, given her childhood history of psoriatic arthritis, the decision was made to refer to rheumatology for a comprehensive evaluation.

### Nonsurgical Management of Temporomandibular Joint Arthropathy

#### Review of rationale of treatment
TMJ arthropathy is a broad category that represents intra-articular pathologic processes that may be systemic, mechanical, or metaplastic in nature. The goal of treatment of any TMJ arthropathy is the establishment of a diagnosis and reduction in symptoms. Given the complexity of the anatomy, kinematics, and interdependence of the bilateral TMJs, establishing a diagnosis can be difficult, because multiple and/or conflicting signs and symptoms may be present. Ultimately, numerous studies have demonstrated equivalent outcomes between nonsurgical and surgical treatment options, and thus, nonsurgical treatment is recommended as the first-line treatment of TMJ arthropathies.[1] In the most recent American Association of Oral and Maxillofacial Surgeons parameters of care guidelines, the indicated therapeutic parameters for nonsurgical management are identical for masticatory myalgias, internal derangements, osteoarthritis, and immune-based arthropathies (ie, rheumatoid arthritis).[15] The initial nonsurgical management recommended is mentioned in **Box 1**.[15]

Treatment outcome measures recommended by the International Association of Oral and Maxillofacial Surgeons for the assessment of treatment success include

---

**Box 1**
**Recommendations for first-line, nonsurgical management of temporomandibular joint arthropathies**

*Recommended First-Line Nonsurgical Treatment Options for TMJ Arthropathies*

Patient education (eg, jaw rest, stress reduction, dietary recommendations)

Pharmacotherapy (eg, NSAIDs, analgesics, muscle relaxants)

Physical medicine (eg, manual therapy, ultrasound, trigger point injections)

Behavioral modification (eg, stress reduction, work modification, counseling, biofeedback, psychotherapy)

Orthopedic appliance therapy

Occlusal therapy in indicated cases of occlusal instability

Diagnostic records to determine progression of the disease (eg, serial bite registration and models, imaging studies in selected cases)

Intracapsular diagnostic and therapeutic injections

Nonsurgical treatments are not listed in order of preference or recommendation.
*Abbreviation:* NSAID, nonsteroidal anti-inflammatory drug.

*Adapted from* American Academy of Orofacial Pain Guidelines for Assessment, Diagnosis, and Management (Differential Diagnosis and Management of TMDs. In: de Leeuw R KG, ed. Oro-facial pain: guidelines for assessment, diagnosis, and management. Quintessence Publishing Co, Inc; 2018.) and 2017 AAOMS Parameters of Care Guidelines (Bouloux G, Koslin MG, Ness G, Shafer D. Temporomandibular Joint Surgery. J Oral Maxillofac Surg. Aug 2017;75(8S):e195-e223. https://doi.org/10.1016/j.joms.2017.04.027).

---

pain absent or so mild that it does not concern the patient; pain being significantly reduced in intensity and frequency; mandibular range of motion of at least 35 mm interincisally and 6 mm laterally and protrusively; absence or reduction of TMJ sounds; regular diet that, at worst, avoids tough or hard foods or that the patient is minimally inconvenienced by their diet; return of normal imaging appearance of the TMJ, or stabilization of the degenerative changes noted in the imaging studies; absence of significant complications; and/or absence of symptoms for at least 2 years.[1]

The 4 tenets of nonsurgical management of arthropathies are medical management, oral appliance therapy, physical medicine modalities, and behavioral therapy. It should be noted that a response to nonsurgical management in isolation does not allow for the definitive diagnosis of TMJ arthropathies. Histopathologic diagnosis is the method of definitive diagnosis, with some oral and maxillofacial surgeons supporting the use of TMJ arthroscopy for direct visualization and arthroscopic findings aiding in diagnosis.[2] Nonsurgical treatment courses should be reassessed for patient-specific response. Furthermore, nonsurgical treatment should be of finite duration in the setting of severe refractory symptoms or dysfunction and may not be appropriate in the setting of diagnostic findings concerning for an aggressive and/or neoplastic conditions.[2,15]

### Medical Management

In patients with TMJ arthralgia, nonsteroidal anti-inflammatory drugs (NSAIDs) represent a class of widely available medications that alleviate mild to moderate pain, and in particular, pain of an inflammatory origin, such as osteoarthritis or rheumatoid arthritis. Although systematic reviews of NSAIDs for TMJ arthropathies have shown

**Table 2**
Comparison of various nonsteroidal anti-inflammatory drugs, including recommended dosing and maximum daily dose

| Name | Brand Name (USA) | Dose | Maximum Daily Dose | Mechanism | Comments |
|---|---|---|---|---|---|
| Ibuprofen | Advil, Motrin | 400–800 mg every 6–8 h | 3200 mg | Nonselective COX inhibitor | Consider maximum dose of 2400 mg for chronic use* |
| Naproxen | Aleve, Naprosyn | 250–500 mg every 12 h | 1500 mg | Nonselective COX inhibitor | Consider maximum dose of 1000 mg for chronic use* |
| Meloxicam | Mobic | 7.5–15 mg once daily | 15 mg | Nonselective COX inhibitor | More potent COX-2 inhibitor; milder GI side effects |
| Celecoxib | Celebrex | 100–200 mg twice daily | 400 mg | COX-2 selective inhibition | Indicated in patients with history of intolerance of NSAIDs due to GI side effects or history of peptic ulcer |
| Indomethacin | Indocin | 25 mg 3 times daily | Immediate release: 200 mg Extended release: 150 mg | Nonselective COX inhibitor | High GI toxicity; recommended primarily in management of paroxysmal hemicrania or hemicrania continua |
| Diclofenac | Cataflam | 50 mg every 8–12 h | 150–200 mg | Nonselective COX inhibitor | |
| Diclofenac (topical) | Voltaren 1% gel | 2 g to affected site up to 4 times daily | Maximum dose per joint: 8 g/d | Nonselective COX inhibitor | Topical formulation ideal for patients who prefer to avoid systemic medication |

* In general, the lowest effective dose for the shortest duration of time is recommended to avoid risk of side effects, although patients with chronic inflammatory conditions may require a trial of greater than or equal to 2 weeks.[18] Caution should be used in patients presenting with any comorbid conditions (eg, renal, cardiovascular, or gastrointestinal disease) or medications (eg, anticoagulants) that increase the risk for toxicity.
Abbreviations: COX, cyclooxygenase; GI, gastrointestinal.

inconclusive results due to the variability in study design, evidence supporting the use of NSAIDs can be drawn from similar chronic pain conditions such as back pain and tension-type headaches.[16,17] A variety of NSAIDs are available either as a prescription or over the counter, each with different dosing regimens and tolerability profiles. **Table 2** reviews the most common NSAID medications and their doses.

Because NSAIDs have both anti-inflammatory and analgesic properties, they can be helpful for both reducing inflammation and pain in the TMJ as well as the associated masticatory muscles. All NSAIDs work with a similar mechanism of action—by reversibly inhibiting the cyclooxygenase (COX) enzymes, COX-1 and COX-2, to reduce the production of prostaglandins and leukotrienes, thereby reducing inflammation as well as pain. NSAIDs that act as nonselective COX inhibitors are not recommended for long-term use due to side effects associated with inhibition of COX-1. COX-1 is present throughout the body and plays a role in protecting the gastric mucosal lining and maintaining renal and hepatic function, among other functions. Inhibition of COX-1 is associated with increased risk for gastrointestinal ulcers and bleeding. Thus, patients on NSAIDs for an extended period should be monitored for any symptoms of gastrointestinal pain or bleeding. Other complications of long-term NSAID use include increased risk for cardiovascular events and kidney disease. COX-2, on the other hand, is present throughout the body in lower concentrations and is facultatively expressed in response to injury and inflammation. Utilization of NSAIDs that selectively target and inhibit COX-2 enzymes, such as celecoxib (Celebrex), can effectively reduce inflammation and pain, while sparing patients from the organ toxicity associated with other NSAIDs. However, COX-2-selective NSAIDs are not risk free and, similar to nonselective COX-inhibiting NSAIDs, are associated with increased risk for cardiovascular events.[19] Thus, to reduce risk of side effects, providers should work with their patients to find the lowest effective dose of NSAIDs to be used for the shortest duration of time. In addition, NSAIDs should be taken by the patient with food to reduce the risk of gastrointestinal side effects. In cases of severe TMJ arthralgia or in those with contraindications to use of NSAIDs, a brief course of steroids may be indicated for its potent anti-inflammatory properties.[20]

For patients suffering from chronic TMJ pain, nociception can become more complex, with pain spreading to neighboring regions along with the development of hyperalgesia and allodynia. A thorough history and examination is indicated to identify associated diagnoses, such as myofascial pain of the masticatory and cervical muscles or neuropathic pain, to best tailor the treatment to the patient. For example, many patients with TMJ arthralgia will present with associated masticatory myalgia related to cocontraction of the muscles working across the painful joint. Muscle relaxants (eg, cyclobenzaprine, methocarbamol) may be indicated to be used as needed or nightly to reduce nocturnal bruxism as well as promote restful sleep.[17,21–23] For patients presenting with chronic pain with a component of central sensitization, medications such as tricyclic antidepressants (eg, amitriptyline, nortriptyline), serotonin-norepinephrine reuptake inhibitors (eg, duloxetine, venlafaxine), or anticonvulsants (eg, gabapentin, pregabalin) can help in modulating pain pathways to reduce symptoms.[22] In select cases in which patients present with severe intractable pain despite all other treatment modalities, chronic opioid use may be indicated, provided that the patient undergoes an adequate screening for risk factors for opioid abuse.[24]

### Appliance Therapy

Oral appliances have been used in the management of TMJ arthropathies to reduce the load placed on the TMJ, which is especially useful for patients with parafunctional bruxism.[25] Systematic reviews evaluating the efficacy of oral appliances in reducing jaw pain in patients with TMD have been largely inconclusive due to low-quality studies or variable study designs, but in general, the use of oral appliances shows modest improvement in their pain relief when compared with a placebo control.[25–27] Appliance therapy also has the benefit of being a noninvasive, reversible procedure when compared with occlusal treatments, injection therapy, or TMJ surgeries.

Oral appliances can vary widely in their design, including the materials used, full or partial coverage of the dentition, fitted for the maxillary or mandibular arch, the thickness of the appliance, and where the occlusal contacts are placed. In general, a full-coverage appliance that fits over all of the teeth (an "occlusal splint") in which the dental arch is recommended to avoid the risk of bite changes or dental pain seen in partial coverage appliances.[25] Harder materials, such as methyl methacrylate or a thermoplastic material, are generally recommended, because softer materials are more deformable and allow for more clenching and muscle activity.[25] Thermoplastic appliances have the benefit of being a hard appliance that is easily adjustable by the dentist, while anecdotally being more comfortable for patients than an acrylic appliance. For patients with a TMJ arthropathy, a stabilization appliance with balanced bilateral posterior occlusion is the most effective design in reducing the load on the TMJs.[25] In contrast, an anterior bite plane, with anterior-only occlusion, has been shown to help reduce the load on the masticatory muscles. Anterior bite planes have also been shown to have modest efficacy in the management of headache disorders.[26] It is important to note that a full-coverage appliance is recommended to avoid the risk of developing tooth pain and/or occlusal changes.

For patients who have painful TMJ clicking and/or intermittent locking, an anterior repositioning appliance may be indicated. Anterior repositioning appliances are full-coverage appliances typically fabricated for the maxillary arch, with an acrylic ramp on the anterior aspect that guides the mandible forward into a protruded position. By protruding the mandible, the mandible translates forward to recapture the disk to reduce symptoms of pain and improve jaw function. However, studies with MRI imaging have shown that even if clinical symptoms of clicking and pain are improved, the disk may not be fully recaptured with appliance. In addition, long-term studies have shown that the disk often slips anteriorly into a displaced position again within 6 months.[28] Most patients were shown to remain pain free even if the disk becomes displaced again. Similarly, studies evaluating the long-term success of patients undergoing TMJ disk repositioning surgery also report a reduction in pain despite relapse of the disk into a displaced position.[29] These appliances are not risk free, because there have been reports of occlusal and skeletal changes associated with continuous use of an anterior reposition appliance, even with only nighttime wear.[25,30] Thus, patients using such appliances should be discouraged against full-time (eg, 24 hours daily) use. Patients should also be monitored closely over time for any changes in occlusion based on clinical examination and baseline dental casts. Patients most typically present with decreases in overbite and overjet as well as development of a bilateral posterior open bite.[30] If recognized at an early stage, patients can be guided to use a morning repositioning appliance to help reposition the mandible to its habitual, pretreatment position.[31]

### Occlusal Management

For patients with signs and symptoms of a TMJ disorder who also present with a malocclusion, occlusal therapies have been suggested to correct the malocclusion, improve chewing efficacy, and improve the biomechanics of the TMJ. Occlusal therapy can refer to a variety of interventions, including occlusal adjustments, restorative dentistry, orthodontic treatment, and orthognathic surgery. However, a systematic review examining the efficacy of occlusal therapies in reducing symptoms of TMJ arthropathy showed inconclusive results when compared with placebo or other more conservative measures for treating TMJ disorders.[26,27] In addition, there is insufficient evidence to support that any occlusal adjustment or orthodontic correction of malocclusion can prevent the development of a TMJ arthropathy.[26] Thus, given the fact that occlusal therapies are typically irreversible and often invasive and costly procedures, careful patient selection is recommended before proceeding with occlusal therapy. For example, for patients with jaw pain suspected to be secondary due to malocclusion (whether arthrogenous or myogenous), an occlusal appliance to correct the malocclusion should be trialed to see if this improves or resolves their pain with nightly use of the occlusal appliance. If the patient returns stating that the appliance only resolves their symptoms when the appliance is being worn during daytime use, then a more permanent procedure to correct the malocclusion could be considered.

### Physical Therapy

Physical therapy is a noninvasive treatment option that can be used for patients with either a chronic or an acute TMJ disorder, including both TMJ arthropathies and myofascial pain disorders. The goals of physical therapy are to improve the patient's pain-free range of motion and jaw function and reduce pain. The most effective techniques used in physical therapy include therapeutic jaw stretching exercises and manual (manipulative) therapy.[32] Manual therapy refers to hands-on techniques such as joint mobilization and manipulation and soft tissue massage to improve range of motion and reduce pain.[33] The benefit of manual therapy and therapeutic exercises has been difficult to assess systematically due to the high heterogeneity between randomized controlled trials as well as small sample sizes and broad inclusion criteria of patients with TMDs that include both muscle- and joint-based TMDs. However, systematic reviews have shown that manual therapy provides a clinically significant reduction in pain and increase in maximum mouth opening in the short term (3 months) and medium term (3–6 months) for patients with the broad diagnosis of TMD.[34–36] Only 1 systematic review examined the benefits of manual therapy and jaw stretching exercises on patients with specifically arthrogenous TMD.[33] The investigators found that manual therapy combined with jaw exercises reduced symptoms and increased range of motion, with significant results seen in patients diagnosed with disk displacement without reduction ("closed lock"), when compared with groups treated with splint therapy, medications, and arthroscopy and arthroplasty.[33]

Alternative modalities of treatment used in physical therapy include electrical nerve stimulation, low-level laser therapy (LLLT), ultrasound, and iontophoresis. The principle of electrical nerve stimulation is to apply electrical pulses to the skin to modify blood flow and neurologic behavior to modulate the perception of pain. The most well-studied form of electrical nerve stimulation uses transcutaneous electrical nerve stimulation (TENS), which uses electricity to cause an involuntary contraction of the muscles. TENS is proposed to reduce pain by several mechanisms, such as by activating large-diameter afferent fibers to activate descending inhibitory systems (gate control theory of pain), reducing the release excitatory neurotransmitters like substance P and glutamate, and promoting release of enkephalins and β-endorphins.[37] Another form of electrical nerve stimulation is microcurrent electrical nerve stimulation (MENS), which uses a low level of electricity with microcurrents less than 1000 μA. The application of MENS does not produce a contraction in the muscle and therefore is not felt by the patient, but has been shown to be effective in reducing muscle-based pain.[38] Although most studies on MENS and TENS investigate its effects on reducing pain and improving range of motion in patients with myogenous TMD, there is limited evidence to support TENS in the treatment of TMJ articular disk disorders.[39–41]

LLLT, otherwise known as *photobiomodulation*, involves the application of wavelengths of red (600–700 nm) and near-infrared (780–1110 nm) wavelengths. LLLT has been shown to reduce inflammation and promote wound healing and has thus been investigated in the treatment of various painful inflammatory conditions. A meta-analysis of LLLT in the treatment of any TMD has revealed a superior, albeit modest, effect of LLLT compared with placebo in reducing pain, with the best and longest lasting effects at higher wavelengths of 910 to 1100 nm.[42] Although most studies focus on the indication of LLLT in treating myogenous TMD-related pain, in vivo studies of TMJ osteoarthritis induced in rats show that application of LLLT inhibits leukocyte infiltration and reduces the expression of proinflammatory cytokines tumor necrosis factor-$\alpha$ and interleukin (IL)-1B while increasing activity of anti-inflammatory cytokines IL-10.[43] Clinically, 1 retrospective study found that patients with TMJ osteoarthritis who underwent arthrocentesis and LLLT had improved mouth range of motion and reduced pain when compared with those treated with arthrocentesis alone.[44]

Iontophoresis refers to a technique of medication delivery that avoids invasive treatments such as intra-articular injections or surgery; it relies on the application of low-grade electric currents to the skin to push medications into deeper anatomic structures. For example, negatively charged medications, such as dexamethasone sodium phosphate, could be applied to the negative pole (anode), such that the medication is repelled from the anode and into the skin. Because the TMJ is a joint that is relatively superficial beneath the skin surface, iontophoresis using dexamethasone and NSAIDs has been investigated to treat TMJ arthropathy. For example, one case series of 28 patients with TMJ involvement of juvenile idiopathic arthritis found that 8 treatments of dexamethasone iontophoresis improved maximal interincisal opening from an average of 35 ± 14 to 39.5 ± 10.5 mm following treatment.[45] Similarly, a double-blind study investigating dexamethasone and lidocaine iontophoresis in 27 adult patients with TMJ capsulitis and TMJ disk displacement without reduction showed improvement in range of motion, although without improvement of symptoms of pain.[46] Of note, iontophoresis is contraindicated in patients with implanted metallic devices in the area where the electric current flows, which includes patients with total joint prostheses of the TMJ or hardware in the jaw.[47]

Therapeutic ultrasound is another noninvasive modality that uses vibrations greater than 16,000 vibrations per second or 16 Hz, which when applied to the jaw produces thermal effects of deep heating as well as mechanical effects of cavitation in the soft tissue.[20] This modality has been purported to improve mandibular range of motion and reduce pain, muscle spasm, and joint stiffness. Although early studies found therapeutic ultrasound to be effective in improving symptoms associated with a myogenous TMD, more recent studies have shown that therapeutic ultrasound can reduce inflammation and promote wound healing, making it useful for patients with bony and intra-articular pathology. Recent animal models of TMJ osteoarthritis have shown promising results with the use of low-intensity pulsed ultrasound therapy promoting the repair and regeneration of bone and soft tissue, including articular cartilage.[48]

### Complementary Medicine

Patients living with chronic pain conditions such as TMDs often seek out treatments that avoid systemic medications or invasive procedures, thus leading them to complementary and alternative medicine (CAM). Survey-based studies of patients with TMD have revealed that up to 35.9% of patients with TMD will seek out CAM, with the most common types of CAM being hands-on treatments similar to physical therapy such as massage therapy and chiropractic therapy.[49] Patients reported varying outcomes with these treatments, with 54.3% of patients finding massage to be "very helpful" and 47.6% of patients finding chiropractic care to be very helpful.[49]

Acupuncture is a commonly sought-after CAM treatment for TMD, with 1 survey-based study showing that up to 15.9% of patients with TMD sought treatment with acupuncture, although only 27.3% of these patients reported it as "very helpful."[49] Acupuncture is a form of traditional Chinese medicine that uses thin needles inserted into the skin and muscles at specific points along the meridian system, which refers to the channels through which the life energy, or qi, flows in the body. Systematic reviews of randomized controlled trials of acupuncture compared with sham acupuncture show largely favorable effects with reduced pain and muscle tenderness, with superior results in the groups treated with acupuncture when compared with sham acupuncture.[50,51] However, there is a paucity of literature on the benefits of acupuncture in patients with specific joint-based TMDs and TMJ arthropathy.

### Behavioral Therapy

For patients suffering from a chronic TMD, there may be a significant role of psychological factors contributing to their symptoms, such as a stressful life event or a psychiatric disorder such as depression, anxiety, or posttraumatic stress disorder. With psychological distress, there is increased arousal of the central nervous system that can lead to parafunctional bruxism and consequent chronic microtrauma to the TMJ.[52] Cognitive behavioral therapy, administered under the guidance of a clinical psychologist, can help patients cope with their pain using a combination of relaxation techniques and pain management coping skills, such as distraction and exercise, to increase their mental self-control over their perceived pain.[53] In patients with persistent TMD present for 3 months or greater in duration, one systematic review concluded that cognitive behavioral therapy showed reduced pain, improved function, as well as reduced interference of their pain on their life.[54]

Acceptance and commitment therapy (ACT) is a form of cognitive behavioral therapy that is evidence based to help patients learn coping skills to live with chronic pain. The goal of ACT is to reframe negative thoughts and feelings, such as pain, and accept them without judgment, ultimately allowing a person to focus on personal values and life goals.[55] Although studies using ACT in the treatment of TMD are sparse, studies in chronic pain conditions such as fibromyalgia and migraines show improvement of anxiety, depression, pain acceptance, and quality of life, and in some cases, a reduction in pain and reduced reliance on medications.[56]

Other behavioral therapy techniques include biofeedback, which are predominantly targeted toward reducing parafunctional jaw clenching and grinding habits that can contribute to a TMJ arthropathy.[57,58]

### SUMMARY

Nonsurgical management of TMJ arthropathies is always recommended as an initial treatment strategy, with the exception being absolute indications for surgery, such as ankylosis or a neoplasm, and can be expected to yield good outcomes. A list of TMJ arthropathies can be found in **Fig. 1**. Recommendations on noninvasive treatments can be found in **Table 1**, which includes patient education, fostering self-directed care, nonjudgmental awareness and reduction of parafunctional habits, jaw rest, exercises to restore pain-free range of motion, pharmacotherapy, and consideration for referral to physical therapy and/or an occlusal appliance.[6] Patients should be educated that the primary goal of management of a TMJ arthropathy is establishing a diagnosis and restoration of function and form, but complete pain relief cannot be expected.[59] The decision to progress a patient through the nonsurgical treatment algorithm and pursue surgical intervention should be based on individualized response to treatment. Initiation of a nonsurgical treatment course does not preclude the patient from obtaining advanced diagnostics and ultimately receiving a referral to an oral and maxillofacial surgeon. A referral is warranted in settings in which pathology, ankylosis, or neoplasm is suspected; in cases with symptoms refractory to nonsurgical treatment; and in cases in which the provider or patient is seeking confirmation or further specification of a working diagnosis. Specific guidance of duration of nonsurgical treatment despite refractory symptoms is a provider-specific and patient-specific clinical judgment; however, a nonsurgical treatment course of 2 to 6 months allows for sufficient time for efficacy of conservative treatments to take effect. Factors to consider before surgical intervention include response to nonsurgical treatment, severity of dysfunction, perceived interference with quality of life, and the stage of the suspected disease.[60] Of note, chronic and/or persistent facial pain that is refractory to nonsurgical treatment is not an automatic indication for surgical intervention; however, appropriate referral to an oral and maxillofacial surgeon for evaluation and possible treatment is recommended for patients who fail nonsurgical treatments.

## CLINICS CARE POINTS

- The primary goal in managing a TMJ arthropathy is to first establish a diagnosis and educate the patient on their condition.
- The simultaneous pursuit of further diagnostic work-up with the initiation of non-surgical treatment is recommended in order to address the patient's symptoms while ensuring an accurate diagnosis.
- Reassessment of signs and symptoms should be completed at defined time intervals.
- The majority of TMJ arthropathies do not require surgical intervention for alleviation of symptoms.
- If signs, symptoms, or diagnostic findings are concerning for a neoplastic or ankylosing arthropathy, an expedited referral to an oral and maxillofacial surgeon is recommended for further evaluation and possible intervention.

## DISCLOSURE

None of the authors have any disclosures.

## REFERENCES

1. Schiffman E, Ohrbach R, Truelove E, et al. Diagnostic criteria for temporomandibular disorders (DC/TMD) for Clinical and Research Applications: recommendations of the International RDC/TMD Consortium Network* and Orofacial Pain Special Interest Groupdagger. J Oral Facial Pain Headache 2014;28(1):6–27.
2. Mercuri LG, Abramowicz S. Arthritic conditions affecting the temporomandibular joint. In: Farah CS, Balasubramaniam R, McCullough MJ, editors. Contemporary oral medicine: a comprehensive approach to clinical practice Switzerland: Springer International Publishing; 2019. p. 1919–54.

3. Dworkin S. Psychological and Psychosocial Assessment. In: Laskin DG, CS; Hylander, WL, ed. Temporomandibular Disorders: An Evidence-Based Approach to Diagnosis and Treatment 2006.

4. Greene CS. Concepts of TMD Etiology: Effects on Diagnosis and Treatment. In: Laskin DG, CS; Hylander, WL, ed. Temporomandibular Disorders: An Evidence-Based Approach to Diagnosis and Treatment 2006.

5. Patterson EKR, Hernandez-Nuno de la Rosa MF, Roselli M, et al. Psychological assessment of pain and headache. In: Ballantyne JC, editor. The Massachusetts general hospital handbook of pain management (lippincott Williams & Wilkins handbook). 3rd edition. Philadelphia, PA: Wolters Kluwer; 2019. p. 60–78.

6. Bouloux G. Chapter 10: temporomandibular joint disorders. In: Bagheri S, editor. Clinical review of oral and maxillofacial surgery: a case-based approach. Elsevier Mosby; 2013.

7. Bag AK, Gaddikeri S, Singhal A, et al. Imaging of the temporomandibular joint: an update. World J Radiol 2014;6(8):567–82.

8. Mallya SMAM, Cohen JR, Kaspo G, et al. Recommendations for imaging of the temporomandibular joint. Position statement from the American Academy of Oral and Maxillofacial Radiology (AAOMR) and the American Academy of Orofacial Pain (AAOP). Oral Surg Oral Med Oral Pathol Oral Radiol 2022. https://doi.org/10.1016/j.oooo.2022.06.007.

9. Larheim TA, Hol C, Ottersen MK, et al. The role of imaging in the diagnosis of temporomandibular joint pathology. Oral Maxillofac Surg Clin North Am 2018; 30(3):239–49.

10. Hegab AF, Al Hameed HI, Karam KS. Classification of temporomandibular joint internal derangement based on magnetic resonance imaging and clinical findings of 435 patients contributing to a nonsurgical treatment protocol. Sci Rep 2021;11(1):20917.

11. Shaefer JR, Riley CJ, Caruso P, et al. Analysis of criteria for MRI Diagnosis of TMJ disc displacement and arthralgia. Int J Dent 2012;2012:283163. https://doi.org/10.1155/2012/283163.

12. Wilkes CH. Internal derangements of the temporomandibular joint. Pathological variations. Arch Otolaryngol Head Neck Surg 1989;115(4):469–77.

13. de Leeuw R, Klasser GD. Differential Diagnosis and Management of TMDs. In: de Leeuw R, Klasser GD, editors. Orofacial pain: guidelines for assessment, diagnosis, and management. Hanover Park, IL: Quintessence Publishing Co, Inc; 2018. p. 143–207.

14. Sidebottom AJ, Salha R. Management of the temporomandibular joint in rheumatoid disorders. Br J Oral Maxillofac Surg 2013;51(3):191–8.

15. Bouloux G, Koslin MG, Ness G, et al. Temporomandibular joint surgery. J Oral Maxillofac Surg 2017;75(8S):e195–223.

16. List T, Jensen RH. Temporomandibular disorders: old ideas and new concepts. Cephalalgia 2017;37(7):692–704.

17. Mujakperuo HR, Watson M, Morrison R, et al. Pharmacological interventions for pain in patients with temporomandibular disorders. Cochrane Database Syst Rev 2010;(10):CD004715.

18. Solomon DH. NSAIDs: Therapeutic use and variability of response in adults. In: Furst DE, Curtis MR, editor. UpToDate. 2022.

19. Nissen SE, Yeomans ND, Solomon DH, et al. Cardiovascular safety of celecoxib, naproxen, or ibuprofen for arthritis. N Engl J Med 2016;375(26):2519–29.

20. Murphy GJ. Physical medicine modalities and trigger point injections in the management of temporomandibular disorders and assessing treatment outcome. Oral Surg Oral Med Oral Pathol Oral Radiol Endod 1997;83(1):118–22.

21. Andre A, Kang J, Dym H. Pharmacologic Treatment for Temporomandibular and Temporomandibular Joint Disorders. Oral Maxillofac Surg Clin North Am 2022; 34(1):49–59.

22. Heir GM. The efficacy of pharmacologic treatment of temporomandibular disorders. Oral Maxillofac Surg Clin North Am 2018;30(3):279–85.

23. Haggman-Henrikson B, Alstergren P, Davidson T, et al. Pharmacological treatment of oro-facial pain - health technology assessment including a systematic review with network meta-analysis. J Oral Rehabil 2017;44(10):800–26.

24. Dowell D, Haegerich TM, Chou R. CDC Guideline for Prescribing Opioids for Chronic Pain - United States, 2016. MMWR Recomm Rep 2016;65(1):1–49.

25. Greene CS, Menchel HF. The use of oral appliances in the management of temporomandibular disorders. Oral Maxillofac Surg Clin North Am 2018;30(3): 265–77.

26. Fricton J. Current evidence providing clarity in management of temporomandibular disorders: summary of a systematic review of randomized clinical trials for intra-oral appliances and occlusal therapies. J Evid Based Dent Pract 2006; 6(1):48–52.

27. Forssell H, Kalso E. Application of principles of evidence-based medicine to occlusal treatment for temporomandibular disorders: are there lessons to be learned? J Orofac Pain 2004;18(1):9–22 [discussion: 23-32].

28. Chen HM, Liu MQ, Yap AU, et al. Physiological effects of anterior repositioning splint on temporomandibular joint disc displacement: a quantitative analysis. J Oral Rehabil 2017;44(9):664–72.

29. Montgomery MT, Gordon SM, Van Sickels JE, et al. Changes in signs and symptoms following temporomandibular joint disc repositioning surgery. J Oral Maxillofac Surg 1992;50(4):320–8.

30. Pliska BT, Nam H, Chen H, et al. Obstructive sleep apnea and mandibular advancement splints: occlusal effects and progression of changes associated with a decade of treatment. J Clin Sleep Med 2014;10(12):1285–91.

31. Sheats RD. Management of side effects of oral appliance therapy for sleep-disordered breathing: summary of American Academy of Dental Sleep Medicine recommendations. J Clin Sleep Med 2020;16(5):835.

32. Rashid A, Matthews NS, Cowgill H. Physiotherapy in the management of disorders of the temporomandibular joint–perceived effectiveness and access to services: a national United Kingdom survey. Br J Oral Maxillofac Surg 2013; 51(1):52–7.

33. Armijo-Olivo S, Pitance L, Singh V, et al. Effectiveness of manual therapy and therapeutic exercise for temporomandibular disorders: systematic review and meta-analysis. Phys Ther 2016;96(1):9–25.

34. Asquini G, Pitance L, Michelotti A, et al. The effectiveness of manual therapy applied to craniomandibular structures in temporomandibular disorders: a systematic review. J Oral Rehabil 2021. https://doi.org/10.1111/joor.13299.

35. Martins WR, Blasczyk JC, Aparecida Furlan de Oliveira M, et al. Efficacy of musculoskeletal manual approach in the treatment of temporomandibular joint disorder: a systematic review with meta-analysis. Man Ther 2016;21:10–7.

36. Herrera-Valencia A, Ruiz-Munoz M, Martin-Martin J, et al. Effcacy of Manual therapy in temporomandibularjoint disorders and its medium-and long-termeffects on

pain and maximum mouth opening:a systematic review and meta-analysis. J Clin Med 2020;9(11). https://doi.org/10.3390/jcm9113404.

37. Vance CG, Dailey DL, Rakel BA, et al. Using TENS for pain control: the state of the evidence. Pain Manag 2014;4(3):197–209.

38. DuPont JS Jr, Graham R, Tidwell JB. Trigger point identification and treatment with microcurrent. Cranio 1999;17(4):293–6.

39. Ekici O, Dundar U, Buyukbosna M. Comparison of the efficiency of high-intensity laser therapy and transcutaneous electrical nerve stimulation therapy in patients with symptomatic temporomandibular joint disc displacement with reduction. J Oral Maxillofac Surg 2021. https://doi.org/10.1016/j.joms.2021.07.014.

40. Zhang Y, Zhang J, Wang L, et al. Effect of transcutaneous electrical nerve stimulation on jaw movement-evoked pain in patients with TMJ disc displacement without reduction and healthy controls. Acta Odontol Scand 2020;78(4):309–20.

41. Ferreira AP, Costa DR, Oliveira AI, et al. Short-term transcutaneous electrical nerve stimulation reduces pain and improves the masticatory muscle activity in temporomandibular disorder patients: a randomized controlled trial. J Appl Oral Sci 2017;25(2):112–20.

42. Ren H, Liu J, Liu Y, et al. Comparative effectiveness of low-level laser therapy with different wavelengths and transcutaneous electric nerve stimulation in the treatment of pain caused by temporomandibular disorders: A systematic review and network meta-analysis. J Oral Rehabil 2021. https://doi.org/10.1111/joor. 13230.

43. Mazuqueli Pereira ESB, Basting RT, Abdalla HB, et al. Photobiomodulation inhibits inflammation in the temporomandibular joint of rats. J Photochem Photobiol B 2021;222:112281.

44. Yanik S, Polat ME, Polat M. Effects of arthrocentesis and low-level laser therapy on patients with osteoarthritis of the temporomandibular joint. Br J Oral Maxillofac Surg 2021;59(3):347–52.

45. Mina R, Melson P, Powell S, et al. Effectiveness of dexamethasone iontophoresis for temporomandibular joint involvement in juvenile idiopathic arthritis. Arthritis Care Res (Hoboken) 2011;63(11):1511–6.

46. Schiffman EL, Braun BL, Lindgren BR. Temporomandibular joint iontophoresis: a double-blind randomized clinical trial. J Orofac Pain 1996;10(2):157–65.

47. Iontophoresis contraindications. Bindner Medical. Available at: https://www. iontodevice.com/iontophoresis/contraindications.html. Accessed July 29, 2022.

48. Tanaka E, Liu Y, Xia L, et al. Effectiveness of low-intensity pulsed ultrasound on osteoarthritis of the temporomandibular joint: a review. Ann Biomed Eng 2020; 48(8):2158–70.

49. DeBar LL, Vuckovic N, Schneider J, et al. Use of complementary and alternative medicine for temporomandibular disorders. J Orofac Pain 2003;17(3):224–36.

50. Jung A, Shin BC, Lee MS, et al. Acupuncture for treating temporomandibular joint disorders: a systematic review and meta-analysis of randomized, sham-controlled trials. J Dent 2011;39(5):341–50.

51. La Touche R, Goddard G, De-la-Hoz JL, et al. Acupuncture in the treatment of pain in temporomandibular disorders: a systematic review and meta-analysis of randomized controlled trials. Clin J Pain 2010;26(6):541–50.

52. Maslak-Beres M, Loster JE, Wieczorek A, et al. Evaluation of the psychoemotional status of young adults with symptoms of temporomandibular disorders. Brain Behav 2019;9(11):e01443.

53. Dura-Ferrandis E, Ferrando-Garcia M, Galdon-Garrido MJ, et al. Confirming the mechanisms behind cognitive-behavioural therapy effectiveness in chronic

pain using structural equation modeling in a sample of patients with temporomandibular disorders. Clin Psychol Psychother 2017;24(6):1377–83.

54. Randhawa K, Bohay R, Cote P, et al. The effectiveness of noninvasive interventions for temporomandibular disorders: a systematic review by the ontario protocol for traffic injury management (OPTIMa) Collaboration. Clin J Pain 2016;32(3): 260–78.

55. Acceptance and Commitment Therapy (ACT). Available at: https://dictionary.apa. org/acceptance-and-commitment-therapy. Accessed May 28, 2022.

56. Galvez-Sanchez CM, Montoro CI, Moreno-Padilla M, et al. Effectiveness of Acceptance and Commitment therapy in central pain sensitization syndromes: a systematic review. J Clin Med 2021;(12):10. https://doi.org/10.3390/ jcm10122706.

57. Mesko ME, Hutton B, Skupien JA, et al. Therapies for bruxism: a systematic review and network meta-analysis (protocol). Syst Rev 2017;6(1):4.

58. Bergmann A, Edelhoff D, Schubert O, et al. Effect of treatment with a full-occlusion biofeedback splint on sleep bruxism and TMD pain: a randomized controlled clinical trial. Clin Oral Investig 2020;24(11):4005–18.

59. Mercuri LG. Temporomandibular joint disorder management in oral and maxillofacial surgery. J Oral Maxillofac Surg 2017;75(5):927–30.

60. Renapurkar SK. Surgical versus nonsurgical management of degenerative joint disease. Oral Maxillofac Surg Clin North Am 2018;30(3):291–7.

# Burning Mouth Syndrome

Shehryar Nasir Khawaja, BDS, MS[a,c,*], Omar F. Alaswaiti, DDS[b],
Steven J. Scrivani, DDS, DMedSc[c]

## KEYWORDS

- Burning mouth syndrome • Chronic pain • Dysesthesia • Pain • Neuropathic

## KEY POINTS

- Burning mouth syndrome (BMS) is a chronic, intraoral burning or dysesthetic sensation that recurs daily.
- For diagnosis of BMS, it is essential to rule out any local or systemic causes of burning pain or dysesthesia.
- The pathophysiology of BMS remains elusive. However, it seems to have neuropathic, endocrinological, and psychosocial components.
- There are no universally accepted guidelines for the management of BMS. Clonazepam, as topical and/or systemic intervention with alpha-lipoic acid, can be offered as first-line therapy.

## CASE REPORT

A 67-year-old woman presented to the clinic with the chief complaint "I have a burning pain in my mouth." The patient reported constant burning pain over the tip of her tongue, lower and upper lips, and behind her upper teeth (anterior hard palate). Her symptoms started around 4 months ago without any apparent reason. In the beginning, the intensity of symptoms was minimal; however, gradually the severity of symptoms has increased. She has no pain when she wakes up in the morning, but the symptoms start and reach full severity within a couple of hours. Hereafter, they remain constant until bedtime. She rates her pain as 7 on a 0 to 10 numeric verbal pain rating scale, where 0 indicates no pain and 10 suggests the worst pain experience. The pain is aggravated by alcohol, acidic or spicy foods, and anything hot or mint flavored. She gets relief from sucking on ice or having anything cold. In addition to pain, she feels that her tongue is raw or burnt, and the texture of anterior teeth feels rough. She has an intermittent spontaneous metallic taste, and her mouth always feels dry.

[a] Orofacial Pain Medicine, Shaukat Khanum Memorial Cancer Hospitals and Research Centres, Lahore and Peshawar, Pakistan; [b] Orofacial Pain Program, Tufts University, School of Dental Medicine, 1 Kneeland St, Boston, MA 02111, USA; [c] Tufts University, School of Dental Medicine, Boston, MA, USA
* Corresponding author. Shaukat Khanum Memorial Cancer Hospital and Research Center, 7A Block R-3, Phase 2, M.A. Johar Town, Lahore, Punjab 54782, Pakistan.
E-mail address: khawajashehryar@gmail.com

Dent Clin N Am 67 (2023) 49–60
https://doi.org/10.1016/j.cden.2022.07.004
0011-8532/23/© 2022 Elsevier Inc. All rights reserved.

dental.theclinics.com

There were no additional associated sensory or motor alterations or autonomic symptoms.

Her medical history was significant for hypercholesterolemia for which she takes rosu-vastatin 10 mg once a day. She was not aware of any allergies to medications. Her family history was significant for diabetes mellitus and heart disease. She had discontinued drinking alcohol 2 months ago because it aggravated her oral symptoms. She had no history of smoking or substance abuse. There was no history of psychiatric disease. She had retired from an office job 2 years ago and lived with her husband and 2 dogs.

On physical examination, her pulse rate was 72 beats/min, and her blood pressure was 125/76 mm Hg. Her respiratory rate was 17 breaths per minute, and her temperature was 36.4°C. During the examination, she was oriented to time, place, and person. There was no asymmetry, atrophy, swelling, lymphadenopathy, or lesions on inspection of the head, face, and neck regions. The vertical and horizontal mandibular range of motion was within normal limits and was achieved without pain. The patient reported no pain on palpation of the masticatory muscles, temporomandibular joint, posterior mandibular area, or submandibular region. No palpable joint sounds or abnormal movement patterns were observed during mandibular motion. The cervical range of motion was within normal limits, and the patient did not report any pain on palpation of the cervical muscles.

Intraoral examination revealed normal, moist, and pink-colored oral mucosa. Tongue movements were normal, the uvula was in the midline, and the soft palate was mobile. No lesions, discolorations, or swelling were observed, and salivary flow was clear and adequate. There was mild pooling of saliva on the floor of the mouth. There were no calculi or plaque deposits. The right mandibular and maxillary third molars were missing. Class I amalgam restorations were present in the right mandibular first molar, left mandibular first and second molars, and left maxillary first molar. The rest of the dentition was sound.

Cranial nerve (CN II-XII) examination revealed no gross discrepancies. The spinal nerves (C2-T1) were grossly intact. Testing of complex motor skills revealed normal coordination. Deep tendon reflexes of the biceps, triceps, and brachioradialis were normal. The panoramic radiograph in the closed-mouth position did not show any disease. A working diagnosis of burning mouth syndrome was made. Before presenting to the pain clinic for assessment, the patient had a thorough evaluation by her primary care physician. She had a complete blood cell count, thyroid function test, liver function test, vitamin D, HbA$_{1c}$ (glycated hemoglobin), cholesterol assessment, and serum electrolyte test. In addition, she had completed a 10-day course of fluconazole 100 mg once a day for a presumptive diagnosis of oral candida infection. The tests were within normal physiologic limits, and fluconazole therapy did not improve her symptoms.

The patient was prescribed clonazepam 0.5 mg at night. She was advised to suck the tablet for 5 minutes and expectorating the tablet afterward. Likewise, the patient was advised to start alpha-lipoic acid 300 mg twice a day. Laboratory studies (vitamin B$_{12}$ and serum folate) were ordered and were within normal limits. A definitive diagnosis of burning mouth syndrome was made.

At the 6-week follow-up, the patient reported that the severity of symptoms had reduced, and she had mild pain. The spontaneous episodes of metallic taste perception had diminished, and the roughness she felt over the teeth had improved. She was advised to start swallowing the clonazepam tablet after sucking on it for 5 minutes. At the subsequent 6-week follow-up, the patient reported that she had been pain free for nearly 3 weeks. However, she continued to have sensitivity to spicy foods. She was advised to continue using clonazepam and alpha-lipoic acid and avoid spicy foods or any other potential irritants.

## INTRODUCTION

Burning mouth syndrome (BMS) is a chronic pain disorder affecting the oral cavity. BMS has previously been referred to as stomatodynia, glossodynia, oral dysesthesia, or primary BMS.[1,2] The inclusion of the word "syndrome" in the nomenclature is controversial. In a recent expert-based Delphi-style investigation, 88% of the field experts believed that BMS was not a syndrome.[3] Nonetheless, the International Classification for Orofacial Pain (ICOP) has used the nomenclature of BMS.[4] For uniformity of understanding and care, this is the terminology used in this article.

Likewise, there have been multiple operational definitions and diagnostic criteria proposed for BMS, making for a diagnostic challenge. It has been reported that it may take on average 13 months from the reported onset of symptoms to a definitive diagnosis. Likewise, a patient may seek care from 3.1 caregivers during this period.[5]

More recently, a committee from the International Network for Orofacial Pain and Related Disorders Methodology developed a set of Research Diagnostic Criteria for Burning Mouth Syndrome (RDC/BMS) based on the ICOP guidelines.[6] These criteria are currently in beta version and undergoing field testing.

This variation in definition and diagnostic criteria between studies has resulted in limited understanding of the epidemiology, pathophysiology, and management of BMS.

## EPIDEMIOLOGY

The prevalence of BMS has been reported to range from 0.1% to 4.6% in the general population.[1,7] This range is likely due to dissimilarities in the operational definitions of BMS, differences in the diagnostic criteria, and the population investigated.[6,7] In general, BMS is most prevalent in postmenopausal women. The estimated men to women ratio of prevalence is between 1:3 and 1:7. Nonetheless, the prevalence increases in both genders with age.[1,2]

## DIAGNOSTIC CRITERIA AND CLASSIFICATION

In the ICOP, BMS has been defined as pain or dysesthesia recurring every day for more than 2 hours for 3 months or more with no evident causation on clinical examination and/or investigation. The ICOP diagnostic criteria of BMS are summarized in **Box 1**. The classification system further divides BMS into BMS without somatosensory changes and BMS with somatosensory changes. These changes can be assessed using either qualitative or quantitative somatosensory testing.[4]

Recently, a Delphi-style expert-based standardized approach to diagnose BMS through a research diagnostic framework was published. RDC/BMS are based on the ICOP definition. The purpose of these guidelines is to operationalize the ICOP BMS definition by creating a structured assessment and clinical examination.

Previously, the presence of symptoms of burning pain or dysesthesia in the oral cavity attributed to any underlying systemic or local causes was referred to as secondary BMS. However, this term is no longer valid or acceptable.[4] Nonetheless, conditions that may mimic BMS are listed in **Box 2**.

## PATHOPHYSIOLOGY

The exact cause of BMS remains elusive. Clinical and animal-based investigations examining etiologic and pathophysiological associations suggest that the cause of BMS has neuropathic, endocrinological, and psychosocial components.

Box 1
The International Classification of Orofacial Pain, 1st edition, diagnostic criteria for burning mouth syndrome

Diagnostic criteria:
A. Oral pain fulfilling criteria B and C.
B. Recurring daily for greater than 2 h/d for greater than 3 months.[a]
C. Pain has both the following characteristics:
   1. Burning quality
   2. Felt superficially in the oral mucosa
D. Oral mucosa is of normal appearance, and local or systemic causes have been excluded.
D. Not better accounted for by another ICOP or Internal Classification of Headache Disorders-3 diagnosis.[b]

[a] Before 3 months, if all other criteria are fulfilled, code as *Probable burning mouth syndrome.*[b] A diagnosis of *burning mouth syndrome* implies that quantitative sensory testing has not been performed. Once it has, either of the 2 subtypes: *burning mouth syndrome without somatosensory changes* or *burning mouth syndrome with somatosensory changes* should be diagnosed.

*Data from* International Classification of Orofacial Pain, 1st edition (ICOP). *Cephalalgia.* 2020;40(2):129-221.

## NEUROPATHIC MECHANISMS

It has been proposed that the sensory portions of trigeminal and glossopharyngeal nerves interact with the gustatory fibers of the chorda tympani nerve. This interaction takes place via both peripheral and central mechanisms.[8–10]

In BMS, there is evidence that small fibers in the epithelium of the tongue undergo atrophy.[9,11,12] Similarly, it has been reported that the number of fibers innervating the taste buds are reduced and that trigeminal innervation of the fungiform papillae varies, which can cause the afferent nerve impulses to decrease.[9,10]

Box 2
List of conditions that may mimic burning mouth syndrome

- Psychosomatic disorders (anxiety, somatization)
- Systemic illness (diabetes, Sjögrens, or thyroid or hepatic illness)
- Nutritional deficiencies such as, iron, zinc, magnesium, or vitamin B ($B_1$, $B_2$, $B_6$, and $B_{12}$)
- Medications (antihypertensive agents such as angiotensin-converting enzyme inhibitors, hormonal replacement therapies, antihistamines)
- Dry mouth
- Inflammatory disorders (stomatitis, lichen planus, geographic tongue)
- Trauma or injury (noniatrogenic)
- Surgical or iatrogenic injury
- Radiation- or chemotherapy-induced pain
- Infections (fungal, bacterial, or viral)
- Autoimmune disorder or systemic illness (diabetes, or thyroid or hepatic illness)
- Hypersensitivity or allergic reaction
- Pain attributed to malignant lesion (cancer-related pain)

The loss of input from the chorda tympani nerve fibers diminishes the disinhibitory action on the trigeminal or glossopharyngeal nerve, which results in overcompensation from the latter; causes modification in the mutual modulation at the level of nucleus tractus solitarius, amygdala, and medial pain system; and triggers deafferentation-hyperactivity changes in the somatosensory regions of the trigeminal system.[8,9,13,14] Likewise, studies using quantitative sensory testing have suggested that the thermal and pain detection thresholds vary among patients with BMS. However, the pain tolerability has consistently been reported to be reduced, suggesting temporal summation (induced by central sensitization).[9,15]

## ENDOCRINOLOGICAL MECHANISMS

Gonadal hormones are essential for maintaining tongue epithelium thickness and keratinization.[9] After menopause, a reduction in the synthesis of ovarian steroids may cause adrenal steroid deficiency or dysfunction.[16] This deficiency or dysfunction can diminish the neuroprotective effects of steroids on neural tissues, which may directly or indirectly generate pain-related behaviors through peripheral and central mechanisms.[9,16] In patients with BMS, tongue epithelium thickness is reduced, and there may be a loss of keratinization.[9] Furthermore, as stated earlier, the clinical symptoms of BMS suggest that patients have peripheral and central sensitization.

Ovariectomy has been shown to result in upregulation of glial cell line-derived neurotrophic factor (GDNF) family ligands and their receptors.[17] Levels of artemin, a member of the GDNF family, was reported to be raised in the tongue epithelial cells of patients with BMS.[18] Moreover, transgenic overexpression of artemin resulted in increased expression of TRPV1 (transient receptor potential cation channel, subfamily V, member 1) and TRPA1 (transient receptor potential cation channel, subfamily A, member 1), which was associated with increased sensitivity to capsaicin and mustard oil and lingual nerve atrophy. These changes are similar to the characteristics of nerve atrophy seen among patients with BMS.[9,18,19]

It has been hypothesized that the lack of neuroprotective steroids leads to hypofunction of minor salivary glands, which may induce latent oral dryness and preclinical inflammation of oral mucosa. These peripheral changes may generate burning pain and dysesthesia and account for the subjective feeling of oral dryness.[9]

## PSYCHOSOCIAL MECHANISMS

The prevalence of anxiety and depression increases postmenopause, and there is a high comorbidity of anxiety and depression in BMS.[20] Among patients with depression and anxiety, there is reduced synthesis of neuroprotective steroids in the hippocampus, amygdala, and medial prefrontal cortex. Similar areas have been reported to have altered brain activity in patients with BMS.[9]

The high prevalence of psychological distress among patients with BMS may be explained by the role of neuroprotective steroids on mood. Dysregulation of gonadal hormones can lead to psychological distress.[9,21] Neuroprotective steroids, such as progesterone metabolites, modulate $\gamma$-aminobutyric acid (GABA$_A$) receptors and result in mood changes.[22] Allopregnanolone can exert an anxiolytic effect by positive modulation of GABA$_A$ receptors and negative modulation of the hypothalamic-pituitary-adrenal (HPA) axis.[9] Similarly, progesterone and estrogen can regulate the endogenous anxiolytic effects of serotonin and allopregnanolone.[9] Overall, in postmenopause, there is reduced serotonergic neurotransmission, reduced GABAergic inhibition, and less efficient HPA axis activity, which increases the risk of developing anxiety and depression. Correspondingly, mental stress induces downregulation of

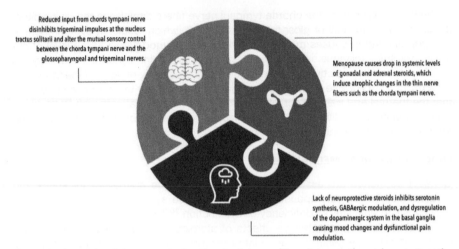

Reduced input from chords tympani nerve disinhibits trigeminal impulses at the nucleus tractus solitarii and alter the mutual sensory control between the chorda tympani nerve and the glossopharyngeal and trigeminal nerves.

Menopause causes drop in systemic levels of gonadal and adrenal steroids, which induce atrophic changes in the thin nerve fibers such as the chorda tympani nerve.

Lack of neuroprotective steroids inhibits serotonin synthesis, GABAergic modulation, and dysregulation of the dopaminergic system in the basal ganglia causing mood changes and dysfunctional pain modulation.

**Fig. 1.** A schematic of the suspected pathophysiology of burning mouth syndrome. A pathologic event, such as infection, trauma, or an allergic reaction can theoretically induce atrophic changes in the thin nerve fibers such as the chorda tympani nerve.

the hypothalamic-pituitary-gonadal (HPG) and HPA axes by modulating the $GABA_A$ receptor, further reducing gonadal hormone levels.[9]

## SUMMARY

A pathologic event, such as infection, trauma, or an allergic reaction, or a physiologic phenomenon such as menopause that reduces systemic levels of gonadal and adrenal steroids, can induce atrophic changes in the thin nerve fibers such as the chorda tympani nerve, innervating the oral mucosa; this causes predominance of the trigeminal nerve, which may clinically produce dysgeusia. Moreover, reduced input from the chorda tympani nerve fibers can disinhibit trigeminal impulses at the nucleus tractus solitarii and alter the mutual sensory control between the trigeminal, the chorda tympani, and the glossopharyngeal nerves, which may clinically present as burning pain or dysesthesia. Furthermore, lack of neuroprotective steroids inhibits serotonin synthesis, GABAergic modulation, and dysregulation of the dopaminergic system in the basal ganglia. These alterations produce mood changes and dysfunctional pain modulation. Collectively, persistent pain (and concurrent psychological distress) suppresses the function of the pain modulation system (**Fig. 1**).

## CLINICAL FEATURES AND SYSTEMIC ASSESSMENT

BMS diagnosis requires a comprehensive history and clinical examination, including laboratory investigations to rule out any local and systemic causes of symptoms.

Most patients report pain rather than dysesthesia.[1,2,23] However, in some cases, both may be present. The quality of pain or dysesthesia is often described as burning, tender, tingling, hot, stinging, scalding, numbness, discomfort, raw, unpleasant, or annoying.[2,23] The intensity of pain varies from mild to severe. On average, it can be approximately $6 \pm 2$ (on a 0 to 10 numeric verbal pain rating scale). However, in some cases, pain can be 10 of 10 in intensity. In some patients, oral intake of food or liquids and talking help alleviate pain intermittently for a few minutes. However, in others, foods or beverages and hot, spicy, acidic, minty, or alcoholic drinks may exacerbate the symptoms.[2,23]

In BMS, symptoms are distributed bilaterally, and the most common locations of pain are the tip and the anterior two-thirds of a tongue. Nonetheless, in most of the patients, more than one site of pain is present. Other areas involved are the hard palate, labial, or buccal mucosa.[1,2,23] The pain is often spontaneous in onset and can last for years. The likelihood of spontaneous remission is rare.[1,2] The pattern of pain varies among patients. In some patients, pain increases toward the end of the day. In others, the intensity of the pain remains constant, or the pain may present intermittently for minutes/hours throughout the day. Nonetheless, it occurs daily for at least 2 hours.[1,2,23]

In more than two-thirds of the patients, primary symptoms of pain or dysesthesia are associated with at least one secondary symptom.[23] The patient may report alteration of taste perception in the presence of taste stimulation (dysgeusia) or an abnormal taste (bitter or metallic) occurring in the absence of stimulation of taste (phantom taste). Similarly, primary symptoms may present with a subjective feeling of oral dryness (xerostomia) or alteration in sensory perception, such as feeling that the tongue or oral mucosa has a sandpaperlike texture or that the surfaces or size of teeth are different.[1,2,23]

The clinical examination is normal and does not correspond to the symptoms. There are no local or systemic causes that may explain the symptoms in the oral mucosa.[1,2] The RDC/BMS has proposed an extensive list of investigations at baseline to rule out secondary causes (**Box 3**).[6] This list is not exclusive, and other tests may be added depending on the outcome of the history and examination. In addition, recent guidelines have proposed quantitative or qualitative sensory testing of the oral cavity to subclassify BMS. However, the clinical significance of this is unknown.

The presence of BMS has a negative effect on the patient's quality of life.[24] Furthermore, patients with BMS have a high prevalence of psychiatric disorders such as anxiety, depression, and somatization; significantly higher adverse early life experiences; cancer phobia; gastrointestinal problems; and chronic fatigue syndrome.[1,2,20]

## MANAGEMENT

There are no universally accepted guidelines for the management of BMS. Nonetheless, over the last couple of years, multiple systematic reviews and meta-analyses have been published, which have provided a better understanding of the effectiveness of the interventions.

Management should commence with a detailed review and explanation of BMS. Patients should be given detailed instructions regarding the possible pathophysiology and management strategies for BMS in a manner that they can understand. Furthermore, expectations of therapy should be addressed. This educational session alone may help alleviate primary and secondary symptoms associated with BMS.[25]

Clonazepam is a benzodiazepine that is an effective topical and systemic intervention for the management of BMS.[23] It is often used as the first-line therapy. Until recently, most of the evidence for the effectiveness of clonazepam was based on case series and retrospective analyses. However, recent systematic reviews and meta-analyses have shown that clonazepam has a significant therapeutic effect in BMS.[7,25] Clonazepam is routinely used between 0.5 and 2 mg single dose at night because of the sedative effect.[23] The beneficial effect of topical therapy has been shown to take place without any systemic absorption. Likewise, in studies in which clonazepam was used both as topical and systemic therapy, it was observed to have a synergistic effect. Similar observations have been reported in studies in which

---

**Box 3**
**List of investigations proposed by the research diagnostic criteria for burning mouth syndrome to be completed at baseline for all patients**

- Complete blood cell count/full blood count (mean corpuscular hemoglobin/mean corpuscular volume/white cell count/hemoglobin)
- Vitamin $B_1$, $B_2$, $B_6$, and $B_{12}$; iron; folate
- Serum iron, ferritin, total iron-binding capacity
- Zinc and magnesium
- Glycated hemoglobin ($HbA_{1c}$)
- Thyroid function test
- Liver function test
- Erythrocyte sedimentation rate or C-reactive protein
- Autoantibodies test (Anti-Ro and anti-La, anti-nuclear antibodies, and extractable nuclear antigen antibodies)
- Serum homocysteine level
- Swab or smear for gram staining

*Data from* Currie CC, Ohrbach R, De Leeuw R, et al. Developing a research diagnostic criteria for burning mouth syndrome: Results from an international Delphi process. *J Oral Rehabil.* 2021;48(3):308-331.

---

clonazepam has been used with other therapies, such as alpha-lipoic acid (ALA), *N*-acetyl cysteine, and gabapentin.[7,25,26] Clonazepam has an agonistic effect on peripheral and central $GABA_A$ receptors subunits $\alpha 1$ and $\alpha 2$. In chronic mental distress, the $GABA_A$ receptor configuration changes, which results in the expression of the $\alpha 4$, $\alpha 5$, and $\gamma$ subunits to undergo a significant increase and the expression of the $\alpha 1$ and $\alpha 2$ subunits to decrease significantly. Benzodiazepines have a poor affinity for the $\alpha 4$, $\alpha 5$, and $\gamma$ subunits, which are highly sensitive to neuroprotective steroids.[27] Correspondingly, in the studies in which the participants had a poor response to clonazepam the patients were found to have a significant level of psychological distress (anxiety and/or depression).[28] The use of clonazepam is commonly associated with drowsiness, dizziness, feeling tired or depressed, memory issues, or gait problems.[29] Furthermore, the use of benzodiazepines accounts for nearly half of the total emergency visits due to toxicity associated with the use of sedatives. Owing to its high potential for misuse and overdose, it is categorized as a schedule IV drug under the Controlled Substance Schedule.[29,30] Furthermore, investigations have suggested that benzodiazepine and opioid cotreatment is associated with increased long-term mortality risk.[29] It may be valuable to involve the patient's primary care physician in caring for such patients.

The systemic use of gabapentinoids, tricyclic antidepressants, and serotonin-norepinephrine reuptake inhibitors (SNRI) has been reported to be beneficial in the management of BMS.[2,23] SNRIs have been used to manage cases refractory to clonazepam, which might be due to the neurosteroidergic effects of these medications at low nonserotonergic doses in the brain. Like clonazepam, gabapentinoids are classified as schedule IV (and schedule V in some states) controlled substances.[31] The use of gabapentinoids, tricyclic antidepressants, and SNRIs is commonly associated with drowsiness, dizziness, memory clouding, and gastrointestinal and genitourinary side effects.[32–34]

ALA, an antioxidant, has extensively been investigated either alone or as an adjunct to a pharmacologic agent or cognitive behavioral therapy for the management of BMS. The regimen consists of 200 to 800 mg in single or divided doses a day for up to 8 weeks. The short-term ($6 \pm 2$ weeks) results are inconsistent; some studies showed significant relief in symptoms, and others suggested a nonsignificant effect. On the contrary, studies that investigated long-term (10 weeks or more) effects of using ALA reported significant benefits. The use of ALA may result in minor side effects, including but not limited to gastrointestinal complaints such as heartburn and headaches.[35]

Herbal Catuama, a herbal compound, has been shown to be helpful in the management of BMS. This compound has been shown to result in a significant reduction in burning after 8 and 12 weeks.[7,36] Herbal Catuama is, relative to controlled substances, a safe intervention and has a low risk of causing sleep issues or weight gain. When used topically or systematically, capsaicin, a TRVP1 (transient receptor potential vanilloid subtype 1) agonist, has been reported to significantly improve symptoms associated with BMS. However, the topical use of the modality was associated with aggravation in burning sensation, and systemic therapy was associated with gastric pain.

Psychotherapy alone or in combination with ALA has been shown to result in pain reduction in patients with BMS. Recently, a systematic review and meta-analysis on the effectiveness of photobiomodulation (low-level laser therapy) in BMS management determined that photobiomodulation results in pain reduction.[37] However, the investigators concluded that more evidence was still required.

There is anecdotal evidence for symptomatic relief using a 1:1 mixture of diphenhydramine (elixir) and kaolin-pectin (solution), local anesthetic (viscous or jelly lidocaine, or benzocaine gel), or Magic mouthwash/Miracle mouthwash (a combination of local anesthetic, antihistamine, antacid, simethicone, or corticosteroid).[30] Beneficial effects of treating subjective oral dryness in BMS have not been studied.

## SUMMARY

BMS is a chronic intraoral pain disorder that is associated with burning pain or dysesthesia. The prevalence of secondary symptoms such as alteration in taste perception, phantom taste, xerostomia, or alteration in sensory perception differs between patients, resulting in a varying clinical presentation. In BMS, there are no organic local or systemic causes for symptoms. BMS has a negative impact on the quality of life, and the patients often have comorbid psychological disorders. Clonazepam is often used as the first-line therapy. However, other modalities have been shown to have a beneficial effect. There are no universal guidelines on the management of BMS primarily due to the lack of standardized definition, diagnostic criteria, and reporting of outcomes in published studies. Nonetheless, recent advances such as the release of the ICOP and RDC/BMS, and the development of an expert and patient-driven set of core outcome measures for randomized controlled trials for BMS may help answer these important questions in the future.

## CLINICS CARE POINTS

- The patient reported near-constant burning pain over the tip of her tongue, lower and upper lips, and behind upper teeth (anterior hard palate) for nearly 4 months.
- The pain was associated with feelings of the tongue being raw or burnt, the texture of anterior teeth feeling rough, intermittent spontaneous metallic taste, and dry mouth.

- The oral mucosa was of normal appearance, and no local or systemic causes for burning pain were identified.
- The patient partially responded to topical clonazepam and systemic ALA therapy. However, after switching her to systemic clonazepam therapy, the patient reported significant pain relief.

## DISCLOSURE

The authors have nothing to disclose.

## REFERENCES

1. Fortuna G, Napenas J, Su N, et al. Oral dysesthesia. In: Farah CS, Balasubramaniam R, McCullough MJ, editors. Contemporary oral medicine. Cham, Switzerland: Springer International Publishing; 2018. p. 1–25.
2. Klasser GD, Grushka M, Su N. Burning Mouth Syndrome. Oral Maxillofacial Surg Clin North Am 2016;28(3):381–96.
3. Chmieliauskaite M, Stelson EA, Epstein JB, et al. Consensus agreement to rename burning mouth syndrome and improve ICD-11 disease criteria: an international Delphi study. Pain 2021;162(10):2548–57.
4. International Classification of Orofacial Pain, 1st edition (ICOP). Cephalalgia 2020;40(2):129–221.
5. Mignogna MD, Fedele S, Lo Russo L, et al. The diagnosis of burning mouth syndrome represents a challenge for clinicians. J Orofac Pain 2005;19(2):168–73.
6. Currie CC, Ohrbach R, De Leeuw R, et al. Developing a research diagnostic criteria for burning mouth syndrome: Results from an international Delphi process. J Oral Rehabil 2021;48(3):308–31.
7. Farag AM, Kuten-Shorrer M, Natto Z, et al. WWOM VII: Effectiveness of systemic pharmacotherapeutic interventions in the management of BMS: A systematic review and meta-analysis. Oral Dis 2021. https://doi.org/10.1111/odi.13817. odi.13817.
8. Felizardo R, Boucher Y, Braud A, et al. Trigeminal projections on gustatory neurons of the nucleus of the solitary tract: A double-label strategy using electrical stimulation of the chorda tympani and tracer injection in the lingual nerve. Brain Res 2009;1288:60–8.
9. Imamura Y, Shinozaki T, Okada-Ogawa A, et al. An updated review on pathophysiology and management of burning mouth syndrome with endocrinological, psychological and neuropathic perspectives. J Oral Rehabil 2019;46(6):574–87.
10. Eliav E, Kamran B, Schaham R, et al. Evidence of chorda tympani dysfunction in patients with burning mouth syndrome. J Am Dent Assoc 2007;138(5):628–33.
11. Yilmaz Z, Renton T, Yiangou Y, et al. Burning mouth syndrome as a trigeminal small fibre neuropathy: Increased heat and capsaicin receptor TRPV1 in nerve fibres correlates with pain score. J Clin Neurosci 2007;14(9):864–71.
12. Beneng K, Yilmaz Z, Yiangou Y, et al. Sensory purinergic receptor P2X3 is elevated in burning mouth syndrome. Int J Oral Maxillofac Surg 2010;39(8):815–9.
13. Boucher Y, Simons CT, Faurion A, et al. Trigeminal modulation of gustatory neurons in the nucleus of the solitary tract. Brain Res 2003;973(2):265–74.
14. Corson JA, Erisir A. Monosynaptic convergence of chorda tympani and glossopharyngeal afferents onto ascending relay neurons in the nucleus of the solitary

tract: A high-resolution confocal and correlative electron microscopy approach: Convergence in the rNTS. J Comp Neurol 2013;521(13):2907–26.

15. Grushka M, Sessle BJ, Howley TP. Psychophysical assessment of tactile, pain and thermal sensory functions in burning mouth syndrome. Pain 1987;28(2): 169–84.

16. Woda A, Dao T, Gremeau-Richard C. Steroid dysregulation and stomatodynia (burning mouth syndrome). J Orofac Pain 2009;23(3):202–10.

17. Hernández-Aragón LG, García-Villamar V, Carrasco-Ruiz M, et al. Role of Estrogens in the Size of Neuronal Somata of Paravaginal Ganglia in Ovariectomized Rabbits. Biomed Res Int 2017;2017:1–12.

18. Shinoda M, Takeda M, Honda K, et al. Involvement of peripheral artemin signaling in tongue pain: possible mechanism in burning mouth syndrome. Pain 2015; 156(12):2528–37.

19. Elitt CM, Malin SA, Koerber HR, et al. Overexpression of artemin in the tongue increases expression of TRPV1 and TRPA1 in trigeminal afferents and causes oral sensitivity to capsaicin and mustard oil. Brain Res 2008;1230:80–90.

20. Kim JY, Kim YS, Ko I, et al. Association Between Burning Mouth Syndrome and the Development of Depression, Anxiety, Dementia, and Parkinson Disease. JAMA Otolaryngol Head Neck Surg 2020;146(6):561.

21. Walf AA, Frye CA. A Review and Update of Mechanisms of Estrogen in the Hippocampus and Amygdala for Anxiety and Depression Behavior. Neuropsychopharmacol 2006;31(6):1097–111.

22. Gunn BG, Cunningham L, Mitchell SG, et al. GABAA receptor-acting neurosteroids: A role in the development and regulation of the stress response. Front Neuroendocrinol 2015;36:28–48.

23. Khawaja SN, Bavia PF, Keith DA. Clinical Characteristics, Treatment Effectiveness, and Predictors of Response to Pharmacotherapeutic Interventions in Burning Mouth Syndrome: A Retrospective Analysis. J Oral Facial Pain Headache 2020;34(2):157–66.

24. Souza FT, Santos TP, Bernardes VF, et al. The impact of burning mouth syndrome on health-related quality of life. Health Qual Life Outcomes 2011;9(1):57.

25. Kim M, Kim J, Kho H. Treatment outcomes and related clinical characteristics in patients with burning mouth syndrome. Colorectal Dis 2021;27(6):1507–18.

26. Han S, Lim JH, Bang J, et al. Use of a combination of N-acetylcysteine and clonazepam to treat burning mouth syndrome. Oral Surg Oral Med Oral Pathol Oral Radiol 2021;132(5):532–8.

27. Locci A, Pinna G. Neurosteroid biosynthesis down-regulation and changes in GABAA receptor subunit composition: a biomarker axis in stress-induced cognitive and emotional impairment. Br J Pharmacol 2017;174(19):3226–41.

28. Grémeau-Richard C, Dubray C, Aublet-Cuvelier B, et al. Effect of lingual nerve block on burning mouth syndrome (stomatodynia): A randomized crossover trial. Pain 2010;149(1):27–32.

29. Xu KY, Hartz SM, Borodovsky JT, et al. Association Between Benzodiazepine Use With or Without Opioid Use and All-Cause Mortality in the United States, 1999-2015. JAMA Netw Open 2020;3(12):e2028557.

30. Kaufmann CN, Spira AP, Alexander GC, et al. Emergency department visits involving benzodiazepines and non-benzodiazepine receptor agonists. Am J Emerg Med 2017;35(10):1414–9.

31. Peckham AM, Ananickal MJ, Sclar DA. Gabapentin use, abuse, and the US opioid epidemic: the case for reclassification as a controlled substance and the need for pharmacovigilance. Risk Manag Healthc Policy 2018;11:109–16.

32. Hillhouse TM, Porter JH. A brief history of the development of antidepressant drugs: from monoamines to glutamate. Exp Clin Psychopharmacol 2015; 23(1):1–21.
33. Gillman PK. Tricyclic antidepressant pharmacology and therapeutic drug interactions updated. Br J Pharmacol 2007;151(6):737–48.
34. Quintero GC. Review about gabapentin misuse, interactions, contraindications and side effects. J Exp Pharmacol 2017;9:13–21.
35. Femiano F, Gombos F, Scully C, et al. Burning mouth syndrome (BMS): controlled open trial of the efficacy of alpha-lipoic acid (thioctic acid) on symptomatology. Oral Dis 2000;6(5):274–7.
36. Spanemberg JC, Cherubini K, de Figueiredo MAZ, et al. Effect of an herbal compound for treatment of burning mouth syndrome: randomized, controlled, double-blind clinical trial. Oral Surg Oral Med Oral Pathol Oral Radiol 2012;113(3):373–7.
37. Spanemberg JC, Segura-Egea JJ, Rodríguez-de Rivera-Campillo E, et al. Low-level laser therapy in patients with Burning Mouth Syndrome: A double-blind, randomized, controlled clinical trial. J Clin Exp Dent 2019;11(2):e162–9.

# Continued persistent facial pain despite several surgical interventions in the temporomandibular joint

Annika Rosèn, DDS, Dr Med Sci[a,b,*], Espen Helgeland, DDS, PhD[a,b], Torbjørn Ø. Pedersen, DDS, PhD[a,b]

KEYWORDS

- Temporomandibular joint • Postoperative pain • Risk factors
- Multiple surgical procedures • Chronic pain

KEY POINTS

- Be aware of risk factors that may contribute to the development of persistent postoperative pain.
- Screening for risk factors preoperatively is important to prevent persistent postoperative pain.
- Making plans for pain management before, during, and after surgery is essential for patients' recovery.
- Multiple surgical procedures should be avoided.

## CASE PRESENTATION
### Identification

A 41-year-old woman was referred from her general medical practitioner for an assessment of her temporomandibular disorder (TMD) to the National Interdisciplinary Orofacial Pain Clinic in Bergen, Norway. Previously, the Norwegian Government Health Directorate had initiated an interdisciplinary program for TMD patients, the National TMD project. A collaboration between the Department of Oral and Maxillofacial Surgery and the Pain Clinic at Haukeland University Hospital formed this interdisciplinary team with specialists from both the dental and the medical health services .[1]

[a] Department of Clinical Dentistry, Faculty of Medicine, University of Bergen, Bergen, Norway;
[b] Department of Oral and Maxillofacial Surgery, Haukeland University Hospital, Bergen, Norway
* Corresponding author. Department of Clinical Dentistry, Faculty of Medicine, University of Bergen, Bergen, Norway.
*E-mail address:* Annika.Rosen@uib.no

Dent Clin N Am 67 (2023) 61–70
https://doi.org/10.1016/j.cden.2022.07.005
0011-8532/23/© 2022 Elsevier Inc. All rights reserved.

### Chief Complaint

Her chief complaint was pain on the left side of her face and in the region of the left temporomandibular joint (TMJ).

### History of Present Illness/Problem

Her complaints started following double-jaw orthognathic surgery performed 19 years ago for a class III malocclusion (**Fig. 1**). She described a persistent reduced sensation in the scalp and skin on the left side of her face immediately following the operation that normalized after approximately 3 years. Also, at that time, she experienced a skeletal relapse. Fifteen years after the surgery, she developed spontaneous onset of acute pain on the left side of the face and temporal region. Intracranial pathologic condition was excluded by MRI, and as the pain persisted, conservative treatment with occlusal splints was initiated by her general dental practitioner. She was at the same time referred to a specialist in oral and maxillofacial surgery (OMFS) at Oslo University Hospital for investigation of her complaints. An arthroscopy of the left TMJ was performed owing to the pain complaints and disc derangements shown on MRI. The arthroscopy had limited effect, and the pain intensity increased in the following years. Several additional treatments were initiated before the patient presented at the authors' clinic. She had tried a regimen of neuropathic pain medication (gabapentin) and baclofen, a spasmolytic, administration of anesthesia blocks (lidocaine) intravenously once per week, injection of botulinum toxin type A (Botox; Allergan, Dublin, Ireland) in the masticatory muscles and in the back of her head, corticosteroid injections into the left TMJ, all with little or no effect on the pain. Next, an anterior mandibular repositioning splint was made, which she used 24 hours per day for many years, resulting in a bilateral posterior open bite. She also had weekly treatment by a physical therapist.

### Pain History

The patient described chronic pain on both sides of her face, but more prominently on her left side. She also described a generalized pain all over her body (**Fig. 2**). The pain was described as constant, with an intensity on a Visual Analogue Scale (0–10, 0 = no pain and 10 = maximum pain) of 7 to 8, every day and night all year around.

### Medical History

The patient had a Morton's neuroma on her left foot and was allergic to several foods, animals, pollen, and penicillin. She has had regular follow-up since 2010 at a private department of pain medicine in Oslo owing to the local and global pain. She was taking gabapentin (360 mg/d), baclofen (10 mg/d), and combination analgesics (codeine and

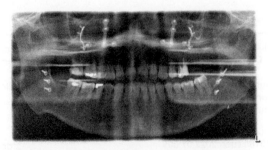

**Fig. 1.** Osteosynthesis after bimaxillary surgery.

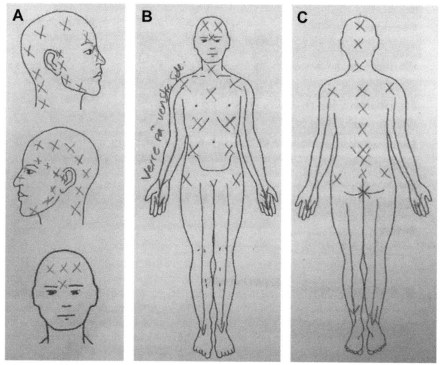

**Fig. 2.** The patient's reported pain at the time of referral. (*A*) Bilateral pain in the head and neck region. (*B*) Ventral pain in the upper and lower extremities, chest, abdomen, and hips. Text written in Norwegian meaning "worse on my left side." (*C*) Dorsal pain in the upper and lower extremities, spine, shoulders, and neck.

acetaminophen) if necessary. Administration of anesthesia blocks (bupivacaine and lidocaine), injection of botulinum toxin type A (Botox) in the masticatory muscles and in the back of her head as well as intravenous ketamine infusions are administered every 2 weeks. The patient has claimed that she could not be alive without this analgesic regimen.

### Social History

The patient lived alone and had a functional relationship with her parents and 5 siblings. She was raised in a small village in the countryside and finished elementary school before starting work in a kindergarten. She had been on sick leave since 2010 owing to her pain condition.

### Psychosocial and Functional Assessments

Before the examination in the National TMD project, all the patients completed comprehensive psychosocial and functional assessments that were routine in the pain clinic at the hospital.[2] The questionnaires consisted of the Roland-Morris scale (RMS) concerning general disability,[3] questions about sleep disorders, the Hospital Anxiety and Depression scale (HADS),[4] and the 2-item version of the Coping Strategies Questionnaire (CSQ) regarding catastrophizing.[5] The results for this patient showed RMS = 8 (maximum score, 24), sleep disorders = 2 (maximum score, 3; wakes up

2–3 times per night owing to pain), HADS 1 + 6 = 7 (maximum score, 21 + 21), and the CSQ/catastrophizing 0 + 3 = 3 (maximum score, 6 + 6). She also completed a Mandibular Function Impairment Questionnaire[6] with a score of 17 (maximum score, 28) (**Table 1**). Most values were within the normal range, except she had a high score on sleep disorders, an increased score on catastrophizing, and reduced mandibular function. A visual description of her pain distribution showed self-reported generalized pain all over her body (see **Fig. 2**).

## Review of Systems

The multidisciplinary assessment included clinical evaluations by an oral and maxillofacial surgeon, an orofacial pain specialist, an anesthesiologist (pain specialist), a psychologist, and a physical therapist over a period of 3 weeks, 1 day a week, of examinations and included imaging, blood, and saliva analyses. At the final consultation, a dynamic feedback meeting was arranged to present the results and treatment recommendations for the patient and her relatives.

## Diagnostic Studies/Imaging

A panoramic radiograph showed her status following orthognathic surgery with osteosynthesis material in both jaws (**Fig. 1**) She had short-rooted teeth, possibly owing to previous orthodontic treatment, which she had both before and after orthognathic surgery. The maxillary left second molar (FDI 27/ADA 15) was missing, and the maxillary left first molar (FDI 26/ADA 14) had a root canal treatment. Also, large dental fillings were present in the remaining molars. MRI showed minor degenerative changes in the left TMJ, on the surface of the condyle, and anterior disc displacement (ADD) with reduction (**Fig. 3**). No pathologic condition or derangement was identified in the right joint.

## Physical Examination

The patient was above average height (189 cm, 6'2") with large hands and mandibular prognathism. Blood tests revealed a vitamin D deficiency.

## Maxillofacial Examination

She presented with a maximum interincisal opening (MIO) of 38 mm, bilateral excursions of 8 mm, and protrusion of 5 mm. Mild tenderness to palpation was noted in the masticatory muscles and neck muscles, including the sternocleidomastoid and the trapezius muscles. She had a bilateral posterior open bite, skeletal class III malocclusion, and a bilateral posterior cross bite. The tongue was above average size, and impressions of the teeth were noted, suggesting a habit of pressing the tongue anterolaterally. Skin sensation was more for both brush-and-pinch sensation in all 3 branches of the trigeminal nerve, more on the left side compared with the right side.

**Table 1**
**Psychosocial and functional assessments**

| Questionnaire | Score | Max-Min | Cut Off |
|---|---|---|---|
| Roland-Morris scale (RMS) | 8 | 0–24 | 7 |
| Sleep disorders (*wakes up at night owing to pain*) | 2 | 0–3 | |
| Hospital Anxiety and Depression scale (HADS) | 1 + 6 = 7 | 0–41 | ≥8+ ≥8 |
| Coping Strategies Questionnaire (CSQ)/catastrophizing | 0 + 3 = 3 | 0–6 | >1+ >1 |
| Mandibular Function Impairment Questionnaire (MFIQ) | 17 | 0–28 | >7 |

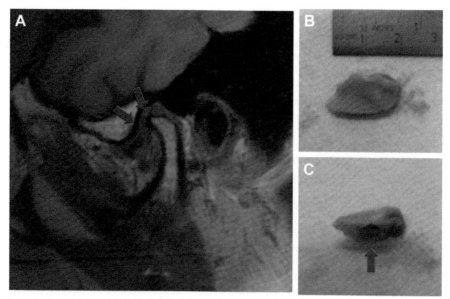

**Fig. 3.** Destruction of the TMJ disc. (*A*) T1-weighted MRI of the left TMJ. The arrows show internal derangement with anterior disc displacement without reduction (ADD). (*B*) Gross image of the left TMJ disc with intact superior surface. (*C*) Impression of the mandibular condyle almost causing a central perforation. The arrow shows impression of the mandibular condyle almost causing a central perforation.

### Diagnoses

The patient was diagnosed with TMD/myalgia. She had general impairment owing to global pain, and local dysfunction-mandibular impairment owing to myalgia. In addition, she had slightly catastrophizing thoughts about pain.

### Differential Diagnosis

Because of the progressive growth of the mandible after the age of 22 years and the patient's physical characteristics, acromegaly and Marfan syndrome were considered as potential differential diagnoses. However, endocrinological and cardiac examinations were performed without pathologic findings. The diagnosis of TMD/myalgia was therefore confirmed.

### Treatment

The posterior open bite was gradually reduced by reducing the height of the occlusal splints, which on average takes about 2 years. Jaw exercises were continued and decreased muscle pain and improved mandibular function. A gradual decrease in the use of analgesics (baclofen and codeine/acetaminophen) was initiated and replaced with acetaminophen and nonsteroidal anti-inflammatory drugs. The patient started using amitriptyline to improve her sleep and a vitamin D supplement. She was told to stop the ketamine infusions and lidocaine and bupivacaine blocks as well as botulinum toxin injections.

Six months later, she presented with a chronic closed lock (CCL) in the left TMJ. MIO was measured at 30 mm, with slightly decreased lateral excursions, and an MRI, which showed internal derangement (ID), ADD without reduction, a Wilkes stage III.[7]

It was decided to perform another arthroscopy of the left TMJ. During the procedure, osteoarthritis grade 2, synovitis grade 2, and ID were noted.[8]

No improvement in function of the jaw or pain symptoms was obtained after the arthroscopy procedure, and 6 months later, it was decided to perform a discectomy of the left TMJ. The surgical procedure exposed a central ingrowth on the superior surface of the condyle and a thinned area in the central part of the articular disc, which appeared to be almost perforated (see **Fig. 3**).

Following this procedure, she had several follow-up appointments. After 6 months, the jaw function increased to an MIO of 38 mm, and the lateral excursions showed 7 mm to the left and 11 mm to the right side. She was now medicated with 10 mg oxycodone × 2 and OxyNorm when she needed it. In addition, she had not stopped visiting the private pain clinic and continued to receive ketamine infusions and analgesics blocks.

However, the pain intensity was the same as before surgery. At this point, the patient described a feeling of general exhaustion and suicidal thoughts. She was convinced that a TMJ prosthesis was the best treatment option for her after consulting a surgeon in Denmark found via a Web search. Her OMFS in Bergen was not convinced and did not agree with her opinion. She had also sought a second opinion from another OMFS in Oslo but neither did this surgeon agree with the patient's suggestion of a prothesis. Instead, the OMFS in Oslo suggested an arthroplasty with an interpositional temporal muscle fascia flap. The patient disagreed and decided to travel to Denmark to have a TMJ prothesis implanted.

In Denmark, an arthroscopy was performed, possibly for diagnostic purposes, 2 years after her initial consultation. According to the operative report, the joint was fully fused, with no identifiable joint surfaces and fibrillar adhesions throughout. It was then decided to implant a TMJ prosthesis 5 months later. It was a custom-made (using Dicom data) titanium TMJ prothesis.

One and a half years after implantation of the TMJ prosthesis, she reported improved occlusion but slightly reduced MIO (32 mm). However, her pain condition persisted in both her face and the rest of her body.

The patient has been contacted twice for follow-up studies, but she has not responded.

## DISCUSSION

Facial pain is relatively common, reported by up to 15%[9] in the population. The exact occurrence is difficult to quantify, because of the variable quality of studies, and socioeconomic and cultural differences around the world. Untreated pain that becomes chronic is a burden for the individual and results in reduced quality of life. It is also a burden for the environment surrounding the patient, including relatives, employers, the health care system, and society in general.[10] The head and neck area are frequently affected, and the second most common cause of pain is following trauma or surgery.[11] Untreated pain may spread to surrounding structures, which can lead to anxiety and increased levels of tension in the body in general. Overactivation of the sympathetic nervous system can affect sleep, causing a downward spiral for impaired well-being.

The Orofacial Pain Prospective Evaluation and Risk Assessment study has reported a 4% incidence per year of first onset of TMD.[12] TMD includes pain in the masticatory apparatus and dysfunction of the TMJ.[13] TMD occurs predominantly in women[14] and has been linked to many comorbidities, including fibromyalgia, irritable bowel syndrome, and depression owing to trauma or stress symptoms.[15] It has also shown higher prevalence of psychosocial factors, such as somatic awareness, distress, catastrophizing, and pain amplification.[16–18]

Chronic pain after surgery could be diagnosed as peripheral traumatic trigeminal neuropathy according to the International Criteria for Orofacial Pain.[19] If the pain has persisted for a significant amount of time, tension in the jaw and neck muscles may increase and secondarily lead to TMD.[19]

Neglected or inadequate pain management after surgery is one of the most common reasons for referral to pain clinics.[20] Intraoperative pain management is in most cases straightforward. However, postoperative pain may be more difficult to control, as this depends on the patient's compliance, and therefore, may be more easily neglected. In fact, there is a 10% to 60% risk of patients developing persistent postsurgical pain after any surgical operation.[21–23] This risk is greater than 10% in those with 2 or more risk factors, such as pain in more than 1 area of the body, high pain intensity, previous surgical procedures, general anxiety, and/or catastrophizing. Furthermore, if the patient already has 1 chronic pain condition and is taking opioid analgesics, the risk of developing opioid-induced hyperalgesia is high.[23] The patient described above had previous orthognathic surgery with both preoperative and postoperative orthodontic treatment, and persistent pain could potentially develop postoperatively in patients without a previous history of TMJ symptoms.[24,25] However, in this patient, the onset of symptoms started 19 years after orthognathic surgery, making it less likely to represent the primary cause of her pain condition. Several factors influence the risk of developing persistent postoperative pain after orthognathic surgery, including pain tolerance, psychological status, and the number of surgical procedures involving the TMJ.[26] It is well known that fear of pain and catastrophizing increase the risk of developing persistent postoperative pain, and women are most commonly affected.[27] This patient presented with a high score on catastrophizing as measured by the CSQ, and the combination of multiple surgical procedures in the affected area may have contributed to the development of her chronic pain. In addition, because she was medicated with opioids after the discectomy procedure, she could have developed opioid-induced hyperalgesia as a reason for her continuing pain.

In this case, multiple TMJ operations were performed with little or no improvement in the patient's pain condition. Degenerative changes to the articular disc, which was stuck on the top of the condyle, was found during discectomy, but the symptoms could not be correlated with the radiographic and clinical findings. Others have also shown that radiographic findings do not necessarily correlate to the patient's symptoms.[28] Computed tomography (CT) scan and MRI before the last arthroscopy showed destruction of the condyle compared with how it was initially (**Fig. 4**), and according to the operative report, it was found to be a totally fused joint. A relevant question is whether the ultimate pathologic condition of the joint was due to progression of the initial disease or if it was due to the multiple surgical procedures. Both are plausible explanations with perhaps a combination of the 2 most likely. The global pain condition of this patient cannot however be explained by the TMJ pathologic condition alone.

Poor outcome of TMJ surgery occurs, and the causes could be misdiagnosis of the original pathologic condition, incorrect selection of surgical technique, technical failures, complications, systemic disease, and unrealistic expectations.[29] It is also important to prescreen the patient before surgery for not only physical but also psychological conditions, especially when it comes to replacement of the TMJ with prosthesis. A most important factor is persistent pain preoperatively. Severe

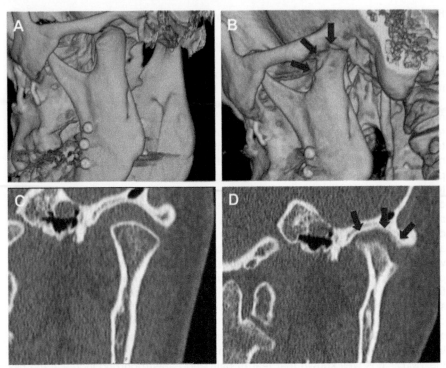

**Fig. 4.** Degenerative changes in the TMJ. (*A*) Initial 3-dimensional (3D) -reconstructed CT image of the left TMJ. (*B*) 3D reconstruction of the left TMJ 4 years later. The arrows show increased destruction of the joint surface. (*C*) Initial CT section with coronal view of the left joint showing an intact mandibular condyle and glenoid fossa. (*D*) CT section with coronal view 4 years later. The arrowa show an irregular surface of the condyle and bony apposition of the glenoid fossa.

preoperative pain, regular opioid use, or multiple previous open TMJ surgeries should be regarded as predictive risk factors for even worse pain after surgery.[30]

## CLINICS CARE POINTS

- It is important to prescreen patients before surgery in order to prevent unnecessary postoperative pain.
- To prevent chronic pain after surgery, identify patients at risk, make plans for pain management before surgery, and closely follow up the patient after surgery.
- Postoperative pain control is essential for the patient's recovery.
- Psychological factors, such as neurotic personal traits, low coping ability, and catastrophizing, are strongly correlated with increased incidence of chronic pain.
- Multiple temporomandibular joint surgical procedures should be avoided, as it is not clear how these procedures will affect the tissues.

## DISCLOSURE

The authors have nothing to disclose.

## REFERENCES

1. Berge T, Schjødt B, Bell RF, et al. Assessment of patients with severe temporomandibular disorder in Norway – a multidisciplinary approach. Nor Tannlegeforen Tid 2016;126:114–21.
2. Bell FR, Borzan J, Kalso E, et al. Food, pain and drugs: Does it matter what pain patients eat? Pain 2012;153:1993–6.
3. Roland M, Morris R. A study of the natural history of back pain. Part I: development of a reliable and sensitive measure of disability in low-back pain. Spine (Phila Pa 1976) 1983;8(2):141–4.
4. Zigmond AS, Snaith RP. The hospital anxiety and depression scale. Acta Psychiatr Scand 1983;67(6):361–70.
5. Robinson ME, Riley JL 3rd, Myers CD, et al. The Coping Strategies Questionnaire: a large sample, item level factor analysis. Clin J Pain 1997;13(1):43–9.
6. Stegenga B, de Bont LG, de Leeuw R, et al. Assessment of mandibular function impairment associated with temporomandibular joint osteoarthrosis and internal derangement. J Orofac Pain 1993;7(2):183–95.
7. Wilkes CH. Internal derangements of the temporomandibular joint. Pathological variations. Arch Otolaryngol Head Neck Surg 1989;115:469–77.
8. Holmlund AB, Axelsson S. Temporomandibular arthropathy: correlation between clinical signs and symptoms and arthroscopic findings. Int J Oral Maxillofac Surg 1996;25(3):178–81.
9. Haggman-Henrikson B, Liv P, Ilgunas A, et al. Increasing gender differences in the prevalence and chronification of orofacial pain in the population. Pain 2020; 161(8):1768–75.
10. Breivik H, Eisenberg E, O'Brien T. Openminds. The individual and societal burden of chronic pain in Europe: the case for strategic prioritisation and action to improve knowledge and availability of appropriate care. BMC Public Health 2013;13:1229.
11. Breivik H, Collett B, Ventafridda V, et al. Survey of chronic pain in Europe: prevalence, impact on daily life, and treatment. Eur J Pain 2006;10(4):287–333.
12. Slade GD, Ohrbach R, Greenspan JD, et al. Painful Temporomandibular Disorder: Decade of Discovery from OPPERA Studies. J Dent Res 2016;95(10): 1084–92.
13. Scrivani SJ, Keith DA, Kaban LB. Temporomandibular disorders. N Engl J Med 2008;359(25):2693–705.
14. Bueno CH, Pereira DD, Pattussi MP, et al. Gender differences in temporomandibular disorders in adult populational studies: A systematic review and meta-analysis. J Oral Rehabil 2018;45(9):720–9.
15. Hoffmann RG, Kotchen JM, Kotchen TA, et al. Temporomandibular disorders and associated clinical comorbidities. Clin J Pain 2011;27(3):268–74.
16. Willassen L, Johansson AA, Kvinnsland S, et al. Catastrophizing Has a Better Prediction for TMD Than Other Psychometric and Experimental Pain Variables. Pain Res Manag 2020;2020:7893023.
17. Staniszewski K, Lygre H, Bifulco E, et al. Temporomandibular Disorders Related to Stress and HPA-Axis Regulation. Pain Res Manag 2018;2018:7020751.
18. De La Torre Canales G, Câmara-Souza MB, Muñoz Lora VRM, et al. Prevalence of psychosocial impairment in temporomandibular disorder patients: A systematic review. J Oral Rehabil 2018;45(11):881–9.
19. International Classification of Orofacial Pain, 1st edition (ICOP). Available at: https://doi.org/10.1177/0333102419893823.

20. Peters ML, Sommer M, de Rijke JM, et al. Somatic and psychologic predictors of long-term unfavorable outcome after surgical intervention. Ann Surg 2007;245(3): 487–94.
21. Johansen A, Romundstad L, Nielsen CS, et al. Persistent postsurgical pain in a general population: prevalence and predictors in the Tromso study. Pain 2012; 153(7):1390–6.
22. Macrae WA. Chronic pain after surgery. Br J Anaesth 2001;87(1):88–98.
23. Kehlet H, Jensen TS, Woolf CJ. Persistent postsurgical pain: risk factors and prevention. Lancet 2006;367(9522):1618–25.
24. Agbaje J, Luyten J, Politis C. Pain complaints in patients undergoing orthognathic surgery. Pain Res Manag 2018;2018:4235025.
25. Kim YK. Complications associated with orthognathic surgery. J Korean Assoc Oral Maxillofac Surg 2017;43(1):3–15.
26. Wolford LM, Rodrigues DB, Limoeiro E. Orthognathic and TMJ surgery: postsurgical patient management. J Oral Maxillofac Surg 2011;69(11):2893–903.
27. Papaioannou M, Skapinakis P, Damigos D, et al. The role of catastrophizing in the prediction of postoperative pain. Pain Med 2009;10(8):1452–9.
28. Eriksson L, Westesson PL. Discectomy as an effective treatment for painful temporomandibular joint internal derangement: a 5-year clinical and radiographic follow-up. J Oral Maxillofac Surg 2001;59(7):750–8 ; discussion 8-9.
29. Vega LG, Gutta R, Louis P. Reoperative temporomandibular joint surgery. Oral Maxillofac 3839 Surg Clin North Am 2011;23(1):119–132, vii.
30. Gerber S, Saeed N. Predictive risk factors for persistent pain following total prosthetic temporomandibular joint replacement. Br J Oral Maxillofac Surg 2021; S0266-4356(21):00404–6.

# Persistent Idiopathic Dentoalveolar Pain

## Is It a Central Pain Disorder?

Gary M. Heir, DMD[a,*], Sowmya Ananthan, BDS, DMD, MSD[b], Mythili Kalladka, BDS, MSD[c], Manvitha Kuchukulla, BDS, MDS[d], Tara Renton, BDS, MDSc, PhD[e,**]

**KEYWORDS**

- Nociplastic pain • Idiopathic facial pain • Atypical facial pain
- Persistent dentoalveolar pain (PDAP) • Atypical odontalgia (AO)

**KEY POINTS**

- Nociplastic pain, formerly known as idiopathic or centralized pain, can present in the face and mouth as Persistent Idiopathic Pain (extraoral or intraoral) as designated by the International Classification of Orofacial Pain. There may a familial and genetic predisposition.
- Diagnosis is by exclusion and a thorough history, and a holistic approach is of the utmost importance.
- Screening for comorbid pain conditions, mood, and sleep disorders is essential in optimizing the management of the patient presenting with nociplastic pain, as this type of pain is generally refractory to most treatments.

## INTRODUCTION

Defined by the International Classification of Orofacial Pain (ICOP) 6.3, persistent idiopathic dentoalveolar pain (PIDP) is a persistent unilateral intraoral dentoalveolar pain, rarely occurring at multiple sites, with variable features but recurring daily for more than 2 hours per day for more than 3 months, in the absence of any preceding causative agent (**Tables 1–3**).[1] The description is as vague as its cause or causes. For this

Disclosures: The authors have nothing to disclose.
Funding: None to report.
[a] Department of Diagnostic Sciences, Center for Temporomandibular Disorders and Orofacial Pain, Rutgers School of Dental Medicine, 110 Bergen Street, Room D835, Newark, NJ 07101, USA; [b] Department of Diagnostic Sciences, Center for Temporomandibular Disorders and Orofacial Pain, Rutgers School of Dental Medicine, USA; [c] Institute for Oral Health, University of Rochester, Rochester, NY, USA; [d] Private Practice, Vermont; [e] Department of Oral Surgery, King's College London Dental Institute, London, United Kingdom
* Corresponding author.
** Corresponding author.
*E-mail addresses:* heirgm@sdm.rutgers.edu (G.M.H.); tara.renton@kcl.ac.uk (T.R.)

Dent Clin N Am 67 (2023) 71–83
https://doi.org/10.1016/j.cden.2022.07.006 

| Table 1 Abbreviations | |
|---|---|
| CWP | Chronic widespread pain |
| DPT | Dental panoramic tomography |
| FM | Fibromyalgia |
| PDAP | Persistent dentoalveolar pain |
| PIDP | Persistent idiopathic dentoalveolar pain |

reason, this entity has been ascribed numerous identities, including psychosomatic pain, symptom somatoform disorder, atypical odontalgia, phantom pain, persistent dentoalveolar pain (PDAP), and now its current persona as persistent idiopathic dentoalveolar pain[3] (PIDP).

The cause or causes of PIDP are elusive and, as of now, have defied identification. Causality must be investigated for the patient presenting with unilateral chronic pain that is long lasting and nonresponsive to treatment. Necessary information includes the history of the following:

- The onset of symptoms as spontaneous or related to specific events.
- An assessment of psychological factors, such as grief, related to a significant life event or physical stress related to onset.
- A history of posttraumatic neuropathic pain or other nontraumatic causes for neuropathic pain is also required, including chemotherapy, heavy metal poisoning, radiation therapy, thermal injury, hematological/vitamin D/magnesium deficiencies, connective tissue disorders, and congenital neuropathies.
- Neurovascular pain often presents with neuropathic features, including migraines, and trigeminal autonomic cephalalgias must also be excluded.
- Comorbid pains; a common feature of nociplastic pain is chronic widespread pain as seen with fibromyalgia (FM) that may be part of a persistent idiopathic presentation.

The authors present a case of presumed PIDP meeting the ICOP criteria. It is hoped this case report will raise discussion as to whether we are truly dealing with an idiopathic entity or have merely failed to discover the "causative agent."

## THE PERIPHERAL NOCICEPTIVE SYSTEM

The peripheral nociceptive system serves a singular purpose. Monitoring the external environment, it warns of actual or potential tissue damage. It constantly reports changes in the environment, which may or may not represent a threat, through a complex system of transduction, transmission, modulation, and perception of noxious inputs. The brain interprets peripheral stimuli and activates or inhibits the descending pain inhibitory system accordingly. The presence of an actual or potential threat activates the immune system. Endocrinological changes consistent with fight or flight response[4] increase sensitivity to stimulation. The central nervous system processes noxious stimuli in various centers of the brain consistent with pain interpretation by the limbic system.[5] The final result is the perception of pain, or not pain.

Noxious stimuli can be inhibited or facilitated depending on how these signals are interpreted. In some instances, the processing of noxious stimuli within the central nervous system may be subject to misinterpretation.[6] Nonnoxious stimulation may result in the perception of a painful input through a variety of mechanisms, such as

| Table 2 Glossary of terms | |
|---|---|
| Nociplastic pain (IASP) | Nociplastic pain or central sensitization is a type of pain that is mechanically different from the normal nociceptive pain caused by inflammation and tissue damage or the neuropathic pain that results from nerve damage. It may occur in combination with other types of pain or in isolation |
| Persistent idiopathic dentoalveolar pain (ICOP) | Persistent unilateral intraoral dentoalveolar pain, rarely occurring at multiple sites, with variable features but recurring daily for more than 2 hours per day for more than 3 months, in the absence of any preceding causative event<br>Diagnostic criteria:<br>A. Intraoral dentoalveolar pain fulfilling criteria B and C<br>B. Recurring daily for >2 h/d for >3 mo<br>C. Pain has both of the following characteristics:<br>• Localized to a dentoalveolar site (tooth or alveolar bone)<br>• Deep, dull, pressurelike quality<br>D. Clinical and radiographic examinations are normal, and local causes have been excluded<br>E. Not better accounted for by another ICOP or International Classification of Headache Disorders-3 (ICHD-3) diagnosis<br>ICOP classifies several diagnostic categories of PIDP<br>• PIDP without somatosensory changes<br>• PIDP with somatosensory changes<br>• Probable PIDP |
| Fibromyalgia[2] | Fibromyalgia is characterized by widespread pain and tenderness (sensitivity to touch). Pain and tenderness tend to wax and wane and move about the body. Other symptoms include fatigue, sleep, memory, and mood issues. The diagnosis can be made with a careful examination. Fibromyalgia is most common in women, although it can occur in men. It most often starts in middle adulthood but can occur in the teen years and in old age. There is a higher risk for fibromyalgia in patients with a rheumatologic disease (health problem that affects the joints, muscles, and bones). These include osteoarthritis, lupus, rheumatoid arthritis, or ankylosing spondylitis. Fibromyalgia does not damage the joints or muscles. Comorbid complaints include the following:<br>• Depression or anxiety<br>• Migraine or tension headaches<br>• Digestive problems: irritable bowel syndrome (commonly called IBS) or gastroesophageal reflux disease (often referred to as GERD)<br>• Irritable or overactive bladder<br>• Pelvic pain<br>• Temporomandibular disorder, (TMD) often called TMJ by patients and nonspecialists (a set of symptoms including muscle and/or jaw pain, jaw clicking) |
| Dysesthesia | An abnormal sensation, spontaneous or evoked, that is unpleasant (a sign, not a diagnosis) |

peripheral and central sensitization.[7,8] The pain inhibitory system may be impaired or genetically deficient.[9] Literature suggests that chronic pain, mediated by the trigeminal system, can involve changes in pain inhibition and pronociceptive changes in processing noxious inputs.[10] Even in the presence of denervation, pain may persist in an area of lost sensation through mechanisms described as stimulus-independent pain or central pain mechanisms.[11] For example, pain experienced in a lost limb is the

| Table 3 Common pharmacologic treatment modalities | |
|---|---|
| Tricyclic antidepressants (TCA) | Serotonin reuptake inhibitors are sodium channel stabilizers, inhibit nociceptive input at the dorsal horn, and thereby reduce transmissions of noxious input |
| Serotonin-noradrenaline reuptake inhibitors (SNRI) | Serotonin-noradrenaline reuptake inhibitors are a class of antidepressant drugs that treat major depressive disorder, anxiety disorders, obsessive-compulsive disorder, social phobia, attention-deficit/hyperactivity disorder, chronic neuropathic pain, fibromyalgia syndrome, and menopausal symptoms |
| Gabanoids | Gabanoids, gabapentin, and pregabalin are anticonvulsants but also function as neuromodulators, as they reduce neuronal excitability by inhibiting the $\alpha$-2-$\delta$ subunit of calcium-gated channels on presynaptic axons |

result of the image of that pain interpreted by the brain as phantom limb pain, or pain felt in the missing appendage commonly recognized as neuropathic pain. One of the leading difficulties in diagnosis is pain presenting with neuropathic features. For example, known lesions or disease may present with positive features, such as allodynia, hyperalgesia, paresthesia, and hyperpathia, or negative features, including hypoesthesia, the absence of pain with sleep with worsening during the day, with stress or illness, but without a demonstrable neuropathic cause, preventing a diagnosis of neuropathic pain. ICOP recognizes PIDP with neuropathic findings, which may be a neuropathic pain with demonstrable positive and or negative signs; however, this variation requires further scrutiny and analysis. One of the most challenging obstacles is obtaining an adequate pain history from the patient. Differentiating preexisting nociceptive pain, such as inflammatory odontogenic pain, from de novo neuropathic or nociplastic pain before the inevitable root canal treatment can be challenging; thus, a clinician can be easily misguided when identifying the precipitating event. The cause and mechanisms of nociplastic pain remain elusive.

## HISTORY OF THE PROBLEM AND DIFFICULTIES WITH NOSOLOGY
### Pain Mechanisms: Local and Referred

The clinical presentation of PIDP runs the gamut from dysesthesia to clinical features consistent with a neuropathic quality, that is, alteration in sensation, which may be spontaneous or provoked. For the purpose of this discussion, PIDP will be classified as a complaint of mild discomfort, aching and throbbing, sensorial changes, including burning, tingling, and occasional sharp pain. There is a disagreement in the literature regarding the presence or absence of a trauma to a tooth or teeth; as mentioned above, many patients will have had multiple medical and surgical interventions in trying to appease their pain. The key is establishing if pretreatment pain was odontogenic or neuropathic, or neurovascular or nociplastic, and if the pain changed after intervention. Thus, many references are made to the ICOP classification that includes a reference to the absence of an adverse event resulting in patient complaints. Despite this, many references are made in the literature to postimplant pain or postendodontic pain as PIDP, which are likely categorized as such owing to a lack of neuropathic cause in the region of pain.

One of the problems faced in arriving at a differential diagnosis is the classification of the clinical entity, or identification of a pain mechanism. The vague and confusing diagnostic terms make the process of diagnosis and targeted therapies more diffi-cult.[12] Although diagnostic terms in many fields of dentistry and medicine have evolved to the point where there may be little doubt regarding the patient's condition, terms such as atypical and idiopathic persist.

A review of the literature finds numerous references to atypical odontalgia,[13,14] psy-chogenic or symptom somatoform disorders,[15,16] phantom tooth pain,[17,18] idiopathic toothache, ill-defined neuropathic pain disorders, and now, PIDP. Treatment recom-mendations run the gamut from neuropathic pain to psychiatric care.[19] Adding to the diagnostic conundrum is confusion in the literature that suggests unknown causes while at the same time recommending specific treatments.

The International Association for the Study of Pain defines orofacial pain as "pain derived from local sources, dysfunction of the nervous system or referral from distant sites."[20] As stated, pain may be referred to a distant site even though the perception of pain is in an area with impaired innervation or which can be, in fact, missing. There is a new descriptive term that coincides with PIDP, nociplastic pain. "Nociplastic pain arises from altered nociception despite no clear evidence of actual or threatened tissue damage causing the activation of peripheral nociceptors or evidence for disease or lesion of the somatosensory system causing the pain."[21] This new definition, suggested by the International Association for the Study of Pain in 2017, seems to encompass all prior de-scriptors of PIDP. This diagnostic concept has been applied to chronic widespread pain disorder, such as FM, and used to identify patients with either diffuse or focal hypersen-sitivities in the absence of a diagnosis of neuralgia, neuropathy, or other causes.[22]

The hypothesis is strong for a central mechanism whereby discomfort or pain arises from central sensitization or central pain generators. In seminal research, the OPPERA study identified a group of individuals who were pain prone or pronociceptive with a predisposition to pain, or an exaggerated perception of nonnoxious stimuli as painful. This fits within the rubric of central pain mechanisms or nociplastic pain as a viable explanation of PIDP, especially for those individuals with comorbid chronic pain com-plaints who are more likely to experience pain to nonnoxious stimulation. Demograph-ically, the population of individuals suffering from FM or FM-like symptoms has similar demographic presentations as those of the PIDP population. This may also explain why similar medications used for FM are effective for this condition.[23,24]

## CASE PRESENTATION
### General Information

A 35-year-old woman presents to a dental clinic with the complaint of dull, diffuse nonspecific burning pain in the mandibular right posterior quadrant.

### Chief Complaint

The pain is constant, burning, and intense and has been present for approximately 6 years, waxing and waning in intensity. "My lower teeth hurt on the right, sometimes on top. I know it's a toothache, but no one can find it. They tell me my teeth are perfect, but I know something is wrong."

## CURRENT PRESENTATION
### Medical History

The patient sustained injuries during a motor vehicle accident that occurred approxi-mately 8 years earlier during which she incurred low back and cervical injuries. She states, "I had six months of physical therapy, but never fully recovered." The patient is also diagnosed with hypothyroidism and complains of always feeling uncomfortable. She cannot clearly define her discomfort but implies global sensitivity and discomfort. She also reports achy joints and muscles, sensitivity to temperature changes, and is easily fatigued. She also reports daily headache and occasional migraine, and "I have TMJ."

### Trauma History

Trauma history includes motor vehicle accident 8 years earlier in which the patient was the restrained driver of the vehicle, which was struck from the rear by another at a high rate of speed. She immediately realized cervical and low back injuries and was taken by ambulance to an emergency department and admitted to the hospital for 3 days for observation of what was perceived as a mild concussion. Imaging was negative, and the patient was discharged to physical therapy with no medications other than over-the-counter pain remedies.

### Review of Systems

Review of systems includes controlled hypothyroidism, borderline diabetes, controlled hypertension, and irritable bowel syndrome.

Current medications include acetaminophen, 325 mg, or naproxen sodium, 220 mg, often taken 2 at a time several times per week. Hydrocodone acetaminophen, 5-325, is used occasionally for more severe pain. Amlodipine, 5 mg, and levothyroxine, 100 μg, are taken daily for management of hypertension and hypothyroidism. Alprazolam, 2.5 mg, is taken at bedtime for sleep.

### Past Treatment

Past treatment includes multiple dental evaluations and routine dental interventions not preceding the pain onset. Medical treatment is with tricyclic antidepressants, gabinoids, nonsteroidal anti-inflammatory drugs (NSAIDs), and acetaminophen. These and many other medication trials have not impacted her pain. The patient has sought multiple consultations with otolaryngology, rheumatology, and endocrinology with no specific findings. She has not received any specific dental treatment for her complaint of what she perceives is of odontogenic origin other than several intraoral orthotics to treat a nonspecific temporomandibular disorder. She returned to physical therapy over the course of the past 6 years at on least 4 occasions. She has received no benefit from any treatment.

### Pain History

Using the SOCRATES acronym, an accurate and comprehensive pain history can be taken:

| | |
|---|---|
| Site | Lower left posterior mandible |
| Onset | Spontaneously 6 y ago |
| Character | Ongoing deep aching burning pain, which is constant but fluctuates |
| Radiation | Occasional radiating up to posterior left maxilla with no pattern |
| Associations | None. The pain does not coincide with headaches or other comorbid pains |
| Timing | Constant with fluctuation |
| Exacerbating factors Alleviating factors | None. The pain "just does its own thing" None |
| Severity (reported on a visual analogue scale of 0–10/10) | The pain ranges between 4 and 6 out of 10 but can escalate to 8 out of 10 occasionally |

## Psychosocial Assessment

The patient is married with 3 children and appears despondent over not finding a solution for her pain. She has missed work because of her chronic pain and is considering applying for disability. She is distressed over the fact that she is constantly ill and its impact on her family, no longer socializes, and is short tempered with her family. She is also worried that her pain is becoming progressive.

- Family history: Mother and both sisters are diagnosed with chronic widespread pain and FM
- Habit history: Previous smoker, quit 10 years ago, drinks 12 units per week of alcohol
- Illegal substance use: None
- Psychological-psychiatric treatment: None

## Clinical Examination

- Neglected personal appearance, seems agitated and stressed
- Mental status: Anxiety, depression
- Maxillofacial examination
  - Facial symmetry
  - Head and neck: Nothing abnormal detected (NAD)
  - Oral cavity: Mucosa seems normal, dentition moderately restored, mild attrition
  - Masticatory system: NAD
  - Mandibular function: NAD
  - Occlusal examination: Angle's class 1
  - TMJ joint nose: None
  - TMJ joint palpation: NAD
  - Cervical muscle examination: NAD
- Neurological examination
  - A cranial nerve screening examination found all cranial nerves intact

## Diagnostic and Assessment Tools

Axis 2 assessment determined significant anxiety as assessed by the Generalized Anxiety Disorder 7-Item (GAD-7) Scale,[25,26] and possible major depression as assessed by the Patient Health Questionnaire (PHQ-9).[27] The patient also demonstrated a significant sleep disorder using the Insomnia Severity Index (ISI),[28] but obstructive sleep apnea was not found using the STOP-BANG Score for Obstructive Sleep Apnea.[29]

- Current affective symptoms
  - Sleep disorder symptoms: Clinical insomnia with no risk for obstructive sleep apnea, subclinical insomnia (ISI and STOP-BANG)
  - Anxiety: High levels of anxiety, somatic disorder (GAD-7)
  - Probable major depression (PHQ-9)

As part of the psychosocial pain history, the patient completed a modified American College of Rheumatology (ACR) preliminary diagnostic criteria form criteria of FM (**Fig. 1**).

It should be understood that scoring of this form represents a continuum rather than a yes or no answer. FM is not a yes or no condition but presents as a range of complaints from none to severe and can be categorized depending on the point score of this form. The higher the score, the more severe the patient's complaints. The higher

**Fibromyalgia Symptoms (Modified ACR 2011 Fibromyalgia Diagnostic Criteria)**

1. Please indicate below if you have had pain or tenderness over the past 7 d in each of the areas listed below. Check the boxes in the diagram below for each area in which you have had pain or tenderness. Be sure to mark right and left sides separately.

☐ No Pain

Left / Right

☐ Jaw  Neck  Jaw ☐
☐ Shoulder  Upper back  Shoulder ☐
☐ Upper arm  Chest/breast  Upper arm ☐
Abdomen
☐ Lower arm  Lower back  Lower arm ☐
Hip ☐   ☐ Hip
Upper leg   Upper leg
☐       ☐
Lower leg  Lower leg
☐       ☐

2. Using the following scale, indicate for each item your severity over the past week by checking the appropriate box.
   **No problem**
   **Slight or mild problems**: generally mild or intermittent
   **Moderate**: considerable problems; often present and/or at a moderate level
   **Severe**: continuous, life-disturbing problems

| | No problem | Slight or mild | Moderate | Severe |
|---|---|---|---|---|
| a. Fatigue | ☐ | ☐ | ☐ | ☐ |
| b. Trouble thinking or remembering | ☐ | ☐ | ☐ | ☐ |
| c. Waking up tired (unrefreshed) | ☐ | ☐ | ☐ | ☐ |

3. During the past 6 months have you had any of the following symptoms?

| | No | Yes |
|---|---|---|
| a. Pain or cramps in lower abdomen | ☐ | ☐ |
| b. Depression | ☐ | ☐ |
| c. Headache | ☐ | ☐ |

4. Have the symptoms in questions 2-3 and pain been present at a similar level for at least 3 months?    No ☐   Yes ☐

5. Do you have a disorder that would otherwise explain the pain?    No ☐   Yes ☐

**Fig. 1.** The 2011 survey criteria for FM.[30] Each positive response to question 1 on the left carries a 1-point score. The response to question 2, a, b, c, carries point scores as follows: no problem = 0; slight or mild = 1; moderate = 2; and severe = 3. Responses to question 3, a and b, score 1 point each. Questions 4 and 5 are for information only and carry no point score. Scoring ranges from 0 to 19, for question 1 on the left, and 12 possible points to questions 2 and 3 on the right. The maximum score is 31 with 12 or below consistent with FM-like symptoms.[31] Scores from 13 to 31 support the diagnosis of FM.

the response score for any individual, the more likely they will report symptoms of increased fatigue, memory loss, headache, comorbidity of chronic pain conditions, and possible overuse or poor response to peripherally acting medications. The higher the score, the more likely is the presence of a centrally mediated pain disorder. Patients with high scores, especially those beyond 13 of this pain scale, indicate likely FM diagnosis.

Although the modified ACR form has not been applied to patients with PIDP, it is hypothesized that the responses will be similar. This patient scored 23 using this assessment, indicating fibromyalgia symptoms (FMS), a nociplastic pain-related disorder owing to centralized sensitization and presentation with multiple responsive pain sites.[32]

***Problem-Oriented Workup***

- Severe pain on function causing difficulty in daily activities
- Anxiety and depression
- Insomnia
- Family history of FMS
- Possible medication overuse headache

***Differential Diagnoses***

Prior motor vehicle accident, hypothyroidism, multiple comorbid pains, anxiety, and depression are all risk factors for chronic widespread pain, which is likely contributory to the idiopathic intraoral pain. The patient also has a family history of FMS, which also increases the risk of nociplastic pain.

Pain has not responded to recurrent dental interventions, antibiotics, NSAIDs, or opioid analgesics; thus odontogenic pain can be excluded. Recent dental radiographs were not contributory. The pain distribution does not fit for temporomandibular disorder. This presentation does not align with neurovascular pain, as her oral pain is constant and unrelated to her migraine headaches. In addition, the intraoral pain does not respond to her migraine treatments. This presentation does not align with a neuropathic pain presentation, as it is not related to onset during trauma or other life events. However, in a recent retrospective review of 160 patients with assumed idiopathic oral pain, only 68 were confirmed with PIDP after scrutiny using ICOP PIDP diagnostic criteria.[3]

This study reported that the most common site of pain was the molar mandibular teeth of 75 of 78 patients, implants in 1 patient, or edentulous postextraction sites in 2 patients. In 54 of the 78 patients, the painful site had been endodontically treated. Mechanical allodynia of the gingival sulcus was found in 68 of 75 teeth and in 1 implant. These features would infer posttraumatic neuropathic pain with a burning quality affecting 42% of the patients. Burning pain was the most common pain characteristic reported, which is also generally described as a characteristic of neuropathic pain.[33] Undisturbed sleep and a pain-free interval after waking were frequently reported in this patient cohort, also a characteristic of neuropathic pain.[34] Delayed onset of pain following irritation reported in 41% of patients has also been described in neuropathic pain. This study highlights the differential diagnostic challenges in these cases, and proposed a differential diagnostic table was suggested to facilitate exclusion of other classified ICOP conditions (**Table 4**).

### Final Diagnoses

- Medical conditions:
  - Nociplastic pain/PIDP, which may be the same entity
  - Possible medication overuse pain
  - FMS with migraine
- Psychological conditions:
  - Anxiety and depression
  - Insomnia

### Treatment Plan

### Management

The clinician must exclude dental pathologic condition and other more common pain pathologic condition and reassure the patient that this pain is real and likely owing to her generalized pain condition and worsened by her mood and sleep disorders. Her family history may suggest a familiar representation of pronociception.

Medication overuse pain must not be overlooked. The patient must be advised to refrain from regularly using NSAIDs and acetaminophen and ideally not take them for 12 weeks to minimize central pain modulation impairment by regular use of over-the-counter pain medications.

Pain management for patients with nociplastic pain presenting as PIDP or FMS is more likely to respond to centrally acting medications.[35] However, the comorbid mood disorders (anxiety and depression), sleep disorders, and history of prior abuse and neglect must not be overlooked, requiring referral to clinical psychology, sleep clinic, and psychiatric specialist care in supporting her pain management.

**Table 4**
**Exclusion of nonpersistent idiopathic dentoalveolar pain conditions[33]**

| Relevant Clinical Findings and Case History | Diagnosis |
|---|---|
| Tenderness to percussion of tooth, apical tenderness, evidence of deep caries, mobile restorations, internal or external resorption, crown or root fractures of the affected teeth or their neighbors or antagonists, pain to heat or cold when applied to the teeth | Odontogenic pain: Symptomatic pulpitis, symptomatic apical periodontitis, bleeding on probing, pathological pocket depths, mucogingival lesions, periodontal and mucogingival pain |
| Myogenic trigger points or active or passive movements that reproduce the typical pain, radiographic signs of maxillary sinusitis, pain in the tuber region or paranasal pressure pain, swollen and sensitive salivary glands, medical history or clinical examination findings relevant to head and neck tumors or sickle-cell anemia | Nonodontogenic inflammatory pain |
| Referred orofacial pain, head and neck tumors, sickle-cell anemia. Symptoms of the autonomic orofacial nervous system (eg, running tears, running nose) associated with the intensity of the pain | Referred pain |
| Occurrence of other typical constellations of findings listed in the ICOP 5.1–5.3 definition (ICOP, 2020) or pain relief by triptans. Various incarnations of facial headache pain | Neurovascular pain or primary headaches |
| Intense shocklike pain within the affected trigeminal distribution and occurrence of typical general medical and specific pain-related history as listed in ICOP 4.1.1 (ICOP, 2020) | Trigeminal neuralgia. A neurological disorder known to be capable of causing, and explaining, the trigeminal neuropathic pain has been diagnosed and occurrence of diagnostic criteria as listed in ICOP 4.1.2.4 (ICOP, 2020). |
| Trigeminal neuropathic pain attributed to other disorders. Pain in a neuroanatomically plausible area within the distribution(s) of one or both trigeminal nerve(s) and a history of trauma to the peripheral trigeminal nerve(s) and other criteria listed in ICOP 4.1.2.3 and 4.1.2.3.1 (ICOP, 2020). Criterion C: History of external trauma and iatrogenic injuries from dental treatments, such as local anesthetic injections, root canal therapies, extractions, oral surgery, dental implants, orthognathic surgery, and other invasive procedures within 6 months before the onset of pain Criterion D: Associated with somatosensory symptoms and/or signs in the same neuroanatomically plausible distribution | Possible or likely posttraumatic trigeminal neuropathic pain |

A trial of serotonin-noradrenaline reuptake inhibitors (SNRIs), the only group of medication not previously tried for this patient, was recommended, along with the other recommended referrals noted above.

*Outcomes*

The patient was well managed on SNRIs, and psychological interventions had significantly reduced her anxiety and depression, and she was sleeping better.

## SUMMARY

PIDP is a dubious entity. This article attempts to establish a connection with other systemic chronic pain conditions, and not as a specific dental issue or a pain manifestation of the head and face. It attempts to change the thought process away from the location of pain and to consider an adverse event that may be driving the patient's complaints. The answer may be found by looking to more central causes, including more than physical findings or the somatic experience, but also the cognitive experience of the patient. It is hoped this will broaden the concept that chronic pain disorders may in actuality have an adverse event that may not be coincidental with the location. As with the case presented, the patient failed all attempts at treatment at the site of pain and only responded to more centrally acting medications combined with psychological support.

## CLINICS CARE POINTS

- Holistic assessment and management of the patient enable the clinician to evaluate the totality of the presenting condition and not just the dental or medical diagnosis.
- Optimal patient management will not be possible without recognizing the functional and psychological components of the patient's presentation.
- The clinician should recognize that patients with persistent idiopathic dentoalveolar pain are long-term chronic pain patients and require continued support. It may not respond to local remedies or procedures.

## REFERENCES

1. International Classification of Orofacial Pain, 1st edition (ICOP). Cephalalgia 2020;40(2):129–221.
2. https://www.rheumatology.org/I-Am-A/Patient-Caregiver/Diseases-Conditions/Fibromyalgia. [Accessed 6 June 2022].
3. Sanner F, Sonntag D, Hambrock N, et al. Patients with persistent idiopathic dentoalveolar pain in dental practice. Int Endod J 2022;55(3):231–9. Epub 2021 Dec 2. PMID: 34792207.
4. Dhabhar FS. Effects of stress on immune function: the good, the bad, and the beautiful. Immunol Res 2014;58(2–3):193–210.
5. James S. Human pain and genetics: some basics. Br J Pain 2013;7(4):171–8.
6. Puretić MB, Demarin V. Neuroplasticity mechanisms in the pathophysiology of chronic pain. Acta Clin Croat 2012;51(3):425–9. PMID: 23330408.
7. Nijs J, Lahousse A, Kapreli E, et al. Nociplastic pain criteria or recognition of central sensitization? Pain phenotyping in the past, present and future. J Clin Med 2021;10(15):3203. Published 2021 Jul 21.

8. Latremoliere A, Woolf CJ. Central sensitization: a generator of pain hypersensitivity by central neural plasticity. J Pain 2009;10(9):895–926.
9. Grouper H, Eisenberg E, Pud D. The relationship between sensitivity to pain and conditioned pain modulation in healthy people. Neurosci Lett 2019;708.
10. Nasri-Heir C, Khan J, Benoliel R, et al. Altered pain modulation in patients with persistent postendodontic pain. Pain 2015;156:2032–41.
11. Woolf CJ, Mannion RJ. Neuropathic pain: aetiology, symptoms, mechanisms, and management. Lancet 1999;353:1959–64.
12. Benoliel R. Atypical odontalgia: quo vadis? Quintessence Int 2013;44(6):383.
13. Baad-Hansen L. Atypical odontalgia - pathophysiology and clinical management. J Oral Rehabil 2008;35(1):1–11.
14. Nixdorf DR, Drangsholt MT, Ettlin DA, et al. Classifying orofacial pains: a new proposal of taxonomy based on ontology. J Oral Rehabil 2012;39:161–9.
15. Somatic and psychic aspects of orofacial dysaesthesia. Hampf G Proc Finn Dent Soc 1987;83(Suppl 2–3):1–72.
16. Fishbain DA, Goldberg M, Rosomoff RS, et al. Münchausen syndrome presenting with chronic pain: case report. Pain 1988;35(1):91–4. PMID: 3200602.
17. Clark GT. Persistent orodental pain, atypical odontalgia, and phantom tooth pain: when are they neuropathic disorders? J Calif Dent Assoc 2006;34(8):599–609.
18. Marbach JJ, Raphael KG. Phantom tooth pain: a new look at an old dilemma. Pain Med 2000;1(1):68–77.
19. https://my.clevelandclinic.org/health/diseases/21822-atypical-face-pain. [Accessed 6 June 2022].
20. https://www.iasp-pain.org/advocacy/global-year/orofacial-pain/. [Accessed 6 June 2022].
21. Merskey H, Bogduk N. Part III: pain terms, a current list with definitions and notes on usage" (pp 209-214) Classification of chronic pain, 2nd edition, IASP task force on taxonomy. Seattle: IASP Press; 1994.
22. Kosek E, Cohen M, Baron R, et al. Do we need a third mechanistic descriptor for chronic pain states? PAIN 2016;157:1382–6.
23. Harper DE; Abnormalities in brainstem inhibitory structures could explain the de cient conditioned pain modulation commonly observed in fibromyalgia; Conference: Society for Neuroscience October 2015; Chicago
24. Ichesco E, Peltier SJ, Mawla I, et al. Prediction of differential pharmacologic response in chronic pain using functional neuroimaging biomarkers and a support vector machine algorithm: an exploratory study. Arthritis Rheumatol 2021; 73(11):2127–37. PMID: 33982890; PMCID: PMC8597096.
25. Spitzer RL, Kroenke K, Williams JBW, et al. A brief measure for assessing generalized anxiety disorder: the GAD-7. Archives of Internal Medicine 2006;166(10): 1092–7.
26. Swinson RP. The GAD-7 scale was accurate for diagnosing generalized anxiety disorder. Evidence-Based Med 2006;11(6):184.
27. Kroenke K, Spitzer RL, Williams JB. The PHQ-9: validity of a brief depression severity measure. J Gen Intern Med 2001;16(9):606–13.
28. Morin CM, Belleville G, Bélanger L, et al. The Insomnia Severity Index: psychometric indicators to detect insomnia cases and evaluate treatment response. Sleep 2011;34(5):601–8.
29. Chung F, Abdullah HR, Liao P. STOP-Bang questionnaire: a practical approach to screen for obstructive sleep apnea. Chest 2016;149(3):631–8. Available at: https://pubmed.ncbi.nlm.nih.gov/26378880/.

30. Wolfe F, Clauw DJ, Fitzcharles MA, et al. Fibromyalgia criteria and severity scales for clinical and epidemiological studies: a modification of the ACR preliminary diagnostic criteria for fibromyalgia. J Rheumatol 2011;38(6):1113–22.
31. Wolfe F. Fibromyalgianess. Arthritis Rheum 2009;61(6):715–6.
32. Fitzcharles MA, Cohen SP, Clauw DJ, et al. Nociplastic pain: towards an understanding of prevalent pain conditions. Lancet 2021;397(10289):2098–110.
33. Colloca L, Ludman T, Bouhassira D, et al. Neuropathic pain. Nat Rev Dis Primers 2017;3:17002. PMID: 28205574; PMCID: PMC5371025.
34. Warfield AE, Prather JF, Todd WD. Systems and circuits linking chronic pain and circadian rhythms. Front Neurosci 2021;15:705173.
35. Woolf CJ. Central sensitization: implications for the diagnosis and treatment of pain. Pain 2011;152(3):S2–15.

# Posttraumatic Trigeminal Neuropathic Pain in Association with Dental Implant Surgery

Check for updates

Tara Renton, BDS, MDSc, PhD[a],
Fréderic Van der Cruyssen, MD, DDS, MHPM[b,c],*

## KEYWORDS

- Posttraumatic trigeminal neuropathy • Neuropathic pain
- Implant-related nerve injury • Trigeminal nerve injury

## KEY POINTS

- Posttraumatic trigeminal neuropathy (PTN) in association with dental implant surgery is preventable.
- PTN has a significant functional and psychological impact on patients with possible life-long reduced quality of life.
- Immediate diagnosis of PTN is of utmost importance; if in doubt, immediate referral for specialist care is recommended in order not to miss the window of opportunity to resolve the damage.
- Appropriate clinical examination and simple neurosensory tests allow for an accurate diagnosis and prognosis.
- Treatment is complex and depends on many factors such as cause, type of damage, and sensory profile.

## CASE PRESENTATION
### General Information

A 55-year-old male.

### Chief Complaint

"Since I had implants fitted in my lower jaw last week, I have a dead fat lip on the side of the surgery, which is extremely painful when I eat, speak, brush my teeth and when I

---

[a] Department of Oral Surgery, King's College London Dental Institute, King's College London, 4th Floor Kings College Hospital, Bessemer Road, Denmark Hill, London SE5 9RS, United Kingdom; [b] Department of Oral & Maxillofacial Surgery, University Hospitals Leuven, Kapucijnenvoer 33, 3000, Leuven, Belgium; [c] Department of Imaging and Pathology, OMFS-IMPATH Research Group, Faculty of Medicine, University Leuven, Leuven, Belgium
* Corresponding author. Department of Oral & Maxillofacial Surgery, University Hospitals Leuven, Kapucijnenvoer 33, Leuven 3000, Belgium.
E-mail address: frederic.vandercruyssen@uzleuven.be

Dent Clin N Am 67 (2023) 85–98
https://doi.org/10.1016/j.cden.2022.07.007
0011-8532/23/Crown Copyright © 2022 Published by Elsevier Inc. All rights reserved.
dental.theclinics.com

| Abbreviations | |
| --- | --- |
| CBCT | Cone beam computed tomography |
| ICHD-3 | International Classification of Headache disorders |
| IAN | Inferior alveolar nerve |
| ICOP | International Classification of Orofacial Pain |
| NAD | Nothing abnormal detected |
| NSAIDs | Nonsteroidal anti-inflammatory drugs |
| PTN | Posttraumatic trigeminal neuropathy |
| PTNP | Posttraumatic trigeminal neuropathic pain |
| PTSD | Posttraumatic stress disorder |
| RCT | Root canal treatment |
| TMJ | Temporomandibular joint |

go out in the cold. I have tried paracetamol (acetaminophen) and ibuprofen, but it makes no difference to the pain. I cannot stand this intense sharp shooting pain when I use my mouth and or open my jaw as I am not able to eat drink without terrible pain. I want to know what is causing this and how it can be fixed."

### History of Present Illness

Patient had six months of intermittent pain associated with his lower right premolar and molar, which after several restorative interventions lead to worsening pain and ultimately to root canal treatment (RCT). The RCT failed and resulted in a necessary extraction. The clinician involved, offered to place immediate implants. During the drilling of the implant bed the patient noticed a sudden intense pain that shot from the surgical site up to his right ear. Drilling was stopped and more local anesthetic was administered. Drilling was recommenced and no further pain was felt.

### Perioperative Scenario

A cone beam computed tomography (CBCT) revealed a very thick lingual cortex with poor cancellous bone, and proximity of the mental foramen in the planned implant sites (**Fig. 1**). For this reason a tooth-supported surgical drilling guide was used. It was decided that the implants would need to be angled toward the lingual cortex to avoid the mental foramen and the inferior alveolar nerve (IAN). It was anticipated that angling the implant lingually in a controlled manner would necessitate a slight deviation of the implant toward the buccal direction.

Tissue-level implants were placed with an intended 2-mm safety zone between the implant and nerve, a postsurgical CBCT taken (see **Fig. 1**), and the patient discharged.

On contacting the patient, the day after surgery, he complained of neuropathic symptoms, and on revisiting the surgeon, a demonstrable neuropathic area was confirmed. As the lower right implant was intruding in the IAN canal on the postsurgical CBCT, the implant was removed.

### Current Presentation

#### Medical history

- Cardiovascular: takes 2.5 mg ramipril daily for hypertension
- Migraine: takes occasional paracetamol, but due to the recent iatrogenic nerve injury his headaches have increased in frequency and intensity
- No other relevant medical history

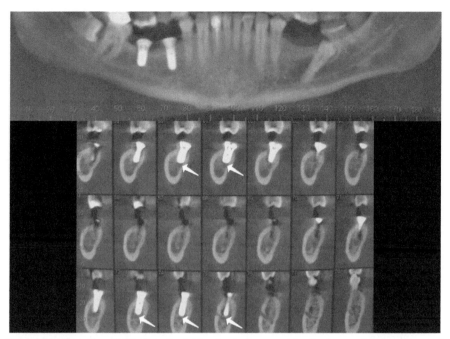

**Fig. 1.** Postoperative CBCT after dental implant placement in the lower right quadrant. A breach of the inferior dental canal is illustrated (*white arrows* indicate the inferior alveolar nerve canal).

### Pain history

Using the *SOCRATES* acronym an accurate and comprehensive pain history can be taken:

| | |
|---|---|
| Site | Lower right lip and gingiva in anterior mandible |
| Onset | Since placement of implant in lower right quadrant |
| Character | Ongoing burning pain with elicited and spontaneous neuralgic pain |
| Radiation | Occasional spontaneous neuralgic pain initiated in gingiva radiating to the right ear. Often the neuralgic pain results in a unilateral headache with migrainous signs; these may include light and sound sensitivity, nausea, scalp and facial sensitivity, and throbbing pain |
| Associations | Neuropathic area in the lip and skin of the chin, gingiva, and mucosa from the implant site onward; it affects 100% of the extraoral dermatome of the mental nerve and 40% of the intraoral dermatome There are no motor deficits or autonomic symptoms. |
| Timing | Ongoing burning pain with elicited neuralgic pain on movement, touch, and cold |
| Exacerbating factors | Any kind of movement including eating, speaking, drinking, and kissing |
| Alleviating factors | Refraining from movement and avoiding cold drafts |
| Severity | Burning pain ranges between 6 and 8 out of 10 The neuralgic pain is 10 out of 10 |

### Psychosocial assessment

- Family history: mother and both sisters have migraine.

- Habit history: previous smoker, quit 20 years ago. Drinks 18 units per week of alcohol.
- Illegal substance use: none.
- Current affective/anxiety symptoms
  - Sleep disorder symptoms: intermediate risk for obstructive sleep apnea, subclinical insomnia
  - Anxiety: high levels of anxiety (Generalised Anxiety Disorder 7 questionnaire), somatic symptom disorder (Patient Health Questionnaire 15), and posttraumatic stress disorder (PTSD) (Primary Care PTSD Screen for DSM-5 [PC-PTSD-5] questionnaire).
  - Social interference: unable to eat in public due to embarrassment and disability with speaking
  - Pain behavior: avoidance behavior to avoid elicited pain
- Psychological-psychiatric treatment: none.

### Clinical examination

- Well-presented but seems agitated and stressed
- Mental health diagnoses: anxiety, somatic disorder, PTSD
- Maxillofacial examination
  - Facial symmetry
  - Head and neck: nothing abnormal detected (NAD)
  - Oral cavity: mucosa seems normal, dentition moderately restored, mild attrition
  - Masticatory system: NAD
  - Mandibular function: NAD
  - Occlusal examination: Angle class 1
  - TMJ joint nose: none
  - TMJ joint palpation: NAD
  - Cervical muscle examination: NAD
- Neurologic examination
  - C2-3, V1, V2: normal
  - V3 right: neuropathic area 100% extraoral and 40% intraoral, mechanical, and thermal allodynia, hyperalgesia
  - Facial nerve: normal (patient was reassured that motor function may feel abnormal but that it is due to the lack of sensory feedback)

### Diagnostic studies

- Postoperative CBCT (see **Fig. 1**).

Problem-oriented workup

- Severe pain on function causing difficulty in daily activities.
- PTSD possibly due to their iatrogenic injury and resultant neuropathic pain causing significant functional disabilities and psychosocial issues.
- Worsening of migraine headaches.

### Differential Diagnoses

Because the onset of sensory neuropathy is directly related to high-risk nerve injury surgery neoplasia does not need to be ruled out.

### Final Diagnoses

- Medical conditions:

  - ○ Posttraumatic trigeminal neuropathic pain (PTNP) with functional interference
  - ○ Worsening of migraine
- Psychological conditions:
  - ○ PTSD
  - ○ Anxiety
  - ○ Sleep disorders

### Treatment Plan

### Posttraumatic trigeminal neuropathy

The clinician should be honest with the patient, confirm his diagnosis, and explain the positive (allodynia and pain) and negative symptoms (numbness). The patient should be advised that the good news is that it will not get worse, but the bad news is that it is unlikely to resolve. The patient should be offered empathy and sympathy on behalf of the surgeon that this has happened, and that they will have tried to prevent the nerve injury from happening and recognized the problem early by removing the offending implant within 30 hours and provided vitamin B complex injections, nonsteroidal anti-inflammatory drugs (NSAIDs), and step-down steroids over five days.

The patient should be reassured that the elicited and ongoing neuropathic pain can be managed with a combination of systemic medications, topical medications and psychological interventions. The patient should be reassured that he will adjust to the symptoms over the long term and that the neuropathy will not cause cancer or any other pathologic condition. In accordance with several international guidelines for management of neuropathic pain in adults, medical management of neuropathic pain may include several categories of medications.[1] The authors usually recommend pregabalin for elicited neuralgic pain and nortriptyline for background neuropathic pain. These medications are well tolerated and have minimal side effects. Topical lidocaine patches can be cut and applied to the face when going out to play sports or ski to prevent cold allodynia.

### Posttraumatic Stress Disorder Anxiety and Sleep Disorders

In the first instance the consultation should be frank and honest providing clarification for the patient of what has happened and the likely prognosis. Referral to a clinical psychologist should be made to address the posttraumatic trigeminal neuropathy (PTN)-related anxiety and PTSD. It is possible that the sleep disorders are related to the PTSD and anxiety and management of these should alleviate these symptoms.

### Migraine

It is recognized that new-onset pain can aggravate background migraines and other primary headaches. The patient's previous episodic migraine has now become chronic (>15 days per month). Consideration should be given to preventative and therapeutic medications for the migraine.

### Course of Care

Three months post injury, early removal of the implant and the acute medication protocol with vitamin B, NSAIDs, and steroids had minimal impact on the patient's neuropathic pain. Nerve repair surgery after this date is demonstrated to have little impact on neuropathic pain. The patient was provided with the clinician's contact details to allow reassurance and contact if necessary. Other resources provided were signposting to trigeminalnerve.org.uk.

*Outcomes*

The patient was well managed on pregabalin 75 mg nocte and nortriptyline 10 mg nocte with significant reduction of his pain (ie, > 50% pain reduction measured on a visual analog scale), and his function was improved. Psychological interventions had significantly reduced his anxiety and PTSD, and he was sleeping better. The lidocaine patches had enabled the patient to resume his tennis and golf in the winter and to tolerate the air-conditioning at work in the summer.

## LITERATURE REVIEW
### Introduction

Dental implants have become an increasingly accepted method to replace nonrestorable dentition. According to the American Academy of Implant Dentistry, around three million people in the United States have dental implants, and the number of people receiving them is increasing by around 500,000 per year. Despite improvement in technology (presurgical planning imaging, computer-guided surgery) and training, the prevention of nerve injury remains elusive. A recent meta-analysis revealed that the short-term (ten days after implant placement) incidence of nerve injury related to implant placement was 13% (95% confidence interval [CI], 6%–25%) and long-term (one year after implant placement) incidence was 3% (95% CI, 1%–7%).[2] Thus most patients return to normal sensation. A second meta-analysis selected 9 of 1589 articles and reported that the risk of neurosensory disturbance related to implant placement was 13.50 per 100 person-years (95% CI, 10.98–16.03), with a greater risk with anteriorly placed mandibular implants.[3] The overall recovery rate was estimated at 51.30 per 100 person-years (95% CI, 31.2–71.4). A recent large cohort study reported that 13% (173 cases) of 1331 cases of postsurgical trigeminal nerve damage were implant related with a permanency rate of 96%. Most implant-related nerve injury cases (95%) presented with neuropathic pain.[4]

Considering the permanency and pain rates related to implant-related neuropathy the functional and psychological impact for the patient cannot be understated. Ongoing and/or elicited pain occurring with every orofacial function including eating, drinking, speaking, kissing, difficulty with cold-induced pain preventing enjoyment of sports and outdoor activity, and sleep disruption adversely affects the patient and their enjoyment of life.[5,6]

The resultant psychosocial impact is considerable as seen in this case with associated anxiety and PTSD and requires recognition, assessment, and clinical psychological intervention and reassurance.[7,8]

### Pathophysiology

The mechanism of implant-related neuropathy remains unclear unless there is significant mechanical disruption of the inferior alveolar canal and nerve, which usually occurs during drill preparation of the implant bed. Different degrees of nerve injury are recognized and are divided into three types based on the severity of the tissue injury, prognosis, and time for recovery: neurapraxia, axonotmesis, and neurotmesis. Neurapraxia is the mildest form, with the best prognosis, whereas neurotmesis is the most severe.[9] It is likely that implant-related nerve injury is a combination of ischemia of the IAN due to hemorrhage around the nerve within the constrained bony canal, and some direct physical trauma allowing intraneural hemorrhage, which massively irritates neural tissue and likely starts within minutes or hours of injury.[10]

### Diagnosis

The aforementioned case history describes a typical story of a patient with PTN and subsequent neuropathic pain, with the diagnosis of PTNP.

Neuropathic pain has recently been redefined as pain arising as a direct consequence of any lesion or disease affecting the somatosensory system.[11,12] Apart from trauma, the most common diseases related with neuropathic pain are diabetes, human immunodeficiency virus, multiple sclerosis, and chemotherapy, which rarely occur in the head and neck region.[12] Recently, the first edition of the International Classification of Orofacial Pain was published accompanied by its diagnostic criteria.[13] PTNP was defined as unilateral or bilateral facial or oral pain caused by trauma to the trigeminal nerves, with other symptoms and/or clinical signs of trigeminal nerve dysfunction and persisting or recurring for more than 3 months. The diagnostic criteria are summarized in **Box 1**.

Recommendations include establishing the diagnosis of posttraumatic neuropathy using a grading scale: unlikely, probable, or definite.[14] These recommendations have been tailored for PTNP.[15]

PTNP is a clinical diagnosis, and mechanosensory tests must assess positive and negative signs; additional tests may include nerve conduction study, laser-evoked potentials, blink tests, skin biopsies showing reduced nerve fiber terminals, and magnetic resonance neurography. However, all clinical and diagnostic aspects should be considered.

### Clinical Assessment

When assessing patients with surgically induced nerve injuries the authors recommend a holistic approach.[16] Many of these patients have experienced an unexpected traumatic event that demands a thorough history taking and examination including attention to sensory testing and psychological assessment, which are necessary both in diagnosis and in the choice of therapy.

The authors believe that the neuropathy develops immediately after trauma, unless related to endodontic procedure in which there may be a 2- or 3-day delay. The

---

**Box 1**
**Diagnostic criteria of posttraumatic trigeminal neuropathic pain according to the recent International Classification of Orofacial Pain (ICOP) version 1**

*Previously used terms: anesthesia dolorosa; painful posttraumatic trigeminal neuropathy*

A. Pain, in a neuroanatomically plausible area within the distribution of one or both trigeminal nerves, persisting or recurring for more than 3 months and fulfilling criteria C and D

B. Both of the following:
1. History of a mechanical, thermal, radiation, or chemical injury to the peripheral trigeminal nerves
2. Diagnostic test confirmation of a lesion of the peripheral trigeminal nerve(s) explaining the pain

C. Onset within 6 months after the injury

D. Associated with somatosensory symptoms and/or signs in the same neuroanatomically plausible distribution

E. Not better accounted for by another ICOP or ICHD-3 diagnosis

*Abbreviation:* ICOP, International Classification of Orofacial Pain. ICHD-3, International Classification of Headache disorders.

hypothesis for this delay is that ischemic and chemical damage due to the chemicals used for RCT take some time to set in and diffuse. A standardized clinical mechanosensory assessment is illustrated in **Fig. 2**. These clinical mechanosensory tests have been shown to have a high specificity; however, they have a low sensitivity.[17] For more accurate sensory profiling, quantitative sensory testing is recommended for selected cases in clinic, including the diagnosis of small fiber neuropathies and for research purposes.[11] Advanced neurophysiologic testing is superior to clinical testing,[18] but this is not always possible intraorally or in large trials. The use of brainstem reflexes and advanced neurophysiologic testing can also accurately establish nerve damage.[19]

Confirming an area of sensory neuropathy, within the same dermatome where the surgery took place, is an important diagnostic feature for sensory neuropathy (**Fig. 2**: neurosensory protocol established by the authors) and establishing the positive and negative signs as specified in the diagnostic criteria (**Fig. 3**).

### Pain Assessment and Functional Impact

Neuropathic pain commonly presents with allodynia (pain on nonnoxious stimuli), hyperalgesia (increased pain to a noxious stimuli), and hyperpathia (continued altered sensation or pain after stimulation ceases). About 50% to 70% of patients report a combination of numbness, altered sensation, and pain, which may be either spontaneous ongoing pain, having a burning character, or spontaneous shooting, electric shocklike sensations. Evoked pain due to touch or cold often leads patients to having difficulties with daily function, such as eating, socializing, kissing, speech, and drinking.[4] Validated neuropathic pain quality measures including Douleur Neuropathique-4, PainDetect, and LANSS questionnaires are able to quantify the presence of

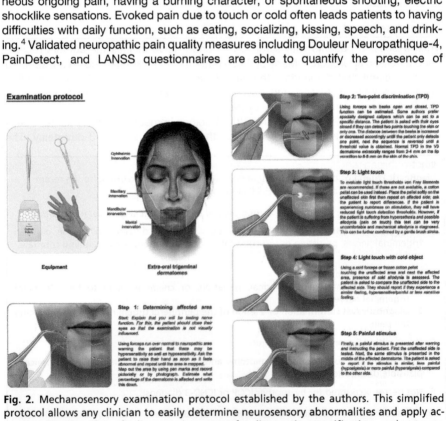

**Fig. 2.** Mechanosensory examination protocol established by the authors. This simplified protocol allows any clinician to easily determine neurosensory abnormalities and apply accurate semantics. These findings are important for diagnostics, stratification, and outcome prediction. (Copyrights to Dr. Fréderic Van der Cruyssen.)

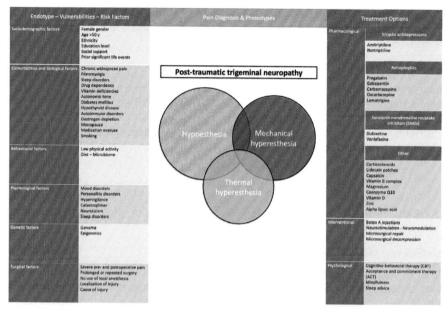

**Fig. 3.** Summary of risk factors in the development of posttraumatic trigeminal neuropathy and subsequent neuropathic pain. Common treatment modalities are summarized as well. Referral to specialist care is recommended. (Copyrights to Dr. Fréderic Van der Cruyssen.)

neuropathic pain, but the sensitivity and specificity are reduced in the trigeminal region due to questions not relevant to oral pain.[7]

### Psychological Assessment

Psychological assessment requires the use of validated questionnaires exploring anxiety, depression, posttraumatic stress disorder, prior abuse and neglect, sleep quality, catastrophizing, and somatization. It is recognized that psychosocial factors including anxiety, depression, hypervigilance, narcissism, introversion, catastrophization, and fear of pain and/or surgery are predictors for persistent postsurgical pain, which is predominantly neuropathic.

Because of nerve injury, patients are often anxious and tearful and exhibit other psychological repercussions. These symptoms were often compounded by the lack of informed consent, which in one study was given to only 30% of patients, most of whom were not specifically warned about potential nerve injury.[7] The presence of anxiety or depression has been suggested to negatively affect treatment outcomes in other pain conditions. In striving for better outcomes, it is therefore advisable to pay attention to the psychological impact in selecting patients for elective implant surgery.

### Phenotyping

Recent studies have used clustering analysis to identify subgroups of neuropathic pain into 3 groups.[4,6,20]

- Sensory loss phenotype (anesthesia, numbness, reduced mechanosensory function)
- Painful with mechanical allodynia and hyperalgesia phenotype
- Painful with thermal allodynia and hyperalgesia phenotype

These subgroups may provide valuable insight into whether the patient will respond to specific treatments, for example, onabotulinum toxin for diabetic painful neuropathy.[21]

### Predicting Outcome

Another study evaluated factors that may predict resolution of trigeminal PTN and reported that nerve site, mechanism, and sensory profile were relevant in predicting resolution or permanency of the nerve injury.[6]

Several factors were associated with likelihood of recovery. We list these factors from more likely to recover to less likely to recover:

- Lingual > inferior alveolar > maxillary nerve
- Local anesthesia > third molar extraction > other extraction > endodontic and implant surgery
- Sensory loss phenotype > pain with mechanical or thermal allodynia and hyperalgesia

### Radiological Investigations

Routine postsurgical radiography is necessary after implant surgery before patient discharge; if the implant or implant bed depth encroaches into the IAN canal this should lead to assessing the patient after the local anesthesia wears off. Dental panoramic tomograms and CBCT scanning are used to assess the relationship between the planned implant site and the mandibular canal containing the IAN. Neither medical computed tomographies nor MRIs are of great assistance in assessing nerve injuries because this is a clinical diagnosis. However, there are some emerging imaging technologies such as magnetic resonance neurography and multimodal assessments that can aid in further diagnosis.[22–24]

### Prevention

It is essential to prevent nerve injuries in all surgery but particularly in elective implant surgery, and patients should be better informed of the benefit and risks.[25,26] The key objective is to plan implant bed depth with a safety zone of at least several millimeters away from the IAN canal based on radiographs.[27–29] The clinician must be aware that many implant drills are 1 to 2 mm longer than the implant and using a 2-mm safety zone will be futile. 3D scanning and computer-assisted surgery with guides have not yet provided evidence-based reduction in nerve injuries. However, a recent study has reported a reduced national incidence of implant-related nerve injuries with increased sales of CBCTs.[30] Many investigators suggest that by "simply" repositioning the IAN that nerve injury will be prevented; however, these techniques are themselves associated with a high incidence of PTN.[31]

### Therapy

Management of PTN will depend on the presentation of the patient (pain, functional and psychological implications), duration, and cause of the nerve injury.[32,33] Urgent patient assessment, confirmation of PTN, and if present removal of the implant within 30 hours is imperative; this will maximize the resolution of implant-related nerve injury and PTNP.[34]

After 30 hours there is no benefit in removing the dental implant, and additional surgery in the region with neuropathic pain can exacerbate the pain. Long-term management of the patient with neuropathic pain will include considerate care and management of the patients' expectations. Use of resources like trigeminalnerve.org.uk may assist both patient and clinician. A combination of psychological and medical interventions will benefit the patient with PTNP.[1]

The evidence base remains limited for managing dental implant-related nerve injuries and related PTNP.[35] If the patient reports numbness, altered sensation, and/or pain, reassurance, acknowledgment of their complaints without minimizing their distress, and further review are basic. The consensus is that prevention of these nerve injuries is possible and optimal. The whole patient with the nerve injury must be treated, not the nerve injury in isolation.

Management may include patient reassurance and education and medical, surgical, and/or psychological treatments (see **Fig. 3**). Patients sustaining local anesthesia, orthognathic, oncology, and trauma-related nerve injuries will mainly be managed therapeutically. Surgical treatment is sometimes indicated and mainly in urgent situation. Urgent surgical intervention should be recommended for known or highly suspected nerve injury, and those related to endodontic or implant nerve injury. Surgical intervention for hypoesthethic injuries does not return the patient to normality, and surgery for patients with pain and hyperesthesia is often not indicated because the pain is not abated. Many patients will need long-term antiepileptics or antidepressants for chronic pain.[36–38] Treatment recommendations are summarized in **Box 2**.

### Psychological Interventions

Counseling is the most useful effective tool for managing patients with problematic permanent sensory nerve injuries. As previously stated, psychological assessment is imperative in holistic patient care. Psychological interventions may include cognitive behavioral therapy, acceptance and commitment therapy, mindfulness, meditation, and group or individual counseling depending on the patient's needs.

### Pharmacologic Treatment

Pharmacologic treatment is indicated for patients with pain or discomfort or with anxiety and/or depression in relation with chronic pain. However, due to the multiple

---

**Box 2**
**Summary of the management and timing of interventions for implant-related trigeminal nerve injuries based on the current evidence base**

Urgent care includes:
- Home check: warn all patients receiving mandibular implants of the potential risk for nerve injury (experiencing a mixture of anesthesia, altered sensation, and pain). At home check within 24 hours of surgery, if the patient reports persistent numbness, altered sensation, and/or pain, then urgent clinical evaluation of the patient should be undertaken to confirm the PTN diagnosis
- Diagnosis includes defining a neuropathic area in the same neurologic dermatome where the surgery took place, negative (anesthesia), and/or positive signs (allodynia and hyperalgesia), which may be spontaneous and/or elicited.
- Apologize: this is not an admission of guilt
- Initiate medical management (recommended for other peripheral sensory nerve injuries)
  ○ Short course of high-dose oral NSAIDs
  ○ Corticosteroids 5-day step-down course
  ○ Vitamin B complex for three months
- Remove the implant as soon as possible unless the neuropathic area is minimal and there is no pain
- Arrange a review and continue to support the patient
- Refer for specialist care when in doubt or when neuropathic complaints persist

noxious side effects of chronic pain medication, less than 18% of patients remain adherent to their medication regime.[1]

## SUMMARY

The symptoms of PTN with associated functional and psychological impact will be the driving force behind the patient seeking treatment.[16] These factors must be assessed and the potential outcomes, positive and negative, should be discussed and agreed with the patient. Decisions on managing the patient with a nerve injury are based on the holistic assessment of the patient. The clinician must assess the degree and impact of the nerve injury and the type of patient. Some patients may present with large painful neuropathies but are happy to continue with minimal life impact, whereas others may present with small areas of neuropathy with no pain but significant related functional and psychological impacts. There are benefits and risks with any intervention, and no reparative surgery or chronic pain medication is devoid of side effects or potential risks. The patient must be made aware of the diagnosis, prognosis, and possible interventions with associated risks and benefits. This is a long conversation and may need to take place over several consultations.

## CLINICS CARE POINTS

- Prevention of trigeminal nerve injury is key because 68% of patients presenting with neuropathic pain and most endodontic and implant-related nerve injuries are permanent

- Interprofessional assessment and management of the patient enables the clinician to evaluate the totality of the presenting condition and not just the medical diagnosis. Without recognizing the functional and psychological aspects of the patient's presentation the clinician will not be able to manage the patient optimally.

- Early intervention within 30 hours for endodontic or implant-related nerve injuries is necessary.

- Early use of medication has been proved to optimize outcome from spinal sensory nerve injuries; this is not yet proven for trigeminal nerve injuries, but at least the patient is reassured that the clinician is trying everything to resolve the nerve injury and prevent neuropathic pain.

- The clinician should recognize that patients with PTN are patients with long-term chronic pain and require continued support.

## DISCLOSURE

Both authors have nothing to disclose.

## FUNDING

None to report.

## REFERENCES

1. Finnerup NB, Attal N, Haroutounian S, et al. Pharmacotherapy for neuropathic pain in adults: A systematic review and meta-analysis. Lancet Neurol 2015; 14(2):162–73.
2. Lin CS, Wu SY, Huang HY, et al. Systematic review and meta-analysis on incidence of altered sensation of mandibular implant surgery. PLoS ONE 2016; 11(4):1–19.

3. Padmanabhan H, Kumar AV, Shivashankar K. Incidence of neurosensory distur-bance in mandibular implant surgery - A meta-analysis. J Indian Prosthodont Soc 2020;20(1):17–26.

4. Van der Cruyssen F, Peeters F, Gill T, et al. Signs and symptoms, quality of life and psychosocial data in 1331 post-traumatic trigeminal neuropathy patients seen in two tertiary referral centres in two countries. J Oral Rehabil 2020;47(10):1212–21.

5. Renton T, Dawood A, Shah A, et al. Post-implant neuropathy of the trigeminal nerve. A case series. Br Dent J 2012;212(11):E17.

6. Van der Cruyssen F, Peeters F, De Laat A, et al. Prognostic factors, symptom evo-lution, and quality of life of posttraumatic trigeminal neuropathy. Pain 2021;163(4): e557–71. Publish Ahead of Print.

7. Smith JG, Elias LA, Yilmaz Z, et al. The psychosocial and affective burden of posttraumatic neuropathy following injuries to the trigeminal nerve. J Orofacl Pain 2013;27(4):293–303.

8. Sullivan MJL, Adams H, Martel MO, et al. Catastrophizing and perceived injus-tice: risk factors for the transition to chronicity after whiplash injury. Spine (Phila Pa 1976) 2011;36(25 Suppl):S244–9.

9. Kaya Y, Sarikcioglu L. Sir Herbert Seddon (1903-1977) and his classification scheme for peripheral nerve injury. Childs Nerv Syst 2015;31(2):177–80.

10. Dahlin LB, Wiberg M. Nerve injuries of the upper extremity and hand. EFORT Open Rev 2017;2(5):158–70.

11. Haanpää M, Attal N, Backonja M, et al. NeuPSIG guidelines on neuropathic pain assessment. Pain 2011;152(1):14–27.

12. Colloca L, Ludman T, Bouhassira D, et al. Neuropathic pain. Nat Rev Dis Primers 2017;3(1):17002.

13. International Classification of Orofacial Pain, 1st edition (ICOP). Cephalalgia : Int J headache 2020;40(2):129–221.

14. Finnerup NB, Haroutounian S, Kamerman P, et al. Neuropathic Pain: an Updated Grading System for Research and Clinical Practice. Pain 2016;157(8):1599–606.

15. Devine M, Hirani M, Durham J, et al. Identifying criteria for diagnosis of post-traumatic pain and altered sensation of the maxillary and mandibular branches of the trigeminal nerve: a systematic review. Oral Surg Oral Med Oral Pathol Oral Radiol 2018;125(6):526–40.

16. Renton T, Van der Cruyssen F. Diagnosis, pathophysiology, management and future issues of trigeminal surgical nerve injuries. Oral Surg 2019. ors.12465.

17. Zuniga JR, Meyer RA, Gregg JM, et al. The accuracy of clinical neurosensory testing for nerve injury diagnosis. J Oral Maxillofac Surg 1998;56(1):2–8. Pub-lished online.

18. Teerijoki-Oksa T, Forssell H, Jääskeläinen SK, et al. Validation of diagnostic methods for traumatic sensory neuropathy and neuropathic pain. Muscle and Nerve 2019;59(3):342–7.

19. Jääskeläinen SK. The utility of clinical neurophysiological and quantitative sen-sory testing for trigeminal neuropathy. J Orofac Pain 2004;18(4):355–9.

20. Baron R, Maier C, Attal N, et al. Peripheral neuropathic pain: a mechanism-related organizing principle based on sensory profiles. Pain 2017;158(2):261–72.

21. Bouhassira D, Letanoux M, Hartemann A. Chronic pain with neuropathic charac-teristics in diabetic patients: a French cross-sectional study. PLoS One 2013;8(9): e74195.

22. Van der Cruyssen F, Peeters F, Croonenborghs TM, et al. A systematic review on diagnostic test accuracy of magnetic resonance neurography versus clinical

neurosensory assessment for post-traumatic trigeminal neuropathy in patients reporting neurosensory disturbance. Dentomaxillofac Radiol 2020;50(1):20200103.

23. Chhabra A, Andreisek G, Soldatos T, et al. MR Neurography: Past, Present, and Future. Am J Roentgenol 2011;197(3):583–91.

24. Van der Cruyssen F, Croonenborghs TM, Renton T, et al. Magnetic resonance neurography of the head and neck: state of the art, anatomy, pathology and future perspectives. Br J Radiol 2021;94(1119):20200798.

25. Yilmaz Z, Ucer C, Scher E, et al. A Survey of the Opinion and Experience of UK Dentists: Part 1: The Incidence and Cause of Iatrogenic Trigeminal Nerve Injuries Related to Dental Implant Surgery. Implant Dent 2016;25(5):638–45.

26. Froum S, Casanova L, Byrne S, et al. Risk assessment before extraction for immediate implant placement in the posterior mandible: a computerized tomographic scan study. J Periodontol 2011;82(3):395–402.

27. Jamil FA, Mohammed JA, Hasan TA, et al. The reliability of surgeons to avoid traumatic insertion of dental implants into high-risk regions: a panoramic radiograph study. BMC Oral Health 2020;20(1):96.

28. Mishra SK, Nahar R, Gaddale R, et al. Identification of anterior loop in different populations to avoid nerve injury during surgical procedures-a systematic review and meta-analysis. Oral Maxillofac Surg 2021;25(2):159–74.

29. Greenstein G, Cavallaro J, Romanos G, et al. Clinical Recommendations for Avoiding and Managing Surgical Complications Associated With Implant Dentistry: A Review. J Periodontol 2008;79(8):1317–29.

30. Marinescu Gava M, Suomalainen A, Vehmas T, et al. Did malpractice claims for failed dental implants decrease after introduction of CBCT in Finland? Clin Oral Investig 2019;23(1):399–404.

31. Castellano-Navarro JM, Castellano-Reyes JJ, Hirdina-Castilla M, et al. Neurosensory issues after lateralisation of the inferior alveolar nerve and simultaneous placement of osseointegrated implants. Br J Oral Maxillofac Surg 2019;57(2):169–73.

32. Renton T, Yilmaz Z. Managing iatrogenic trigeminal nerve injury: A case series and review of the literature. Int J Oral Maxillofac Surg 2012;41(5):629–37.

33. Renton T. Oral surgery: part 4. Minimising and managing nerve injuries and other complications. BDJ 2013;215(8):393–9.

34. Bhavsar I, Khalaf M, Ferrin J, et al. Resolution of Implant-Induced Neurosensory Disturbance: A Procedural Failure. Implant Dent 2015;24(6):735–41.

35. Coulthard P, Kushnerev E, Yates JM, et al. Interventions for iatrogenic inferior alveolar and lingual nerve injury. Cochrane database Syst Rev 2014;4:CD005293.

36. Zuniga JR, Yates DM. Factors Determining Outcome After Trigeminal Nerve Surgery for Neuropathic Pain. J Oral Maxillofac Surg 2016;74(7):1323–9.

37. Zuniga JR, Yates DM, Phillips CL. The presence of neuropathic pain predicts postoperative neuropathic pain following trigeminal nerve repair. J Oral Maxillofac Surg 2014;72(12):2422–7.

38. Kushnerev E, Yates JM. Evidence-based outcomes following inferior alveolar and lingual nerve injury and repair: a systematic review. J Oral Rehabil 2015;42(10):786–802.

# Trigeminal Neuralgia

Shehryar Nasir Khawaja, BDS, MSc[a],*, Steven J. Scrivani, DDS, DMedSc[b]

**KEYWORDS**

- Chronic pain • Pain • Trigeminal neuralgia • Management

**KEY POINTS**

- Trigeminal neuralgia (TN) is a neuropathic pain disorder characterized by recurrent, paroxysmal episodes of short-lasting severe intensity electric shock-like pain along the sensory distribution of trigeminal nerve.
- The diagnosis of TN is established clinically and requires a comprehensive history and examination. This is essential as there is no objective laboratory investigation to confirm the diagnosis.
- It is critical for patient care to make a distinction between classical or idiopathic TN and secondary TN.
- Magnetic resonance imaging (MRI) is the first choice for diagnosing secondary TN. However, if contraindicated or not available, computed tomography (CT) scan with contrast can be considered to rule out tumors.
- The mainstay of management of TN is pharmacologic management. Other modalities include reversible interventions and surgical procedures.

## CASE REPORT

A 62-year-old female presented to the clinic with a chief complaint of "I have been experiencing electric shock-like jolts over the right side of my face." The patient reported that she had been feeling episodes of electric shock-like pain over the lower right side of her face. These started nearly a month ago without any apparent cause. The episodes presented multiple times a day and lasted for a few seconds. The pain was severe in intensity, and it radiated over the lower teeth toward her ear. The pain was triggered by a light touch or a breeze over the skin around the right ala of the nose. Likewise, the pain could be triggered by washing her face and sometimes while laughing or yawning. There were no temporal patterns associated with the pain and the patient reported no associated sensory or motor alterations or autonomic symptoms.

[a] Orofacial Pain Medicine, Department of Internal Medicine, Shaukat Khanum Memorial Cancer Hospital & Research Centers, Lahore, Pakistan; [b] Department of Diagnostic Sciences, Craniofacial Pain Center, Tufts University School of Dental Medicine, Boston, MA, USA
* Corresponding author. Shaukat Khanum Memorial Cancer Hospital and Research Center, 7A Block R-3, Phase 2, M.A. Johar Town, Lahore, Punjab 54782, Pakistan.
*E-mail address:* khawajashehryar@gmail.com

Dent Clin N Am 67 (2023) 99–115
https://doi.org/10.1016/j.cden.2022.07.008
0011-8532/23/© 2022 Elsevier Inc. All rights reserved.

dental.theclinics.com

Her medical history was significant for hypertension and hypercholesterolemia. She used valsartan 80 mg, amlodipine 5 mg and rosuvastatin 10 mg once a day. She was not aware of any allergies to medications. Her family history was significant for heart disease. She had no history of smoking, drinking, or substance abuse. There was no history of psychiatric disease. She was a homemaker, married, and had two daughters.

Her pulse rate was 74 beats/min during the physical examination, and her blood pressure was 130/80 mm Hg. Her respiratory rate was 18 breaths per minute, and her temperature was 36.9 centigrade. She was sitting pain-free at the time of examination and was oriented to time, place, and person. There were no apparent asymmetries, atrophies, swellings, or lesions on the inspection of the head, face, and neck regions. The vertical and horizontal mandibular range of motion was within normal limits and without pain. The patient reported no pain on the palpation of the masticatory muscles, temporomandibular joint, posterior mandibular area, or submandibular region. There were no palpable joint sounds or abnormal patterns of movements observed during mandibular motion. The cervical range of movements was within normal limits and the patient did not report any pain on the palpation of the cervical muscles.

Intraoral examination revealed normal, moist, and pink-colored oral mucosa. Tongue movements were normal, the uvula was in the midline, and the soft palate was mobile. No lesions, discolorations, or swelling were observed, and salivary flow was adequate. Her third molars were missing, and the rest of the dentition was sound. There were mild signs of attrition present along the occlusal surface of the molar teeth. However, no cracks or carious lesions were observed.

Cranial nerve (CN II–XII) examination revealed no gross discrepancies; however, during the assessment of the sensory function of the trigeminal nerve, an episode of pain was triggered from light touching of the skin around the right ala of the nose. The spinal nerves (C2-T1) were grossly intact. Testing of complex motor skills revealed normal coordination. Deep tendon reflexes of the biceps, triceps, and brachioradialis were normal. The panoramic radiograph in the closed-mouth position did not show any disease. A working diagnosis of trigeminal neuralgia (TN) was made, and the patient was prescribed carbamazepine 200 mg three times a day. The patient was advised to start carbamazepine 200 mg once at night for the first 3 days, followed by taking it two times a day for 3 days, and subsequently switching to taking it three times a day after another 3 days. Furthermore, laboratory studies (complete blood count and liver function test) were ordered and were within normal limits. A high spatial resolution three-dimensional (3D) T2-sequence (FIESTA) with 3D T1 postcontrast MRI study was ordered. This did not show any intracranial pathology or neurovascular contact. A definitive diagnosis of idiopathic TN was made.

At the 3-week follow-up, the patient reported that the frequency and intensity of painful episodes had been reduced. Furthermore, occasionally, she felt brief paresthesia over the prior site of pain and reported experiencing drowsiness with carbamazepine, which was manageable by taking a nap for a few minutes after taking medication. For the paresthesia, in addition to carbamazepine, she was advised to start pregabalin 50 mg three times a day. Due to the prior complaint of drowsiness with carbamazepine, pregabalin was titrated from taking it once a day at nighttime to taking one capsule three times a day over a week.

At the 3-month follow-up, the patient reported that she had been pain-free for more than 2 months and had not experienced any paresthesia. She was advised to taper the pregabalin dosage down by 50 mg/wk until she felt recurrent episodes of paresthesia or pain and subsequently do the same with carbamazepine by 200 mg/wk. At the 6-month follow-up, complete blood count and liver function tests were repeated and were within normal limits. At that time the patient was on a maintenance dosage of carbamazepine 400 mg/d.

## CLINICS CARE POINTS

- The patient reported brief episodes of electric shock-like pain along the trigeminal nerve distribution. There were no reports of any other sensory, motor, or autonomic symptoms, which is essential to rule out other episodic pain disorders.
- During the clinical examination, the examiner was able to trigger the episode of pain, which is characteristic of trigeminal neuralgia (TN).
- High-definition magnetic resonance imaging of the brain was obtained to rule out any neurovascular or secondary cause of pain.
- The patient had a partial response with carbamazepine therapy. However, the dosage of the medication was limited due to medication-associated drowsiness. The patient was started on pregabalin (add-on therapy), which provided her with significant pain relief. This highlights the benefits of having a patient on combination therapy.
- After 2 months, when the patient had no episodes of pain, she was gradually tapered off pregabalin, and the dosage of carbamazepine was reduced. It is not uncommon in TN for the pain episodes to go into a refractory phase for weeks, months, or years.

## INTRODUCTION

Trigeminal neuralgia (TN) is a neuropathic pain disorder characterized by recurrent, paroxysmal episodes of short-lasting severe intensity electric shock-like pain along the sensory distribution of the trigeminal nerve.[1,2] These features make it a debilitating condition. This is reflected in the epidemiologic studies, which show significant associations between TN and anxiety, depression, and poor quality of life and sleep.[3] Recent classifications systems and guidelines have helped improve the characterization and understanding of the disorder.[1,2,4,5]

## EPIDEMIOLOGY

Trigeminal neuralgia is a rare condition. A systematic review reported that the prevalence of TN ranged from 0.03% to 0.3%.[6] The annual incidence of TN varies from 4.3 to 8 per 100,000, and the average age of onset is estimated to be 53 to 57 years.[7–9] The incidence of TN begins to increase every decade after 60 years. It is nearly 17.5 per 100,000 in 60 to 69 year olds and estimated to be 25.9 per 100,000 in greater than 80 year olds.[7,9,10] The incidence of TN in children and adolescents is rare.[11] TN is more likely to affect females, and the exact female to male ratio differs between studies. However, it is calculated to be around 3:1.[6–8]

## DIAGNOSTIC CRITERIA AND CLASSIFICATION

Trigeminal neuralgia is a pain disorder characterized by recurrent, paroxysmal, unilateral, short-lasting episodes of electric shock-like pain along the sensory distribution of one or more divisions of the trigeminal nerve. It may be accompanied by concomitant continuous or near-continuous background pain. The new International Classification of Orofacial Pain (ICOP) and the third edition of the International

Classification of Headache Disorders (ICHD 3) have similar diagnostic criteria for TN as the International Association of Study of Pain (IASP) (**Box 1**).[1,2] They have grouped TN into 3 main categories according to the underlying etiology. Classical TN is defined as TN that has developed without apparent cause other than neurovascular compression (with morphologic changes in the trigeminal nerve root) (**Box 2**). If there are no morphologic changes in the trigeminal nerve root (even though contact may exist) or electrophysiological tests show no significant abnormalities, TN will be considered Idiopathic TN (**Box 3**). TN caused by other pathologic characteristics, such as tumors, space-occupying lesions, or multiple sclerosis, is termed secondary TN (**Box 4**). Classical and idiopathic TN are subdivided into purely paroxysmal (recurrent short-lasting pain) and TN with concomitant continuous pain (recurrent short-lasting pain with continuous or near-continuous background pain).

## CLINICAL FEATURES AND DIAGNOSTIC INVESTIGATIONS

The diagnosis of TN is established clinically and requires a comprehensive history and examination. This is essential as there is no objective laboratory investigation to confirm the diagnosis of TN.

The pain associated with TN is severe and paroxysmal, and it is generally electric shock-like in quality. However, the pain can also be described as icepick-like, sharp, stabbing, or shooting in nature. The pain episodes are intermittent and last from a fraction of a second to 2 minutes. The pain initiates and terminates abruptly. The episode frequency varies from a few pain attacks to hundreds of attacks per day. The pain episodes are followed by a refractory period during which the pain cannot be elicited.[1,2,4,12] In addition, up to 50% of the patients may have a less intense (mild–moderate) concomitant continuous or near-continuous (lasting for hours) dull, throbbing, or aching quality pain in the same area as the intermittent intense pain.

---

**Box 1**
**The International Classification of Orofacial Pain, 1st Edition (ICOP) and the International Classification for Headache Disorders, 3rd Edition (ICHD-3) diagnostic criteria for Trigeminal Neuralgia[1,2]**

Diagnostic criteria:
A. Recurrent paroxysms of unilateral facial pain in the distribution (s) of one or more divisions of the trigeminal nerve, with no radiation beyond[a], and fulfilling criteria B and C.
B. The pain has all of the following characteristics:
  1. lasting for a fraction of a second to 2 minutes [b]
  2. severe intensity [c]
  3. electric shock-like, shooting, stabbing, or sharp in quality
C. Precipitated by innocuous stimuli within the affected trigeminal distribution [d]
D. Not better accounted for by another ICOP or ICHD-3 diagnosis.

[a] In a few patients, pain may radiate to another division, but remains within the trigeminal dermatomes[b] Duration can change over time, with paroxysm becomes more prolonged. A minority of patients will report attacks predominantly lasting for greater than 2 minutes.[c] Pain may become more severe over time.[d] Some attacks may be, or appear to be, spontaneous, but there must be a history or finding of pain provoked by innocuous stimuli to meet this criterion. Ideally, the examining clinician should attempt to confirm the history by replicating the triggering phenomenon. However, this may not always be possible because of the patient's refusal, the awkward anatomic location of the trigger, and/or other factors.

---

**Box 2**
**The International Classification of Orofacial Pain, 1st Edition (ICOP) and the International Classification for Headache Disorders, 3rd Edition (ICHD-3) diagnostic criteria for Classical Trigeminal Neuralgia[1,2]**

Diagnostic Criteria for Classical Trigeminal Neuralgia
A. Recurrent paroxysms of unilateral pain fulfilling criteria for trigeminal neuralgia
B. Demonstration in magnetic resonance imaging (MRI) or during surgery of neurovascular compression (not simply contact), with morphologic changes [a] in the trigeminal nerve.

Diagnostic Criteria for Classical Trigeminal Neuralgia, Purely Paroxysmal
A. Recurrent paroxysms of unilateral facial pain fulfilling criteria for Classical trigeminal neuralgia
B. Pain-free between attacks in the affected trigeminal distribution.

Diagnostic Criteria for Classical Trigeminal Neuralgia with Concomitant Continuous Pain
A. Recurrent paroxysms of unilateral facial pain fulfilling criteria for Classical trigeminal neuralgia
B. Concomitant continuous or near-continuous pain between attacks in the ipsilateral trigeminal distribution.

[a] Typically atrophy or displacement.

---

The pain is distributed along one or more sensory divisions of the trigeminal nerve. It most often occurs in maxillary or mandibular division alone or in combination. The occurrence of pain along the ophthalmic division of the trigeminal nerve is rare.[13,14] A pathognomonic feature of TN is the presence of trigger zones or areas. These are

---

**Box 3**
**The International Classification of Orofacial Pain, 1st Edition (ICOP) and the International Classification for Headache Disorders, 3rd Edition (ICHD-3) diagnostic criteria for Idiopathic Trigeminal Neuralgia[1,2]**

Diagnostic Criteria for Idiopathic Trigeminal Neuralgia
A. Recurrent paroxysms of unilateral pain fulfilling criteria for trigeminal neuralgia, either purely paroxysmal or associated with concomitant continuous or near-continuous pain
B. Neither Classical trigeminal neuralgia nor Secondary trigeminal neuralgia has been confirmed by adequate investigations [a,b]
C. Not better accounted for by another ICDH-3 or ICOP diagnosis.

Diagnostic Criteria for Idiopathic Trigeminal Neuralgia, Purely Paroxysmal
A. Recurrent paroxysms of unilateral facial pain fulfilling criteria for Idiopathic trigeminal neuralgia
B. Pain-free between attacks in the affected trigeminal distribution.

Diagnostic Criteria for Idiopathic Trigeminal Neuralgia with Concomitant Continuous Pain
A. Recurrent paroxysms of unilateral facial pain fulfilling criteria for Idiopathic trigeminal neuralgia
B. Concomitant continuous or near-continuous pain between attacks in the ipsilateral trigeminal distribution.

[a] Including electrophysiological tests or magnetic resonance imaging. [b] A contact between a blood vessel and the trigeminal nerve and/or nerve root is a common finding in neuroimaging in healthy subjects. When such a contact is found in the presence of trigeminal neuralgia, but without evidence of morphologic changes (eg, atrophy or displacement) in the nerve root, the criteria for Classical trigeminal neuralgia are not fulfilled and the condition is considered idiopathic.

---

**Box 4**
**The International Classification of Orofacial Pain, 1st Edition (ICOP) and the International Classification for Headache Disorders, 3rd Edition (ICHD-3) diagnostic criteria for Secondary Trigeminal Neuralgia[1,2]**

Diagnostic Criteria for Secondary Trigeminal Neuralgia
A. Recurrent paroxysms of unilateral pain fulfilling criteria for Trigeminal neuralgia, either purely paroxysmal or associated with concomitant continuous or near-continuous pain
B. An underlying disease has been demonstrated[a] that is known to be able to cause, and explain, the neuralgia[b]
C. Not better accounted for by another ICOP or ICHD-3 diagnosis.

[a] Magnetic resonance imaging (MRI) is best equipped to detect an underlying cause of Secondary trigeminal neuralgia. Other investigations may include neurophysiological recording of trigeminal reflexes and trigeminal evoked potentials, suitable for patient who cannot undergo MRI. [b] Recognized causes are tumors in the cerebellopontine angle, arteriovenous malformations, and multiple sclerosis.

---

regions of the face (trigeminal system) that elicit a TN episode on innocuous, mechanical, or tactile stimulation. The most common triggering stimuli have been reported to be light touch and vibration, such as washing face, talking, chewing, brushing teeth, or shaving. Prior studies have suggested that they are present in up to 91% of patients [12,13,15,16]. They often occur in the central part of the face (perioral area), near the ala of the nose and lips, and over time, the trigger region may migrate.[14–16]

TN may begin abruptly or gradually after a preceding syndrome called pre-TN (although controversial), which is characterized by a dull aching pain along the distribution of the trigeminal nerve. This has been reported in up to 18% of the cases.[17] Similarly, the disorder may go into remission for months and years in an unpredictable manner.[18]

The pain associated with TN may be accompanied by involuntary contraction of the face (spasm). Due to this, TN is referred to as tic douloureux.[15] Patients with classical or idiopathic TN have no evidence of clinical sensory abnormalities within the trigeminal distribution unless advanced examination methods such as quantitative sensory testing are used.[19] Nonetheless, subtle sensory abnormalities such as mild hypoesthesia or minimal hyperesthesia may exist.

Clinical evidence of sensory deficit should raise suspicion for an underlying organic cause unless proven otherwise, that is, secondary TN. Likewise, the bilateral presence of pain should raise suspicion for multiple sclerosis (MS). However, these clinical characteristics have poor sensitivity because not all patients with secondary TN will not develop a sensory deficit and most patients with MS report unilateral pain.

The European Academy of Neurology (EAN) guidelines on TN has recommended magnetic resonance imaging (MRI) as the first-choice imaging study for diagnosing secondary TN. Standard 3-T or 1.5-T MRI can reliably exclude secondary intracranial causes of TN (multiple sclerosis, space-occupying lesions, or tumors). However, for evaluating any distortion, displacement, indentation, or trigeminal nerve atrophy by a blood vessel, a combination of 3 high-resolution sequences: three-dimensional (3D) T2-weighted, 3D time-of-flight, and magnetic resonance angiography along with 3D T1-weighted gadolinium may be required. If MRI is contraindicated or not available, computed tomography (CT) scan with contrast can be considered to rule out tumors.

If imaging is unavailable, the guidelines recommend testing trigeminal reflexes to differentiate between secondary TN and primary TN. The pooled diagnostic accuracy of trigeminal reflexes in differentiating primary and secondary TN is excellent (pooled sensitivity 94% and pooled specificity 88%). In contrast, the guidelines have given a strong recommendation against the use of evoked potentials to identify secondary TN because the pooled diagnostic accuracy of these investigations has been calculated to be modest (pooled sensitivity of 84% and a pooled specificity of 52%).[4]

## PATHOPHYSIOLOGY

The pathophysiology of TN is complex. In classical TN, by definition, there is evidence of compression of the trigeminal nerve at or near the dorsal root entry zone (DREZ) by a blood vessel.[20–22] Within this region, peripheral Schwann cell myelination transition to central oligodendroglia myelination occurs, which is hypothesized to make this zone susceptible to pressure. In most cases, the compression is secondary to an arterial vessel of the Circle of Willis, and most frequently, the rostroventral superior cerebellar artery is involved. However, venous and combined compressions have been reported.[5,22,23]

Surgical investigations have reported grooving or indentation in the trigeminal nerve along the compression area. The histologic samples of these regions are often characterized by demyelination, dysmyelination, and remyelination, and close apposition of groups of axons with no intervening glial processes, similar to animal models of nerve injury.[22]

There is significant evidence that partial injury to the trigeminal ganglion or trigeminal nerve root may be an important initiating factor in the onset of TN.[20,21] A partial nerve injury may result in a cascade of changes within the sensory neurons. Injury can result in the formation of focal areas of axonal demyelination, which may regenerate spontaneous action potentials that can travel in either direction along the nerve. Similarly, a single-action potential may evoke sustained after-discharges in a few cases. Furthermore, an injury may cause abnormal coupling between primary afferents, resulting in ephaptic transmission.[20,21] However, there is significant evidence to the contrary hypothesis. Many animal models of complete or partial nerve injury do not present with the clinical phenotype seen in TN in humans. In addition, there are clinical features of TN that cannot be explained by a nerve injury model, such as refractory periods, long periods of spontaneous remission, and the presence of compression on the pain-free contralateral side.

An *"ignition hypothesis"* has been suggested to explain the pathophysiology of TN. It suggests that partial injury to the trigeminal nerve roots or ganglion results in forming a group of hyper-excitable and functionally linked primary sensory neurons. The hypothesis suggests that spontaneous or evoked discharge of individual neurons can rapidly spread by ephaptic and other mechanisms to excite an entire population of adjacent sensory neurons, which may clinically result in a sudden jolt of pain[21].

Ephaptic cross-communication between neurons could explain the mechanism for the trigger zone phenomenon observed in TN. An innocuous cutaneous stimulus (eg, a light touch over a small area of the face, shaving, or washing face) can reliably evoke a typical episode of TN pain attack. The trigger zone phenomenon is consistent with ephaptic interactions between low-threshold large caliber, rapidly conducting cutaneous sensory afferents (A-beta fibers) and the smaller caliber, nociception carrying fibers (A-delta and C-fibers).[24]

The characteristic refractory period that follows the TN attacks can be partially explained by the suppressive effect of A-fiber stimulation on C-fiber responses and C-fiber stimulation on A-fibers through central inhibitory mechanisms.[24] On the contrary, ephaptic cross-communication and ectopic impulse generation cannot explain the presence of concomitant continuous pain. It has been hypothesized that there may be a role of centrally mediated facilitation of nociceptive processing or reduced descending inhibitory mechanism (central sensitization) in such patients.

In secondary TN, there is an identifiable underlying disease that can cause neuralgia, such as a tumor in the cerebellopontine angle, arterio-venous-malformation, or multiple sclerosis.[1,2] Histologic studies have suggested that these systemic conditions can cause damage to the trigeminal nerve like that observed with neurovascular compression.

On the contrary, idiopathic TN has neither any evidence of nerve compression by a neurovascular bundle nor an identifiable local or systemic pathology.[1,2] Multiple pathologies have been proposed, ranging from neuronal voltage-gated ion channel gain-of-function mutations to neural inflammation and nonspecific, nonmultiple sclerosis lesions in the brainstem.

## DIFFERENTIAL DIAGNOSIS

Trigeminal neuralgia has pathognomonic features that differentiate it from other facial pain conditions. The diagnosis should be easily made with a careful and comprehensive history and detailed physical examination. However, TN is often misdiagnosed due to a lack of objective diagnostic tests or, in some cases overlapping symptomatology and the diverse group of health care providers from which patients seek consultation.

TN may mimic dental pain, due to the fact that it is most commonly experienced in the second and third trigeminal distributions and up to 65% of cases have been reported to undergo unnecessary dental interventions. Odontogenic pain, unlike TN, has clinical evidence of pathology, such as broken teeth, exposed dentin, cracks, or carious lesions. In this situation, teeth may be sensitive to cold or hot liquids and/or sweets and may be tender to palpation or percussion, often with the pain of longer duration.

Trigeminal autonomic cephalalgias (TAC) are a primary headache disorder characterized by severe, unilateral episodes of pain along the trigeminal nerve distribution with the corresponding activation of the autonomic nervous system. Short-lasting unilateral neuralgiform headaches with conjunctival injection and tearing (SUNCT) and short-lasting unilateral neuralgiform headaches with autonomic symptoms (SUNA) are a type of TAC that clinically seem very similar to TN.[2] However, paroxysmal pain episodes associated with SUNCT or SUNA are predominantly localized around the orbital and temporal region, lack refractory periods, and are always associated with ipsilateral lacrimation and/or conjunctival redness and respond poorly to carbamazepine.[25]

Glossopharyngeal neuralgia is a painful paroxysmal disorder associated with brief episodes of electric shock-like, shooting, or stabbing pain along the distribution of glossopharyngeal nerve.[2,26] Unlike TN, pain is often triggered after swallowing or speaking loudly. The location of the pain is deep in the oral cavity. However, sometimes it may radiate toward the ear and/or beneath the angle of the jaw.[9,26] Gustatory neuralgia or First-Bite Syndrome is a taste-evoked painful condition characterized by sudden electric shock-like pain in the periauricular region. The pain is triggered during the initial bites of a meal and alleviates with subsequent masticatory movements.

There are no reports of pain in between meals.[27,28] Unlike TN, gustatory neuralgia is always localized in the peri-auricular region, triggered after a gustatory stimulus, and most patients have a history of trauma in the head-and-neck region or postoperatively following the resection of the sympathetic chain or parotid gland or after surgery involving the parapharyngeal space, infratemporal fossa, temporomandibular joint complex, carotid bifurcation, or internal carotid artery.

It is critical for patient care to distinguish between classical or idiopathic TN and secondary TN. The studies investigating the diagnostic accuracy of clinical characteristics for distinguishing primary (classical or idiopathic) TN from second TN were unable to find a significant difference between the 2 disorders in terms of the involvement of the ophthalmic division of trigeminal nerve and response to treatment modalities. The age of the patients with secondary TN (STN) was significantly younger than the age of the patient with primary TN. However, there was considerable overlap between the age ranges. The clinical presentation of sensory discrepancy and bilateral pain occurrence correlates with secondary TN. However, these clinical symptoms have poor sensitivity. The EAN guidelines suggest using MRI for differentiation and subclassification of TN. If MRI is unavailable, CT brain has been suggested as an alternative to rule out an organic cause of TN. The most commonly reported tumors associated with STN are meningioma, acoustic neuroma, epidermoid tumor, pituitary tumor, glioma, lymphoma, arachnoid cyst, and schwannoma.[15,29,30]

## MANAGEMENT

The management of TN consists of medical and surgical therapies. Medical management consists of pharmacologic modalities and reversible interventions such as botulinum toxin type A and local anesthesia injections. The surgical (invasive) therapies consist of various peripheral and intracranial procedures.[13,31] Nonetheless, the mainstay of management is pharmacologic management. The overall prognosis of the management is favorable, and most of the patients report adequate pain relief with medical therapies at long-term follow-up.[7,32]

Due to the nature of this facial pain condition, many patients seek an evaluation by a variety of dental specialists. With the complicated presentation and uncommon incidence of TN, there is often delay in diagnosis, misdiagnosis, and unnecessary treatments provided.

## MEDICAL THERAPY
### Pharmacologic Therapy

The cornerstone of pharmacologic therapy for TN is antiepileptic drugs (AED). In the recent guidelines on TN, the EAN recommends the use of carbamazepine and oxcarbazepine as the drugs of choice for the long-term treatment of TN.[4] The number needed to treat (NNT) for any pain relief for carbamazepine in TN is 1.9 (95% confidence intervals (CI) 1.4–2.8) and for significant pain relief is 2.6 (CI 2–3.4).[33] Oxcarbazepine, a derivative of carbamazepine, has similar effectiveness as carbamazepine in reducing the number of TN attacks and improving global assessment and, it may be associated with a more favorable side-effect profile. Before starting a patient on carbamazepine or oxcarbazepine, it is generally advised to complete initial laboratory monitoring as these medications may cause severe side effects, such as leukopenia, abnormal liver function, and aplastic anemia, and hyponatremia. The tolerability of these medications is lower in females than males, and cross-allergy between the drugs has been reported.[34]

Lamotrigine is an antiepileptic drug that reduces the repetitive firing of sodium channels by slowing the recovery rate of voltage-gated channels. It can be used either as monotherapy or as add-on therapy for the long-term management of TN, TN cases refractory to carbamazepine or oxcarbazepine, and in the management of secondary TN associated with MS.[35]

Gabapentinoids (gabapentin and pregabalin) are antiepileptic drugs that block calcium channels. Even though they may have fewer side effects than sodium channel blocks (carbamazepine, oxcarbazepine, and lamotrigine), field experts believe that the effectiveness of these drugs against TN may be comparatively less. They are recommended for patients who fail or cannot use sodium channel blocks or add-on therapy.[31]

Other antiepileptics that can be beneficial as an add-on therapy consist phenytoin, topiramate, fosphenytoin, and valproic acid.[7,31,36–38] Fosphenytoin and valproic acid, have the advantage of being available for use in intravenous formulation.[38] Infusion of fosphenytoin (and potentially valproic acid) and lidocaine, intravenously, has been recommended in the acute treatment of severe exacerbations during TN.

Baclofen, an analog of the neurotransmitter gamma-aminobutyric acid, has a low side-effect profile and an NNT of 1.4 (CI 1–2.6).[39] It is recommended as add-on therapy, as it has a synergistic effect with both carbamazepine and phenytoin. Clonazepam, a benzodiazepine, has been shown to effectively manage symptoms associated with TN. However, due to its poor tolerability, it can be considered in low doses as an add-on therap.[31]

There is modest evidence of the use of topical local anesthetics for pain control in TN.[7,31] These may be helpful in situations whereby patients have difficulty swallowing or as a bridging therapy until systemic medications begin to work. This therapy may work better in circumstances whereby pain is intraoral as the properties of the oral mucosa allow the medication to be absorbed more easily in comparison to the skin overlying head and face region.[31]

### Reversible Interventions

In the recent EAN guidelines, botulinum toxin type A (BTX-A) has been added as an add-on therapy for the management of TN. Similarly, ropivacaine, a local anesthetic injection, has been suggested to provide relief in TN as an add-on to sodium or calcium channel blocks.

When used concurrently with pharmacotherapeutics, BTX-A in up to 86% of patients has shown at least a 50% reduction in pain. Similarly, studies have reported a significant decrease in the frequency of paroxysmal pain episodes. There is no consensus among studies on the optimal dosage or technique for injecting BTX-A. Investigators have reported using up to 100 international units (IU) of BTX-A. However, in a dose-comparison study, no statistical difference was observed in the effectiveness of botulinum toxin in reducing at least 50% pain between the groups receiving 25 IU and 75 IU. Botulinum toxin has been injected subdermally, subcutaneously, or submucosally at the pain site or trigger zone. Due to the inherent nature of BTX-A, the procedure is associated with a low risk of transient side effects such as facial weakness and edema or hematoma.[40–42]

Local anesthetic injections can be used for diagnostic purposes and provide temporary relief from symptoms. However, the evidence for nerve blocks as a therapeutic modality is weak. Local anesthesia injections have been recommended for patients whereby a therapeutic dosage of medications has not been achieved (as a bridge therapy), TN refractory to treatment, or those waiting for a surgical procedure.[43,44]

### Surgical Therapies

Surgical modalities can be aimed peripherally at the affected nerve distribution or centrally at the trigeminal ganglion or nerve root (site of vascular compression) in the posterior fossa. The EAN guidelines suggest that medical management with adequate dosing and monitoring should be attempted before surgical therapies are conducted for the management of TN. However, there is limited evidence available to suggest the optimal number of medications that should be trialed before surgical therapies are offered to a patient.

### Peripheral Procedures

Peripheral procedures are aimed at inducing trauma to the nerve. These include peripheral neurectomy, cryoablation, or chemical destruction using phenol, glycerol, or alcohol. Peripheral neurectomy is the surgical destruction of the offending branch of the trigeminal nerve.[45,46] It is often reserved for cases whereby medical therapy is ineffective or contraindicated or for patients in whom gangliolysis and microvascular decompression surgery (MVD) are contraindicated due to medical comorbidities. The success rate of peripheral neurectomies is variable, and they are associated with an increased risk of developing painful posttraumatic trigeminal neuropathy (PPTTN).[45,46]

The details of peripheral procedures are summarized in **Table 1**. In summary, peripheral procedures are well tolerated but have high recurrence and complication rates. They should be reserved for patients with significant medical comorbidities that do not allow them to undergo central procedures or whereby the expectations from the procedure are to provide relief for a short or medium term.

### Central Procedures

Central procedures are directed toward the trigeminal ganglion or nerve root in the posterior fossa.

Percutaneous trigeminal ganglion rhizotomies are destructive procedures in which a portion of the trigeminal ganglion is ablated by one of the several techniques (**Table 2**). These procedures are performed under fluoroscopic guidance, and methods include controlled heat (radiofrequency rhizolysis), chemical neurolysis (glycerol injection), or mechanical trauma (balloon compression). In a recent expert-based review, these procedures have been suggested for patients in whom MRI does not show any vascular contact. Similarly, it can be used for patients whereby MVD surgeries are contraindicated.[52] Overall, percutaneous trigeminal ganglion rhizotomy procedures have acceptable outcomes. However, they are associated with sensory discrepancies, such as facial and corneal numbness or hypoesthesia, trigeminal weakness, keratitis, and masticatory muscle weakness.[15]

Gamma knife stereotactic radiosurgery (GKS) is a noninvasive, destructive technique that uses 70–90 Gy radiation units to damage the trigeminal nerve root at the point of vascular compression.[54,55,58] It uses MRI sequencing for mapping the exact location of the compression. However, if there is no evidence of vascular compression, the trigeminal root entry zone is targeted (see **Table 2**). Like GKS, Cyber-knife radiosurgery (CKS) has been used to treat TN. The CKS uses a linear accelerator to induce damage to the trigeminal nerve. This modality has a moderate-excellent response rate of 78% at an 11-month follow-up.[59]

Microvascular decompression surgery (MVD) is the first-choice surgery in patients with classical TN. It is based on the hypothesis that the contact between the intracerebral vessels and the trigeminal nerve root causes chronic demyelination, which

**Table 1**
Summary of characteristics of peripheral surgical procedures for the management of trigeminal neuralgia

| Name of the Procedure | Procedure Details | Comments and Side-effects |
|---|---|---|
| Cryoablation[7,47] | Extreme cold is used to burn a nerve. Cryoablation has shown to result in analgesia for up to 13 mo, after which, in nearly 80% of patients, pain may reoccur at the original site. Repeated procedures often yield better outcomes. | Up to one-third of cases can develop painful posttraumatic trigeminal nerve neuropathy. |
| Phenol chemical neurolysis[48] | Up to 5 mL of phenol is injected around the nerve. It has shown to be significantly effective in providing pain relief in TN-associated symptoms for a median of 9 mo in nearly 87% of the patients. | Phenol has an instant anesthetic effect, and injections are relatively well tolerated. Phenol has a high affinity for blood vessels, due to this, it should be avoided in areas of increased vascularity. Phenol-injections have been associated with sensory changes, motor weakness, and ecchymosis |
| Glycerol chemical neurolysis[49,50] | Up to 5 mL of glycerol is injected around the nerve. Glycerol can result in 7–24 mo of relief in 60% of patients with TN. Repeated injections produce a shorter analgesic response. | Glycerol is highly viscous and requires a large-bore needle for injection, and it has been associated with hematoma, ecchymosis, sensory changes, and transient mandibular hypomobility. |
| Absolute alcohol chemical neurolysis[50,51] | Up to 5 mL of absolute alcohol is injected around the nerve. Absolute alcohol injections can provide 13–19 mo of relief in symptoms. | Injections are painful to administer and have a high risk of complications, including full-thickness skin or mucosal ulceration, regional fibrosis, cranial nerve palsies, herpes zoster reactivation, and bony necrosis. |

**Table 2**
Summary of characteristics of central surgical procedures for the management of trigeminal neuralgia

| Name of the Procedure | Procedure Details | Comments and Side-Effects |
|---|---|---|
| Radiofrequency rhizolysis[13,52] | It uses controlled heat (60–90 centigrades) in short intervals to damage the trigeminal nerve fibers. This technique has 87%–95% initial pain relief, significant long-term (12–80 mo) pain relief of 83%, and a low pain recurrence of 11%–20%. | Radiofrequency rhizolysis is associated with dysesthesias, masticatory muscle weakness, loss of corneal reflex, keratitis, diplopia, anesthesia dolorosa, and meningitis. |
| Chemical rhizolysis[15,52] | Up to 0.4 mL of glycerol is injected into the trigeminal cistern. It can result in initial pain relief for 6 mo in 84% of the cases. However, this percentage drops to 54% at a 3-y follow-up. | It is associated with corneal numbness and keratitis, anesthesia dolorosa, transient masseter muscle weakness, cranial nerve deficits, and vascular injuries. |
| Trigeminal ganglion balloon compression[52,53] | The procedure is performed by placing a catheter into the trigeminal cistern and inflating it with radiocontrast dye to compress the trigeminal ganglion. This technique has shown nearly 90% success in providing initial pain relief. | The procedure requires close monitoring due to the possibility of causing severe bradycardia and hypotension. |
| Gamma knife stereotactic radiosurgery (GKS)[54,55] | GKS is a noninvasive, destructive technique that uses 70–90 Gy radiation units to damage the trigeminal nerve root at the point of vascular compression. However, if there is no evidence of vascular compression, the trigeminal root entry zone is targeted. It may take up to a month for the GKS to show response, and the success rate varies between 65% and 88%. | GKS is ideal for patients who are refractory to medical treatments and are not surgical candidates. Complications include numbness, paresthesias, and dysesthesias. |
| Microvascular decompression surgery (MVD)[56,57] | MVD involves an intracranial procedure performed under general anesthesia, whereby the nerve and vessel are separated and repositioned. The pain relief was 97% at 1-y follow-up and 70% at 10-y follow-up. The best outcome from MVD was shown in cases whereby it was performed within 7 years of onset of TN. On the contrary, female sex, symptoms lasting at least 8 years, venous compression of the trigeminal nerve root entry zone, and the lack of immediate postoperative cessation of pain were significant predictors of eventual recurrence. | MVD is associated with a low risk of serious complications such as death (0.3%), meningitis (0.4%), and edema, hemorrhage, or stroke (0.6%). |

results in the onset of TN.[56,57] The surgery involves an intracranial procedure performed under general anesthesia, whereby the nerve and vessel are separated and repositioned (see **Table 2**).

## SUMMARY

Trigeminal neuralgia is a rare neuropathic pain disorder. Previously, there was confusion in the literature regarding the classification and critical clinical features of the various types. This contributed to a limited understanding of pathophysiology and a lack of consensus on management guidelines. However, the recently published ICOP and ICHD-3 classification systems have aligned with the International Association of Study of Pain (IASP) classification criteria. It has led to clarity among clinicians and investigators on the key clinical features of the disorder and given insights regarding the pathophysiology. The EAN has updated management guidelines, incorporating the data from recent studies.

Nonetheless, more research is needed to understand the etiology of TN, especially idiopathic TN. Similarly, the evidence quality for most treatment modalities is based on retrospective or open-labeled studies, warranting further studies conducted using robust investigation standards.

## DISCLOSURE

The authors have nothing to disclose.

## REFERENCES

1. International Classification of Orofacial Pain, 1st edition (ICOP). Cephalalgia 2020;40(2):129–221.
2. Headache Classification Committee of the International Headache Society (IHS) The International Classification of Headache Disorders, 3rd edition. Cephalalgia 2018;38(1):1–211.
3. Zakrzewska JM, Wu J, Mon-Williams M, et al. Evaluating the impact of trigeminal neuralgia. Pain 2017;158(6):1166–74.
4. Bendtsen L, Zakrzewska JM, Abbott J, et al. European Academy of Neurology guideline on trigeminal neuralgia. Eur J Neurol 2019;26(6):831–49.
5. Bendtsen L, Zakrzewska JM, Heinskou TB, et al. Advances in diagnosis, classification, pathophysiology, and management of trigeminal neuralgia. Lancet Neurol 2020;19(9):784–96.
6. De Toledo IP, Réus JC, Fernandes M, et al. Prevalence of trigeminal neuralgia: A systematic review. J Am Dental Assoc 2016;147(7):570–6.e2.
7. Zakrzewska JM, Linskey ME. Trigeminal neuralgia. BMJ Clin Evid 2009;2009.
8. MacDonald BK, Cockerell OC, Sander JW, et al. The incidence and lifetime prevalence of neurological disorders in a prospective community-based study in the UK. Brain 2000;123(Pt 4):665–76.
9. Katusic S, Williams DB, Beard CM, et al. Epidemiology and clinical features of idiopathic trigeminal neuralgia and glossopharyngeal neuralgia: similarities and differences, Rochester, Minnesota, 1945-1984. Neuroepidemiology 1991;10(5–6):276–81.
10. Katusic S, Beard CM, Bergstralh E, et al. Incidence and clinical features of trigeminal neuralgia, Rochester, Minnesota, 1945-1984. Ann Neurol 1990;27(1):89–95.

11. Brameli A, Kachko L, Eidlitz-Markus T. Trigeminal neuralgia in children and adolescents: Experience of a tertiary pediatric headache clinic. Headache 2021; 61(1):137–42.
12. Cruccu G, Finnerup NB, Jensen TS, et al. Trigeminal neuralgia: New classification and diagnostic grading for practice and research. Neurology 2016;87(2):220–8.
13. Mathews ES, Scrivani SJ. Percutaneous stereotactic radiofrequency thermal rhizotomy for the treatment of trigeminal neuralgia. Mt Sinai J Med 2000;67(4): 288–99.
14. Scrivani SJ, Keith DA, Mathews ES, et al. Percutaneous stereotactic differential radiofrequency thermal rhizotomy for the treatment of trigeminal neuralgia. J Oral Maxillofac Surg 1999;57(2):104–11 [discussion: 111–2].
15. Bajwa ZH, Smith SS, Khawaja SN, et al. Cranial Neuralgias. Oral Maxillofac Surg Clin North Am 2016;28(3):351–70.
16. White JC, Sweet WH. Pain and the neurosurgeon: a Forty-year experience. Springfield, IL: C. C. Thomas; 1969. Available at: https://books.google.com.pk/ books?id=54ZyQgAACAAJ.
17. Mitchell RG. Pre-trigeminal neuralgia. Br Dent J 1980;149(6):167–70.
18. Maarbjerg S, Gozalov A, Olesen J, et al. Trigeminal Neuralgia - A Prospective Systematic Study of Clinical Characteristics in 158 Patients. Headache 2014; 54(10):1574–82.
19. Flor H, Rasche D, Islamian AP, et al. Subtle Sensory Abnormalities Detected by Quantitative Sensory Testing in Patients with Trigeminal Neuralgia. Pain Physician 2016;19(7):507–18.
20. Devor M, Govrin-Lippmann R, Rappaport ZH. Mechanism of trigeminal neuralgia: an ultrastructural analysis of trigeminal root specimens obtained during microvascular decompression surgery. J Neurosurg 2002;96(3):532–43.
21. Devor M, Amir R, Rappaport ZH. Pathophysiology of trigeminal neuralgia: the ignition hypothesis. Clin J Pain 2002;18(1):4–13.
22. Love S, Coakham HB. Trigeminal neuralgia: pathology and pathogenesis. Brain 2001;124(Pt 12):2347–60.
23. Matsushima T, Huynh-Le P, Miyazono M. Trigeminal Neuralgia Caused by Venous Compression. Neurosurgery 2004;55(2):334–9.
24. DaSilva AF, DosSantos MF. The role of sensory fiber demography in trigeminal and postherpetic neuralgias. J Dent Res 2012;91(1):17–24.
25. Cohen AS. Short-lasting unilateral neuralgiform headache attacks with conjunctival injection and tearing. Cephalalgia 2007;27(7):824–32.
26. Patel A, Kassam A, Horowitz M, et al. Microvascular decompression in the management of glossopharyngeal neuralgia: analysis of 217 cases. Neurosurgery 2002;50(4):705–10 [discussion: 710–1].
27. Scrivani SJ, Keith DA, Kulich R, et al. Posttraumatic gustatory neuralgia: a clinical model of trigeminal neuropathic pain. J Orofac Pain 1998;12(4):287–92.
28. Nasir KS, Hussain R, Jamshed A. Pre-operative Occurrence of First Bite Syndrome in Two Cases of Parotid Gland Tumour. J Cancer Allied Spec 2019;6(1). https://doi.org/10.37029/jcas.v6i1.331.
29. Lobato RD, Gonzaáez P, Alday R, et al. Meningiomas of the basal posterior fossa. Surgical experience in 80 cases. Neurocirugia (Astur) 2004;15(6):525–42.
30. Roberti F, Sekhar LN, Kalavakonda C, et al. Posterior fossa meningiomas: surgical experience in 161 cases. Surg Neurol 2001;56(1):8–20 [discussion: 20–1].
31. Cruccu G, Gronseth G, Alksne J, et al. AAN-EFNS guidelines on trigeminal neuralgia management. Eur J Neurol 2008;15(10):1013–28.

32. Di Stefano G, Maarbjerg S, Nurmikko T, et al. Triggering trigeminal neuralgia. Cephalalgia 2018;38(6):1049–56.
33. Wiffen PJ, McQuay HJ, Moore RA. Carbamazepine for acute and chronic pain. Cochrane Database Syst Rev 2005;3:CD005451.
34. Zakrzewska JM, Patsalos PN. Long-term cohort study comparing medical (oxcarbazepine) and surgical management of intractable trigeminal neuralgia. Pain 2002;95(3):259–66.
35. Zakrzewska JM, Chaudhry Z, Nurmikko TJ, et al. Lamotrigine (lamictal) in refractory trigeminal neuralgia: results from a double-blind placebo controlled crossover trial. Pain 1997;73(2):223–30.
36. Gilron I, Booher SL, Rowan JS, et al. Topiramate in trigeminal neuralgia: a randomized, placebo-controlled multiple crossover pilot study. Clin Neuropharmacol 2001;24(2):109–12.
37. Braham J, Saia A. Phenytoin in the treatment of trigeminal and other neuralgias. Lancet 1960;276(7156):892–3.
38. McCleane GJ. Intravenous infusion of phenytoin relieves neuropathic pain: a randomized, double-blinded, placebo-controlled, crossover study. Anesth Analg 1999;89(4):985–8.
39. Fromm GH, Terrence CF, Chattha AS. Baclofen in the treatment of trigeminal neuralgia: double-blind study and long-term follow-up. Ann Neurol 1984;15(3):240–4.
40. Hu Y, Guan X, Fan L, et al. Therapeutic efficacy and safety of botulinum toxin type A in trigeminal neuralgia: a systematic review. J Headache Pain 2013;14(1):72.
41. Wu CJ, Lian YJ, Zheng YK, et al. Botulinum toxin type A for the treatment of trigeminal neuralgia: results from a randomized, double-blind, placebo-controlled trial. Cephalalgia 2012;32(6):443–50.
42. Morra ME, Elgebaly A, Elmaraezy A, et al. Therapeutic efficacy and safety of Botulinum Toxin A Therapy in Trigeminal Neuralgia: a systematic review and meta-analysis of randomized controlled trials. J Headache Pain 2016;17(1):63.
43. Nader A, Kendall MC, De Oliveria GS, et al. Ultrasound-guided trigeminal nerve block via the pterygopalatine fossa: an effective treatment for trigeminal neuralgia and atypical facial pain. Pain Physician 2013;16(5):E537–45.
44. Lemos L, Flores S, Oliveira P, et al. Gabapentin Supplemented With Ropivacain Block of Trigger Points Improves Pain Control and Quality of Life in Trigeminal Neuralgia Patients When Compared With Gabapentin Alone. Clin J Pain 2008; 24(1):64–75.
45. Quinn JH, Weil T. Trigeminal neuralgia: treatment by repetitive peripheral neurectomy. Supplemental report. J Oral Surg 1975;33(8):591–5.
46. Murali R, Rovit RL. Are peripheral neurectomies of value in the treatment of trigeminal neuralgia? An analysis of new cases and cases involving previous radiofrequency gasserian thermocoagulation. J Neurosurg 1996;85(3):435–7.
47. Pradel W, Hlawitschka M, Eckelt U, et al. Cryosurgical treatment of genuine trigeminal neuralgia. Br J Oral Maxillofac Surg 2002;40(3):244–7.
48. Wilkinson HA. Trigeminal nerve peripheral branch phenol/glycerol injections for tic douloureux. J Neurosurg 1999;90(5):828–32.
49. Erdem E, Alkan A. Peripheral glycerol injections in the treatment of idiopathic trigeminal neuralgia: retrospective analysis of 157 cases. J Oral Maxillofac Surg 2001;59(10):1176–80.
50. Fardy MJ, Zakrzewska JM, Patton DW. Peripheral surgical techniques for the management of trigeminal neuralgia–alcohol and glycerol injections. Acta Neurochir (Wien) 1994;129(3–4):181–4 [discussion: 185].

51. McLeod NMH, Patton DW. Peripheral alcohol injections in the management of tri-geminal neuralgia. Oral Surg Oral Med Oral Pathol Oral Radiol Endod 2007; 104(1):12–7.
52. Lopez BC, Hamlyn PJ, Zakrzewska JM. Systematic review of ablative neurosur-gical techniques for the treatment of trigeminal neuralgia. Neurosurgery 2004; 54(4):973–82 [discussion: 982–3].
53. Brown JA, Gouda JJ. Percutaneous balloon compression of the trigeminal nerve. Neurosurg Clin N Am 1997;8(1):53–62.
54. Young RF, Vermeulen SS, Grimm P, et al. Gamma Knife radiosurgery for treatment of trigeminal neuralgia: idiopathic and tumor related. Neurology 1997;48(3): 608–14.
55. Sheehan J, Pan HC, Stroila M, et al. Gamma knife surgery for trigeminal neural-gia: outcomes and prognostic factors. J Neurosurg 2005;102(3):434–41.
56. Barker FG, Jannetta PJ, Bissonette DJ, et al. The long-term outcome of microvas-cular decompression for trigeminal neuralgia. N Engl J Med 1996;334(17): 1077–83.
57. Kondo A. Microvascular decompression surgery for trigeminal neuralgia. Stereo-tact Funct Neurosurg 2001;77(1–4):187–9.
58. Henson CF, Goldman HW, Rosenwasser RH, et al. Glycerol rhizotomy versus gamma knife radiosurgery for the treatment of trigeminal neuralgia: an analysis of patients treated at one institution. Int J Radiat Oncol Biol Phys 2005;63(1): 82–90.
59. Lim M, Villavicencio AT, Burneikiene S, et al. CyberKnife radiosurgery for idio-pathic trigeminal neuralgia. Neurosurg Focus 2005;18(5):E9.

# Pathology Mimicking Orofacial Pain

Shaiba Sandhu, BDS, DDS[a,b,*], Shruti Handa, BDS, DMD[a,b]

## KEYWORDS

- Orofacial pain • Facial swelling • Parotid gland swelling • Salivary gland tumors
- Pleomorphic adenoma

## KEY POINTS

- Pathology arising from structures adjacent to the temporomandibular joint can present with temporomandibular disorder (TMD)-like symptoms including facial pain and trismus.
- The symptoms of salivary gland pathology involving the parotid gland can sometimes mimic TMD.
- A comprehensive history, thorough clinical examination, and appropriate imaging can help make an accurate diagnosis.
- Understanding the various types of pathology that can present with orofacial pain is crucial for timely diagnosis, treatment, and improved prognosis.

## CLINICAL CASE

A 64-year-old retired school teacher presented with the chief complaint of right-sided jaw pain and fullness. She had had this condition for the past 7 years, but a week before presentation, she developed pain in the area without any inciting event, which prompted the referral to see an orofacial pain specialist with the suspicion of a possible temporomandibular joint (TMJ) disorder. She reported that the fullness had neither increased nor decreased over the years, and she had never been evaluated for this condition in the past. The pain was localized to the right TMJ and masseter area, with radiation of pain to the posterior aspect of her right ear. The pain was sharp, shooting in the beginning, with a 9/10 intensity that gradually transitioned into a dull ache of 4/10 over the next few days. The pain was constant and aggravated by coughing, sneezing, yawning, and chewing. She had tried ibuprofen, 400 mg, with no relief. She did not complain of any facial numbness, hypersensitivity, or facial weakness nor of any bite change, jaw joint noises, or jaw locking episodes. She had no systemic

[a] Division of Orofacial Pain, Oral and Maxillofacial Surgery, Department of Surgery, Massachusetts General Hospital, 55 Fruit Street, Boston, MA 02114, USA; [b] Harvard School of Dental Medicine, Boston, MA, USA
* Corresponding author. Division of Orofacial Pain, Oral and Maxillofacial Surgery, Department of Surgery, Massachusetts General Hospital, 55 Fruit Street, Boston, MA 02114.
E-mail address: ssandhu@mgh.harvard.edu

Dent Clin N Am 67 (2023) 117–127
https://doi.org/10.1016/j.cden.2022.07.009
0011-8532/23/© 2022 Elsevier Inc. All rights reserved.

dental.theclinics.com

constitutional features (fever, malaise, night sweats) nor autonomic symptoms. She denied any history of head or neck trauma. She had a long-standing history of migraines but no new headaches, earaches, or neck pain. She did not complain of any toothache or dental sensitivity to hot or cold foods.

Her past medical history was relevant for hypertension, hyperlipidemia, arteriosclerotic vascular disease, bariatric surgery, gastroesophageal reflux disorder, insomnia, and migraines. Her medications included butalbital-acetaminophen-caffeine (50–325–40 mg as needed), trazodone (50 mg once daily), omeprazole (40 mg three times daily), rosuvastatin (20 mg once daily), spironolactone (50 mg once daily), valsartan (160 mg once daily), carvedilol (25 mg), diltiazem (120 mg once daily), hydralazine (25 mg three times daily), and quetiapine (50 mg once daily). She was a former smoker with a 12.5 pack-year history. No pertinent family history of cancer or any autoimmune diseases was reported.

Examination revealed mild facial asymmetry with a firm, tender swelling over the right deep masseter area approximately 3.5 × 4 cm (**Figs. 1**). This tenderness duplicated her chief complaint. There was no associated erythema, fluctuance, or purulent discharge or lymphadenopathy. Cranial nerves V and VII were intact. Slight pain on palpation of the bilateral masseters and neck muscles was noted but this was subclinical. She had a normal mandibular range of motion with 40 mm maximal interincisal opening and 8 mm bilateral excursions without any pain or joint noises. No intraoral lesions, swelling, or any signs of odontogenic infection were noted. The ducts of major salivary glands were patent with adequate salivary flow, and the oral mucosa was pink and moist. Her occlusion was stable with good bilateral posterior contacts.

A panoramic radiograph did not show any signs of condylar flattening, erosion, osteophyte, subcondylar sclerosis, or sclerosis. The cortical margins of the mandible were intact, and there were no signs of dental pathology or any pathology of the maxilla or mandible.

The development of recent onset of pain in an area of long-standing facial fullness raised the concern for a neoplastic process. Our differential diagnosis included parotid gland tumor, odontogenic infection, benign or malignant jaw tumors (such as ameloblastoma, osteosarcoma, Hodgkin disease, multiple myeloma, or metastatic disease),

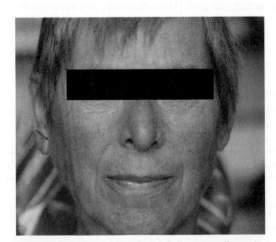

**Fig. 1.** Clinical image depicting right-sided facial fullness/swelling that was diagnosed as pleomorphic adenoma, a benign parotid gland tumor. The arrow indicates rigth-sided facial fullness.

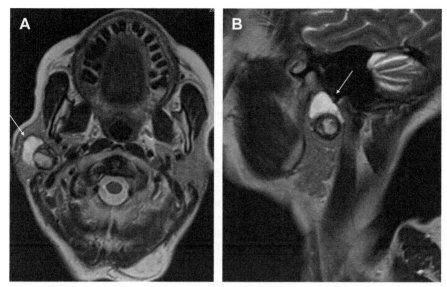

**Fig. 2.** Pleomorphic adenoma. MRI depicting a 2.5 x 2.4 × 2.8-cm avid homogenous enhancement in the superficial lobe of the right parotid gland in (*A*) axial T2 and (*B*) sagittal T2 sections. The arrow indicates the pleomorphic adenoma.

or an immune-mediated condition (such as Sjogren syndrome). In addition, she had subclinical myofascial masticatory and cervical pain.

An MRI was ordered that demonstrated a 2.5 x 2.4 × 2.8 cm heterogeneous cystic lesion in the superficial lobe of the right parotid gland. The patient was referred for fine-needle aspiration, which demonstrated a benign mixed tumor, consistent with pleomorphic adenoma. She underwent right total parotidectomy, and the pathology demonstrated completely excised pleomorphic adenoma. There were no postoperative complications, and her facial pain resolved as she recovered successfully from the surgery. In this case, it is important for clinicians to note that the associated TMD-like symptoms were secondary to the neoplasm of the parotid gland instead of a primary pathology involving the TMJ or the myofascial muscles of the joint space and its associated structures (**Fig. 2**).

## SALIVARY GLAND TUMORS
### *Epidemiology*

Salivary gland tumors constitute about 3% to 6% of head and neck tumors, making them rare neoplasms. The incidence of salivary gland tumors has been reported to be 0.4 to 13.5 cases per 100,000 people, with benign tumors being more common than malignant.[1,2] Thirty-one different types of salivary gland neoplasms have been identified by the 2017 World Health Organization (WHO) classification, of which pleomorphic adenoma and Warthin tumor are the most common benign tumors and, mucoepidermoid carcinoma and adenoid cystic carcinoma are the most common malignant histologic types.[3]

Salivary gland tumors have a high predilection for parotid glands, followed by minor salivary glands, submandibular glands, and sublingual glands in that order.[4] Among the minor salivary glands, there is increased predilection for the palate followed by the upper lip and buccal mucosa.[5] Most of the parotid gland tumors are benign

(69%–88%), and most of the sublingual glands tumors are malignant (75%–100%).[2,4,6–9] There is an equal prevalence of benign and malignant tumors in the submandibular glands, and most tumors of the minor salivary glands (60%) are malignant.[2,4,6]

The 2 most common benign tumors—pleomorphic adenoma and Warthin tumor—have a gender predilection for women and men, respectively.[8,10–13] A consensus is currently lacking regarding gender predilection for malignant salivary gland tumors. Benign salivary gland tumors are more common at around 50 years of age; malignant tumors commonly occur 10 years later.[14–19] No predilection for ethnicity has been reported.

The exact cause of salivary gland tumors is unknown, but these tumors have been identified with high incidence in patients with a history of Epstein-Barr virus–related cancers, immunosuppression, childhood radiation therapy, and in atomic bomb survivors.[20,21] Interestingly, smoking and alcohol use, which are significant risk factors for head and neck cancers, have not been found to influence the risk for salivary gland cancers.[22] Genetic alterations are also implicated in the development of salivary gland tumors. Pleomorphic adenoma gene 1 and high-mobility group AT-hook 2 gene alterations are highly specific for pleomorphic adenomas and carcinoma ex-pleomorphic adenoma.[23,24]

### Clinical Features

Benign tumor of the salivary glands commonly presents as a slow-growing, well-circumscribed painless mass. Pleomorphic adenoma, Warthin tumor (usually present bilaterally), and myoepithelial tumors are the most common benign salivary gland tumors of the parotid gland.[25] Parotid gland tumors commonly involve the superficial lobe where they typically present as asymptomatic, slow-growing, facial swelling without any systemic symptoms. When the deep lobe is involved, patients may present with symptoms such as pharyngeal narrowing, sleep apnea, dyspnea on exertion, trismus, and pain.[25]

Involvement of the facial nerve causing facial weakness, increased tumor growth, onset of pain or paresthesia, trismus, fixation of tumor mass, pharyngeal asymmetry, dysphagia, glossopharyngeal nerve palsy, bleeding from the parotid duct outlet, and lymphadenopathy should raise suspicion for a malignant process.[26,27] A retrospective study including 131 patients with parotid gland carcinoma found facial nerve palsy and skin infiltration to be independent poor prognostic factors for the treatment outcome.[27] Mucoepidermoid carcinoma, adenoid cystic carcinoma, and acinic cell carcinoma are the most common malignant salivary gland tumors affecting the major salivary glands.[28] Adenoid cystic carcinoma has been associated with early and frequent perineural invasion and distant metastases, most commonly to the lungs.[29] The duration of the symptoms may vary from 2 to 48 months before referral to a specialist.[30]

### Diagnosis

A thorough clinical examination can help identify the red flags and prevent a clinician from missing these pathologies. Clinical examination has been shown to have an accuracy of approximately 85% in differentiating benign parotid gland tumors from their malignant counterparts.[31] Imaging (such as ultrasound, MRI, computerized tomography, and PET scans) and histopathology (fine-needle aspiration [FNA] cytology or biopsy) are crucial in making the diagnosis of salivary gland pathology.[32,33]

MRI is the diagnostic modality of choice and can help evaluate the extent of the tumor, local invasion, marrow infiltration, and perineural spread.[32] PET can be used to determine distant metastases.[33] Imaging modalities are extremely helpful, but they lack the ability to differentiate between benign and malignant salivary gland tumors. These tumors can be differentiated with histopathology using either FNA, which has a sensitivity of 73% and specificity of 91%,[34,35] or core needle biopsy where a larger tissue sample is needed.[36.]

## Management

The management of salivary gland tumors varies depending on the benign or malignant nature of the tumor, the staging, and the grade of the tumor. The 3 standard treatment modalities are surgery, radiation therapy, and chemotherapy. Surgical excision remains the cornerstone treatment of most salivary gland tumors, except when the risk to benefit ratio of surgery is high, as in the elderly.[37] Complications of surgery can include facial nerve palsy, Frey syndrome, and first bite syndrome.[38–40] External beam radiation therapy is used in cases with unresectable or macroscopically persistent or recurrent disease.[41] Chemotherapy with Taxol and platinum-based agents has been used for the treatment of unresectable advanced salivary gland cancers and cases with distant metastases[42–44] but the impact of chemotherapy on overall survival remains unclear.

## Prognosis

The recurrence rate of pleomorphic adenoma and Warthin tumor is in the range of 1% to 5% and 7% to 12%, respectively, primarily due to incomplete surgical excision, tumor spillage, and satellite lesions.[45,46] The malignant transformation of pleomorphic adenoma into carcinoma ex-pleomorphic adenoma can occur in 2% to 15% of cases.[47,48]

According to the American Cancer Society, the 5-year relative survival rate for localized salivary gland cancer is 95%, regional salivary gland cancer (local invasion of nearby structures and lymph nodes) is 69%, and for salivary gland cancer with distant metastases is 44%.[49] The 5-year survival rate for high-grade mucoepidermoid cancer has been reported in the range of 0% to 43%, for intermediate-grade in the range of 62% to 92%, and low-grade in the range of 92% to 100%.[50] For adenoid cystic carcinoma, although the 5-year survival rate is high (approximately 89%), the 15-year survival rate reduces significantly to about 40% due to the associated risk of perineural invasion and distant metastases.[51]

## DIFFERENTIAL DIAGNOSIS
### Odontogenic Infection

Pain and swelling in the orofacial region should raise suspicion of odontogenic infection, as it is common. The source of the infection primarily includes dental caries, pulpal and periapical disease, periodontal disease, pericoronitis, and osteomyelitis. Odontogenic infection can result in an abscess or diffuse soft-tissue bacterial infection (cellulitis), further leading to facial pain, swelling, and trismus.[52] Potentially life-threatening conditions such as cavernous sinus thrombosis, brain abscess, airway obstruction, and mediastinitis can result from untreated odontogenic infections.[52] Clinical examination and imaging assume a vital part in recognizing the source and determining the degree of the spread of infection and its associated complications.

The radiographic changes depend on the duration and the type of odontogenic infection as well as the immunity of the patient. The early radiographic changes in pulpal and periapical disease consist of widening of the apical periodontal ligament, disruption of lamina dura, and formation of periapical radiolucency.[53] If the disease remains untreated, it can either lead to formation of apical granuloma/cyst or can result in osteomyelitis (characterized by further osteolytic changes in the bone with the formation of sequestrum) or anatomic space infection (characterized by involvement of soft tissues).[53] However, in odontogenic infections despite the expansion of the radiographic lesion, the epicenter would remain at the apex of the offending tooth. In the present case, the radiographic and clinical examination did not reveal any source of odontogenic infection.

### Jaw Bone Tumors

Tumors arising from numerous structures in and around the TMJ, including the mandibular ramus, can cause TMD-like pain symptoms. Jaw bone tumors can also present as facial swelling depending on the growth and the extent of involvement and may be benign or malignant. Benign jaw tumors are typically slow growing and painless. The 2 most widely recognized odontogenic tumors are keratocystic odontogenic tumor (KCOT) and ameloblastoma. Both these benign tumors cause a cystic expansile mass of the jaw. Because of the locally aggressive behavior, these 2 tumors, if left untreated, could result in extraoral facial swelling. Radiographically, ameloblastoma and KCOT may present as unilocular or multilocular radiolucency predominantly in the posterior mandible and ramus.[54]

Clinical signs and symptoms of malignant jaw tumors may include pain, paresthesia or anesthesia, a rapidly expanding swelling, and mobility of teeth within the field of disease.[54] The primary malignant jaw tumor, osteosarcoma of the jaw, is rare (primarily accounting for approximately 4% of all the primary malignant jaw lesions and 7% of all osteosarcomas) and commonly occurs in the fourth decade of life.[55] It may vary from a radiolucent or radiopaque lesion to a mixed lesion, or it may present as a generalized widening of periodontal ligament spaces.[54] Malignancies of the hematopoietic system such as multiple myeloma and non-Hodgkin lymphoma can also involve the jaws.[55,56] Although multiple myeloma typically has a characteristic radiographic feature of well-defined, multiple, punched-out radiolucent lesions,[55] extranodal non-Hodgkin lymphoma may appear as poorly defined, osteolytic lesions of the jaw.[56] Distant metastasis to the jaw is rare, accounting for less than 1% of all oral cavity malignancies and generally suggests widespread dissemination of cancer.[57] The most common finding is an ill-defined radiolucency, which is typical of osteolytic metastatic breast cancer, but radiopaque changes may also be observed, as with osteoblastic tumors of metastatic prostate cancer.[57] In our patient, the presence of facial swelling along with new-onset pain raised the suspicion for a jaw tumor, but the radiographic examination did not reveal any osteolytic or osteosclerotic process, ruling out this possibility.

### Sjogren Syndrome

Sjogren syndrome (SS) is an autoimmune disease characterized by lymphocytic infiltration of the secretory glands, primarily the lacrimal and salivary glands, leading to dry eyes and dry mouth, respectively.[58] However, lymphocytic infiltration and deposition of immune complexes may occur in extraglandular sites, including the skin, mucosa, lungs, kidneys, peripheral nervous system, and musculoskeletal system, making SS a systemic disease. Systemic features include fatigue (approximately 70%–80% of patients), interstitial lung disease, tubulointerstitial nephritis, neurologic symptoms, and arthritis in about 71% of patients.[58]

Salivary gland enlargement is a sign of lymphoproliferation and typically presents as a facial swelling when involving the parotid glands. The risk of development of non-Hodgkin lymphoma in SS has been reported in the range of 2.7% to 9.8%.[59] Musculoskeletal involvement in SS is characterized by intermittent polyarticular arthropathy chiefly affecting small joints.[60] The involvement of the TMJ and myofascial muscles has not been extensively assessed in patients with SS. An observational study including 72 SS patients found a 91.7% prevalence of TMD symptoms (myofascial pain, reduced range of motion, TMJ arthralgia, headache, and tinnitus) in the SS group versus the control group.[61] Although facial swelling could indicate an underlying autoimmune disease such as SS involving the parotid gland, our patient did not have any clinical features of dry mouth or dry eyes, and the histopathology from the biopsy ruled it out.

### Neurogenic Tumor (Schwannoma)

Schwannomas are benign neoplasms originating from the Schwann cells that sheath a nerve. Facial nerve schwannomas (FNS) are rare but, when present in the parotid gland parenchyma, can present as a painless and slow-developing mass similar to pleomorphic adenoma.[62,63] FNS have been reported in the age range of 43 to 51 years and have been found to show no gender predilection.[63] Facial paralysis is a common symptom in patients with FNS, but it may not be consistently present at the time of diagnosis.[63]

MRI with and without gadolinium contrast is the primary method of imaging for the assessment of FNS. In the parotid gland parenchyma, FNS typically presents as a well-circumscribed, avidly enhancing intra-parotid mass that is T1 isointense and T2 hyperintense to muscle.[62] For a definitive diagnosis, a biopsy is indicated.[63] In our case, the imaging may be suspicious for an intraparotid, but the FNA cytology was consistent with pleomorphic adenoma.

## SUMMARY

TMD represents a significant source of orofacial pain of nonodontogenic origin. When evaluating a patient with orofacial pain, clinicians should consider all the potential differential diagnoses, especially when red flags such as swelling/facial fullness or paresthesia/numbness are present. Comprehensive history taking, thorough examination, and appropriate investigation are crucial for the diagnosis and management of these conditions that can cause considerable harm if left untreated.

## CLINICS CARE POINTS

- Orofacial pain can be a symptom of a myriad of head and neck pathologies; the clinician should be aware of the potential differential diagnoses.
- A thorough review of patient's history, examination, and appropriate investigation are vital to rule out pathologies that can mimic orofacial pain conditions.

## DISCLOSURE

The authors do not have any disclosures. The authors do not have any conflicts of interest associated with this publication, and there has been no financial support for this work that could have influenced its outcome. This manuscript is original, has not been previously published, and is not currently under consideration by another journal.

## REFERENCES

1. Eveson JW, Auclair P, Gnepp DR, et al. Tumours of the salivary glands. In: Barnes L, Eveson JW, Reichart P, et al, editors. Pathol Genet Head Neck

Tumours, Vol. 9, 3rd ed. Lyon (France): IARC Press; 2005. p. 212–5. WHO/IARC classification of Tumours.

2. Gontarz M, Bargiel J, Gąsiorowski K, et al. Epidemiology of primary epithelial salivary gland tumors in southern Poland—a 26-year, clinicopathologic, retrospective analysis. J Clin Med 2021;10(8):1663.

3. El-Naggar AK, Chan JKC, Grandis JR, et al. Tumours of salivary glands. In: WHO Classification of Head and Neck Tumours WHO Classification of Tumours, Vol. 9, 4th edition. Lyon (France): IARC Press; 2017. p. 159–202. WHO/IARC classification of tumours.

4. Gao M, Hao Y, Huang MX, et al. Salivary gland tumours in a northern Chinese population: A 50-year retrospective study of 7190 cases. Int J Oral Maxillofac Surg 2017;46(3):343–9.

5. Galdirs TM, Kappler M, Reich W, et al. Current aspects of salivary gland tumors - a systematic review of the literature. GMS Interdiscip Plast Reconstr Surg DGPW 2019;8:Doc12. https://doi.org/10.3205/iprs000138.

6. Tilakaratne WM, Jayasooriya PR, Tennakoon TM, et al. Epithelial salivary tumors in Sri Lanka: A retrospective study of 713 cases. Oral Surg Oral Med Oral Pathol Oral Radiol Endod 2009;108(1):90–8.

7. da Silva LP, Serpa MS, Viveiros SK, et al. Salivary gland tumors in a Brazilian population: A 20-year retrospective and Multicentric Study of 2292 cases. J Cranio-Maxillofacial Surg 2018;46(12):2227–33.

8. Lukšić I, Virag M, Manojlović S, et al. Salivary gland tumours: 25 years of experience from a single institution in Croatia. J Cranio-Maxillofacial Surg 2012;40(3). https://doi.org/10.1016/j.jcms.2011.05.002.

9. Jones AV, Craig GT, Speight PM, et al. The range and demographics of salivary gland tumours diagnosed in a UK population. Oral Oncol 2008;44(4):407–17.

10. Ito FA, Ito K, Vargas PA, et al. Salivary gland tumors in a Brazilian population: A retrospective study of 496 cases. Int J Oral Maxillofac Surg 2005;34(5):533–6.

11. Fonseca FP, de Vasconcelos Carvalho M, de Almeida OP, et al. Clinicopathologic analysis of 493 cases of salivary gland tumors in a southern Brazilian population. Oral Surg Oral Med Oral Pathol Oral Radiol 2012;114(2):230–9.

12. Tian Z, Li L, Wang L, et al. Salivary gland neoplasms in oral and maxillofacial regions: A 23-year retrospective study of 6982 cases in an eastern Chinese population. Int J Oral Maxillofac Surg 2010;39(3):235–42.

13. Shishegar M, Ashraf MJ, Azarpira N, et al. Salivary gland tumors in maxillofacial region: A retrospective study of 130 cases in a southern Iranian population. Pathol Res Int 2011;2011:1–5.

14. Pons Vicente O, Almendros Marqués N, Berini Aytés L, et al. Minor salivary gland tumors: A clinicopathological study of 18 cases. Med Oral Patol Oral Cir Bucal 2008;13(9):E582–8.

15. Vargas PA, Gerhard R, Araújo Filho VJ, et al. Salivary gland tumors in a Brazilian population: A retrospective study of 124 cases. Revista do Hosp das Clínicas 2002;57(6):271–6.

16. Targa-Stramandinoli R, Torres-Pereira C, Piazzetta CM, et al. Neoplasias de glándulas salivales menores: estudio de 10 años [Minor salivary gland tumours: a 10-year study]. Acta Otorinolaringol Esp 2009;60(3):199–201.

17. Jansisyanont P, Blanchaert RH, Ord RA. Intraoral minor salivary gland neoplasm: A single institution experience of 80 cases. Int J Oral Maxillofac Surg 2002;31(3):257–61.

18. Toida M, Shimokawa K, Makita H, et al. Intraoral minor salivary gland tumors: A clinicopathological study of 82 cases. Int J Oral Maxillofac Surg 2005;34(5): 528–32.
19. Regezi JA, Lloyd RV, Zarbo RJ, et al. Minor salivary gland tumors. A histologic and immunohistochemical study. Cancer 1985;55(1):108–15.
20. Saku T, Hayashi Y, Takahara O, et al. Salivary gland tumors among atomic bomb survivors, 1950-1987. Cancer 1997;79(8):1465–75.
21. Dong C, Hemminki K. Second primary neoplasms among 53 159 haematolymphoproliferative malignancy patients in Sweden, 1958–1996: A search for common mechanisms. Br J Cancer 2001;85(7):997–1005.
22. Sadetzki S, Oberman B, Mandelzweig L, et al. Smoking and risk of parotid gland tumors. Cancer 2008;112(9):1974–82.
23. Martins C, Fonseca I, Roque L, et al. PLAG1 gene alterations in salivary gland pleomorphic adenoma and carcinoma ex-pleomorphic adenoma: A combined study using chromosome banding, in situ hybridization and immunocytochemistry. Mod Pathol 2005;18(8):1048–55.
24. Mito JK, Jo VY, Chiosea SI, et al. HMGA2 is a specific immunohistochemical marker for pleomorphic adenoma and carcinoma ex-pleomorphic adenoma. Histopathology 2017;71(4):511–21.
25. Bradley PJ. Frequency and Histopathology by Site, Major Pathologies, Symptoms and Signs of Salivary Gland Neoplasms. Adv Otorhinolaryngol 2016;78:9–16.
26. Wong DS. Signs and symptoms of malignant parotid tumours: an objective assessment. J R Coll Surg Edinb 2001;46(2):91–5.
27. Stodulski D, Mikaszewski B, Stankiewicz C. Signs and symptoms of parotid gland carcinoma and their prognostic value. Int J Oral Maxillofac Surg 2012;41(7): 801–6.
28. Boukheris H, Curtis RE, Land CE, et al. Incidence of carcinoma of the major salivary glands according to the WHO classification, 1992 to 2006: a population-based study in the United States. Cancer Epidemiol Biomarkers Prev 2009; 18(11):2899–906.
29. Gao M, Hao Y, Huang MX, et al. Clinicopathological study of distant metastases of salivary adenoid cystic carcinoma. Int J Oral Maxillofac Surg 2013;42(8): 923–8.
30. Leverstein H, van der Wal JE, Tiwari RM, et al. Malignant epithelial parotid gland tumours: analysis and results in 65 previously untreated patients. Br J Surg 1998; 85(9):1267–72.
31. McGuirt WF, Keyes JW, Greven KM, et al. Preoperative identification of benign versus malignant parotid masses: A comparative study including Positron Emission Tomography. Laryngoscope 1995;105(6):579–84.
32. Lee YY, Wong KT, King AD, et al. Imaging of salivary gland tumours. Eur J Radiol 2008;66(3):419–36.
33. Jeong H-S, Chung MK, Son Y-I, et al. Role of 18F-FDG PET/CT in management of high-grade salivary gland malignancies. J Nucl Med 2007;48(8):1237–44.
34. Hughes JH, Volk EE, Wilbur DC, Cytopathology Resource Committee, College of American Pathologists. Pitfalls in salivary gland fine-needle aspiration cytology: lessons from the College of American Pathologists Interlaboratory Comparison Program in Nongynecologic Cytology. Arch Pathol Lab Med 2005;129(1):26–31.
35. Das DK, Anim JT. Pleomorphic adenoma of salivary gland: to what extent does fine needle aspiration cytology reflect histopathological features? Cytopathology 2005;16(2):65–70.

36. Schmidt RL, Hall BJ, Layfield LJ. A systematic review and meta-analysis of the diagnostic accuracy of ultrasound-guided core needle biopsy for salivary gland lesions. Am J Clin Pathol 2011;136(4):516–26.

37. Son E, Panwar A, Mosher CH, et al. Cancers of the major salivary gland. J Oncol Pract 2018;14(2):99–108.

38. Eng CY, Evans AS, Quraishi MS, et al. A comparison of the incidence of facial palsy following parotidectomy performed by ENT and non-ENT surgeons. J Laryngol Otol 2007;121(1):40–3.

39. Sanabria A, Kowalski LP, Bradley PJ, et al. Sternocleidomastoid muscle flap in preventing Frey's syndrome after parotidectomy: a systematic review. Head Neck 2012;34(4):589–98.

40. Handa S, Shafik AA, Intini R, et al. First bite syndrome – an underrecognized and underdiagnosed pain complication after temporomandibular joint surgery. J Oral Maxillofac Surg 2022;80(3):437–42.

41. Chen AM, Garcia J, Lee NY, et al. Patterns of nodal relapse after surgery and postoperative radiation therapy for carcinomas of the major and minor salivary glands: What is the role of elective neck irradiation? Int J Radiat Oncol Biol Phys 2007;67(4):988–94.

42. Gilbert J, Li Y, Pinto HA, et al. Phase II trial of taxol in salivary gland malignancies (E1394): a trial of the Eastern Cooperative Oncology Group. Head Neck 2006; 28(3):197–204.

43. Ross PJ, Teoh EM, A'hern RP, et al. Epirubicin, cisplatin and protracted venous infusion 5-Fluorouracil chemotherapy for advanced salivary adenoid cystic carcinoma. Clin Oncol (R Coll Radiol 2009;21(4):311–4.

44. Gebhardt BJ, Ohr JP, Ferris RL, et al. Concurrent Chemoradiotherapy in the Adjuvant Treatment of High-risk Primary Salivary Gland Malignancies. Am J Clin Oncol 2018;41(9):888–93.

45. Laskawi R, Schott T, Schröder M. Recurrent pleomorphic adenomas of the parotid gland: clinical evaluation and long-term follow-up. Br J Oral Maxillofac Surg 1998;36(1):48–51.

46. Ethunandan M, Pratt CA, Morrison A, et al. Multiple synchronous and metachronous neoplasms of the parotid gland: the Chichester experience. Br J Oral Maxillofac Surg 2006;44(5):397–401.

47. Lingam RK, Daghir AA, Nigar E, et al. Pleomorphic adenoma (benign mixed tumour) of the salivary glands: its diverse clinical, radiological, and histopathological presentation. Br J Oral Maxillofac Surg 2011;49(1):14–20.

48. Andreasen S, Therkildsen MH, Bjørndal K, et al. Pleomorphic adenoma of the parotid gland 1985-2010: A Danish nationwide study of incidence, recurrence rate, and malignant transformation. Head Neck 2016;38(Suppl 1):E1364–9.

49. American Cancer Society. Survival rates for salivary gland cancer. American Cancer Society. 2021. Available at: https://www.cancer.org/cancer/salivary-gland-cancer/detection-diagnosis-staging/survival-rates.html. Accessed March 19, 2022.

50. Pires FR, de Almeida OP, de Araújo VC, et al. Prognostic factors in head and neck mucoepidermoid carcinoma. Arch Otolaryngol Head Neck Surg 2004;130(2):174–80.

51. American Society of Clinical Oncology. Adenoid cystic carcinoma - statistics. Cancer.Net. 2021. Available at: https://www.cancer.net/cancer-types/adenoid-cystic-carcinoma/statistics. Accessed March 19, 2022.

52. Bali RK, Sharma P, Gaba S, et al. A review of complications of odontogenic infections. Natl J Maxillofac Surg 2015;6(2):136–43.

53. Mardini S, Gohel A. Imaging of Odontogenic Infections. Radiol Clin North Am 2018;56(1):31–44.
54. Mosier KM. Lesions of the Jaw. Semin Ultrasound CT MR 2015;36(5):444–50.
55. Ghosh S, Wadhwa P, Kumar A, et al. Abnormal radiological features in a multiple myeloma patient: a case report and radiological review of myelomas. Dentomaxillofac Radiol 2011;40(8):513–8.
56. Oliveira CS, de Lima MH, D'Almeida Costa F, et al. Mandible lymphoma: An aggressive osteolytic lesion. Appl Cancer Res 2020;40(1). https://doi.org/10.1186/s41241-020-00087-w.
57. Kumar G, Manjunatha B. Metastatic tumors to the jaws and oral cavity. J Oral Maxillofac Pathol 2013;17(1):71–5.
58. Demarchi J, Papasidero S, Medina MA, et al. Primary Sjögren's syndrome: Extraglandular manifestations and hydroxychloroquine therapy. Clin Rheumatol 2017;36(11):2455–60.
59. Chiu YH, Chung CH, Lin KT, et al. Predictable biomarkers of developing lymphoma in patients with Sjögren syndrome: a nationwide population-based cohort study. Oncotarget 2017;8(30):50098–108.
60. Kassan SS, Moutsopoulos HM. Clinical manifestations and early diagnosis of Sjögren syndrome. Arch Intern Med 2004;164(12):1275–84.
61. Crincoli V, Di Comite M, Guerrieri M, et al. Orofacial Manifestations and Temporomandibular Disorders of Sjögren Syndrome: An Observational Study. Int J Med Sci 2018;15(5):475–83. Published 2018 Mar 8.
62. Teh A, Kumar A, Teh C, et al. Overview of Parotid Gland Masses. J Am Osteopath Coll Radiol 2018;7(4):5–10.
63. Quesnel AM, Santos F. Evaluation and Management of Facial Nerve Schwannoma. Otolaryngol Clin North Am 2018;51(6):1179–92.

# Head and Neck Cancer-Related Pain

Shehryar Nasir Khawaja, BDS, MSc[a],*, Steven J. Scrivani, DDS, DMedSc[b]

## KEYWORDS

- Cancer care • Cancer pain • Neoplasm-related pain • Neuropathic pain
- Pain management • Squamous cell carcinoma

## KEY POINTS

- Head and neck cancers (HNC) are a heterogeneous group of aggressive aerodigestive tract cancers.
- The prevalence of pain in HNC is approximately 70%, which increases to 90% in advanced cases or when the tongue or the floor of the mouth is involved.
- There are no universally accepted classification or diagnostic criteria for HNC-related pain, and currently, this type of pain is classified based on the underlying pathophysiological mechanism, the location of the tumor, and the protagonist of pain.
- The clinical presentation of HNC-related pain can vary, and it may mirror the clinical characteristics (phenotype) of various primary pain disorders. However, unlike primary pain disorders, the pain may be accompanied by sensory or motor deficits.
- The management of HNC-related pain primarily consists of pharmacotherapy and non-pharmacological interventions, such as physical, occupational, and behavioral therapy. However, pain may not respond to conventional modalities on some occasions, and interventions may be needed for pain control.

## CASE REPORT

A 42-year-old maleman was seen in the clinic for constant, right-side lower jaw pain. The pain started nearly 6 months ago; however, the intensity and severity of episodes had increased over the last couple of weeks. The patient reported constant burning and dull ache extending from the right submandibular area and mandible, medially up to the midline (not crossing it), intraorally over the mandibular teeth, tongue, and floor of the mouth, and posteriorly toward the posterior mandibular area and the auricular region. Furthermore, he reported experiencing stabbing electric pain intermittently

[a] Orofacial Pain Medicine, Department of Internal Medicine, Shaukat Khanum Memorial Cancer Hospital & Research Centers, Lahore, Pakistan; [b] Department of Diagnostic Sciences, Craniofacial Pain Center, Tufts University, School of Dental Medicine, Boston, MA, USA
* Corresponding author. Shaukat Khanum Memorial Cancer Hospital and Research Center, 7A Block R-3, Phase 2, M.A. Johar Town, Lahore, Punjab 54782, Pakistan.
E-mail address: khawajashehryar@gmail.com

Dent Clin N Am 67 (2023) 129–140
https://doi.org/10.1016/j.cden.2022.07.010          **dental.theclinics.com**

along the lower right jaw and teeth, multiple times a day, for up to a minute. The intensity of pain was rated 7 out of 10, on a numeric pain rating scale (NPRS), whereby 0 indicated no pain, and 10 suggested the worst pain possible, at baseline. However, during the episodes of stabbing pain, the intensity was rated 10 out of 10.

His medical history was significant for squamous cell carcinoma of the right mandibular alveolar region. He was treatment naïve and expected to undergo induction chemotherapy, followed by surgical jaw resection. He was not aware of any allergies to medications. There was a positive history of gastric and breast cancer in his family. He had a 30 pack-years history of smoking. He did not drink but occasionally chewed betel nut quid. There was no history of psychiatric disease. He worked as a salesman, was married, and had 3 children.

His pulse rate was 80 beats/min during the physical examination, and his blood pressure was 130/80 mm Hg. His respiratory rate was 18 breaths per minute, and his temperature was 36.8 centigrade. He was sitting in distress during the examination. He rated his pain as 8, on a 0 to 10 NPRS.

The patient was oriented to time, place, and person during examination. There was mild-moderate swelling over the right mandibular area, which extended into the submandibular region. The vertical mandibular range of motion was 23 mm with pain in the right jaw and masseteric region. The patient reported pain on the palpation of the right masseter muscle, submandibular area, posterior mandibular region, and mandibular bone. There were no palpable joint sounds or abnormal patterns of movements observed during mandibular motion. The cervical range of movements was within normal limits. The patient reported pain on the palpation of the right anterior, middle, and posterior scalene muscles, suprahyoid muscles, and sternocleidomastoid muscle. The right anterior and deep cervical lymph nodes were enlarged and tender to palpation.

Intraoral examination revealed a 20 mm diameter ulcerative crater-like lesion with necrotic margins, yellow-white center, over the prior sites of the right mandibular first molar and second premolar. The underlying bone was enlarged. The right mandibular second and third molars and first premolar had grade I mobility. The tongue movements were limited due to pain, the uvula was the midline, and the soft palate was mobile. The salivary flow was adequate. The dentition was compromised by generalized calculus deposits and stains.

The patient had complete numbness over the distribution of the right mental nerve. There was hypoesthesia to light and sharp touch over the distribution of the inferior alveolar nerve. The rest of the cranial nerves (CN II–XII) examination revealed no gross discrepancies. The spinal nerves (C2-T1) were grossly intact. Testing of complex motor skills revealed normal coordination. Deep tendon reflexes of the biceps, triceps, and brachioradialis were normal.

The magnetic resonance imaging (MRI) face and neck study with contrast revealed a lobulated infiltrating tumor in the right mandibular area measuring 3.2 cm × 3.1 cm in transverse and anteroposterior dimensions, respectively, which extended into the ipsilateral masticator space and medially into the floor of the mouth. The tumor was causing cortical erosions and marrow infiltration in the mandible Suspicious ipsilateral lymph nodes were noted, and provisional staging on imaging suggested this as a T4a, N1, Mx disease.

The patient was diagnosed with neoplasm-related pain with features of trigeminal neuralgia with concomitant facial pain (*trigeminal neuralgia attributed to the space-occupying lesion*), myofascial pain (*secondary myofascial orofacial pain*), and arthralgia (*jawbone pain attributed to the malignant lesion*). He was prescribed carbamazepine 200 mg three times a day (titrated over a week), amitriptyline 10 mg once at night, celecoxib 200 mg twice a day, paracetamol 1000 mg three times a day, and omeprazole 20 mg once a day. In addition, at the same appointment, the patient was administered right inferior alveolar and lingual nerves block using a solution of 2.5 mL of lidocaine 2% without epinephrine and 1 mL of dexamethasone 4 mg/mL, and right cervical nerves (2, 3, and 4) block using a solution of 4 mL of bupivacaine 0.5% without epinephrine and 1 mL of dexamethasone 4 mg/mL. These injections resulted in complete pain relief at the chairside.

At 1-week follow-up, the patient reported complete relief in the stabbing electric pain episodes and burning pain. However, he continued to have a dull ache in the mandibular bone and pain in the masseteric region with mouth opening. At this point, oxycodone 5 mg two times a day and lactulose 10 mg up to three times a day were added (as a laxative to counter constipation associated with opioid use). The patient subsequently initiated the cancer treatment and underwent induction chemotherapy and surgery. After the surgery, the analgesics were tapered off, and the patient reported no pain at rest.

## CLINICS CARE POINTS

- The pain developed in temporal relation to the neoplastic disease process.
- The patient reported brief episodes of electric shock-like pain with continuous burning pain along the trigeminal nerve distribution, which in the presence of a space-occupying lesion, would suggest that the patient had *trigeminal neuralgia attributed to space-occupying lesion.*
- The patient reported pain in the jawbone, masseter muscle, and submandibular region, which was confirmed and provoked during the examination. The underlying disease extended into the muscles, masticator space, and bone, indicating that the patient had *secondary myofascial orofacial pain* and *jawbone pain attributed to malignancy.*
- The patient was started on medical therapy to manage his various pain conditions, which was aided by administering regional nerve blocks. These injections gave him immediate pain relief. The patient had a good response to the therapy; however, he continued to have pain in the jawbone and the masseter muscle. He was started on oxycodone, which provided complete pain relief.
- After surgery, the patient had no pain episodes, and he was gradually tapered off the medications.

## INTRODUCTION

Head and neck cancers (HNC) are a heterogeneous group of aerodigestive tract cancers that are the ninth most common malignancy in the world.[1] Almost 90% of these cancers are squamous cell carcinoma or variants thereof. These cancers are aggressive in their biological behavior and often result in significant disease-related destruction. The management is assertive and comprises high-dose chemotherapy, radical composite surgeries, and significant cumulative dose radiation therapies. Due to the inherent nature of the disease and the treatment, pain is a common symptom experienced by the patients. The pain correlates with morbidity and negatively impacts the emotional state and debilitating effect on physiologic function and the overall quality of life.[2,3]

## EPIDEMIOLOGY

The prevalence of pain in all cancer types is around 40%. On the contrary, the prevalence of pain in HNC is approximately 70%, which increases to 90% in advanced cases or with the presence of disease in the tongue or floor of the mouth.[3–5] The higher prevalence of pain in HNC is likely secondary to the complex and rich innervation of the head and neck region, associated intricate orofacial and cervical movements, the erosive and aggressive nature of the disease, and a greater prevalence of psychosocial distress in comparison to patients with other cancer types.[3,5]

In most patients, the pain is of mild intensity (<4, on a 0–10 NPRS). However, similar to prevalence, the severity of symptoms worsens in malignant disease, squamous cell carcinoma variants, and involvement of tongue and floor of the mouth[5,6]

### Diagnostic Criteria and Classification

There are no universally accepted classification or diagnostic criteria for HNC-related pain. Previously, HNC-related pain has been classified based on the underlying pathophysiological mechanism (nociceptive or inflammatory, neuropathic, or both), the location of the tumor (local or distant), or the protagonist of pain (tumor-related, treatment-related, or both).[2,7,8]

The latest editions of the head and neck pain classification systems, International Classification of Orofacial Pain, first edition (ICOP), and International Classification of Headache Disorders, third edition (ICHD), have not included HNC-related pain as a diagnostic category.[9,10] The classification systems have included some clinical presentations, such as oral mucosa pain attributed to malignant lesion, gingival pain attributed to malignant lesion, jaw pain attributed to malignant lesion, and trigeminal neuralgia attributed to space-occupying lesion.[9] However, it does not include other common disorders, which may present secondary to malignancy, such as myofascial orofacial pain or temporomandibular joint arthralgia.

To standardize care and improve understanding of HNC-related pain, this article defines HNC-related pain by modifying the ICOP diagnostic criteria for various pain conditions attributed to malignancy and the ICHD criteria for headaches attributed to intracranial neoplasm (**Box 1**). It is important to note that these criteria have not been validated.

## CLINICAL FEATURES

The clinical presentation of HNC-related pain can vary. It depends on multiple factors, including but not limited to the cancer type, size and site of the tumor, depth of invasion, involvement of regional structures (muscle, nerve, or bone), lymph node involvement, concomitant or prior cancer therapy, younger age, and psychosocial factors.[2,3,8]

The pain is primarily ipsilateral to the site of disease; however, in up to 30% of the patients, pain may be bilateral.[5,6] The pain can be localized or spreading, and it may or may not conform to the distribution of regional nerves. In most of the patients, pain is continuous. The quality of pain can be aching, burning, dull, stabbing, throbbing, or electric, and in most patients, it is a combination of multiple descriptors.[2,5,6,11] The pain often worsens with jaw and cervical functional and parafunctional movements, and in some, it may be triggered by innocuous, mechanical, or tactile stimulation.

HNC-related pain can mirror the clinical characteristics (phenotype) of various primary pain disorders. However, unlike primary pain disorders, the pain may also be accompanied by sensory or motor deficits. Furthermore, there may be a history of weight loss, dysphagia, bilateral distribution of neuropathic pain, younger than

---

**Box 1**
**The diagnostic criteria for head and neck cancer (HNC)-related pain disorder, modified from diagnostic criteria given in International Classification of Orofacial Pain (1st Edition) and International Classification of Headache Disorders (3rd edition)[1,2]**

Diagnostic criteria:
A. Pain in the neuroanatomically plausible area within the distribution(s) of at least trigeminal, cervical, facial, glossopharyngeal, or vagus nerve(s), persisting or recurring for greater than 3 months and fulfilling criteria C and D.
B. Cancer of the head-and-neck region has been identified.
C. Evidence of causation demonstrated by at least one of the following:
   a. Pain has developed in temporal related to the HNC or led to its discovery.
   b. Pain has significantly worsened in parallel with the worsening of the HNC.
   c. Pain has significantly improved in parallel with the improvement of the HNC.
D. Pain is associated with somatosensory symptoms and/or signs [a,b] in the same neuroanatomically plausible distribution.
E. Not better accounted for by another ICOP or ICHD-3 diagnosis.

[a] Somatosensory symptoms or signs may be negative (hypesthesia, hypoalgesia, numbness), and/or positive (hyperalgesia, allodynia, paresthesia).[b] There may be a window whereby there may not be an overlap between pain and somatosensory symptoms and/or signs.

---

expected age at presentation, mobile teeth, or presence of swelling, lesion, discoloration, atrophy, or asymmetry.[2,5,6,11] It is prudent to note that HNC-related pain may not always accompany associated symptoms, and pain may often precede the development of other clinical features or be the only feature associated with HNC.[12,13]

In HNC, the patient may have more than one clinical painful disorder phenotype, and these may exist simultaneously, such as in the patient documented in the case report. Furthermore, a given phenotype may change during the course of the disease or management as the disease modifies.

## PATHOPHYSIOLOGY

Pain from cancer is induced through numerous mechanisms. The clinical presentation of HNC-related pain is a consequence of complex interactions between cancer, cancer microenvironment, and systemic physiologic processes occurring during various phases of carcinogenesis.[2,14,15] These interactions continue to evolve through the course of the disease, treatment, and survivorship, which may explain why clinical characteristics change during the various stages of the disease.[15]

The cancer microenvironment is formed by the noncancerous cells surrounding the tumor, such as blood vessels, immune cells, fibroblasts, signaling molecules, and extracellular matrix. Cancer cells can secrete, and induce components of the cancer microenvironment, or secrete chemical mediators that sensitize or activate primary afferent nociceptors. Furthermore, the regional tissue and bone destruction, and subsequent nerve damage, can result in a cascade of responses that may sensitize the nociceptive pathways.[14,16]

The primary chemical mediators that contribute to HNC-pain include endothelin. Squamous cell carcinoma cells in HNC produce high endothelin-1 (ET-1) levels which are responsible for mediating nociceptive effects in the cancer microenvironment. Furthermore, it sensitizes the release of adenosine triphosphate (ATP) which generates pain by activating P2X2/3 receptors on nociceptors.[14] Cancer cells produce various neutrophils, including but not limited to nerve growth factor (NGF), tumor necrosis factor-alpha, and neuturin, which activate regional nociceptors. Likewise, the release of proteases into the cancer microenvironment results in regional destruction and protein catabolism. This results in a subsequent reduction in regional pH and acts synergistically with the cytokine activity and modulation of other mediators, providing a positive feedback loop.[17]

The continuous stimulation of nociceptive pathways subsequently induces plasticity in the peripheral nervous system (reduction in activation threshold, increase in the receptive field, and activation of silent receptors) and central nervous system (adaptive changes in thalamus, cortex, and higher centers, alteration in descending pain control mechanisms, and excitability in trigeminal subnucleus caudalis).[17,18]

## MANAGEMENT

Ineffective cancer pain management is associated with functional decline, increased psychological stress, and reduced quality of life. Yet, up to 80% of all patients with cancer suffer inadequate pain management.[15] The effective management of HNC-related pain primarily consists of pharmacotherapy and nonpharmacological interventions, such as physical, occupational, and behavioral therapy. However, pain may not respond to conventional modalities, and interventions may be needed for pain control in some cases.

## PHARMACOTHERAPY

The mainstay of HNC-related pain management is pharmacotherapy.[19,20] The medication regimen should be directed toward the clinical phenotype, provided on a time-contingent basis, and should be driven by the pain intensity. Furthermore, due to the proximity and nature of the disease in HNC, a patient may have limited oral intake, or have a gastric tube so the medication regimen will have to be adjusted to allow appropriate delivery of medications.

For musculoskeletal pain conditions, the most dependable option is opioid therapy. Opioids act on mu, delta, and kappa receptors in the central and peripheral nervous systems. They are potent, versatile, and effective. Opioids are available in multiple formulations, strengths, and modes of administration (**Table 1**).[21] There has been considerable scrutiny regarding excessive and unnecessary opioid prescriptions in the United States and this has been a source of hesitancy for physicians, and patients alike. The common side-effects of opioids include constipation, nausea, drowsiness, and mental clouding, and tolerance.[8,21]

Nonsteroidal anti-inflammatory drugs (NSAIDs) are a group of analgesics that function by inhibiting the enzymatic activity of cyclooxygenase (COX)-I and COX-II enzymes, which allows them to have analgesic and anti-inflammatory effects properties.[22] They are available in various formulations and strengths (see **Table 1**). NSAIDs can be effective as a part of multimodal therapy to manage HNC-related pain emanating from osseous or muscular origin. Furthermore, COX-II inhibitors have been shown to have a negative impact on cancerirogensis.[23] NSAIDs are commonly associated with gastrointestinal effects, including dyspepsia and peptic ulcer disease.[22] Acetaminophen is a centrally acting analgesic (see **Table 1**). However, the exact mechanism of action is unknown. It has a safe side-effect profile, nonetheless, at high doses, acetaminophen use has been associated with hepatotoxicity. The analgesic efficacy of acetaminophen alone is limited.[17,19,20] However, as an adjunct in multimodal drug therapy for managing osseous or muscular painful HNC-related conditions, it can help potentiate the analgesic response. Acetaminophen is available in various formulations and combinations with opioids, NSAIDs, or muscle relaxants.[24]

**Table 1**
Summary of characteristics of pharmacotherapies for the management of head and neck cancer-related pain

| Medication Type | Examples | Available Formulations | Possible Indications and Comments | Side-Effects |
|---|---|---|---|---|
| Opioids | Morphine, buprenorphine, Oxycodone, hydrocodone, hydromorphone Fentanyl | Oral (tablet, capsule, liquid) Subcutaneous

Transdermal, intranasal spray | Musculoskeletal pain Low efficacy in neuropathic painful conditions | Constipation, nausea, drowsiness, dizziness, pruritus, headache, dry mouth and mental clouding, and tolerance and dependence. |
| Nonsteroidal anti-inflammatory medications | Ibuprofen, diclofenac, naproxen, meloxicam, celecoxib Ketorolac | Oral (tablet, capsule, liquid) Suppository Parenteral (intramuscular, intravenous) | Musculoskeletal pain Celecoxib has anticarcinogenesis properties. | Nausea, abdominal pain, vomiting, dyspepsia, peptic ulcer disease, diarrhea, headache, hypertension, and acute kidney injury |
| Acetaminophen | – | Oral (tablet, liquid), suppository, parenteral (intravenous) | Musculoskeletal pain | Generally, well tolerated but may cause nausea, vomiting, headache, and hepatoxicity |
| Muscle relaxants | Cyclobenzaprine, methocarbamol, metaxalone, tizanidine, carisoprodol, and baclofen | Oral (tablet, capsule) | Muscular pain | Drowsiness, nausea, vomiting, constipation, dry mouth, urinary retention, and dizziness |
| Tricyclic antidepressants | Amitriptyline, nortriptyline, doxycycline | Oral (tablet, liquid) | Muscular pain Neuropathic pain | Dry mouth, weight gain, hypotension, nausea, vomiting, constipation, urinary retention, drowsiness, and dizziness |

*(continued on next page)*

**Table 1**
*(continued)*

| Medication Type | Examples | Available Formulations | Possible Indications and Comments | Side-Effects |
|---|---|---|---|---|
| Anticonvulsants | Gabapentin, pregabalin, carbamazepine, oxcarbazepine, lamotrigine, divalproex sodium | Oral (tablet, capsule, liquid) | Neuropathic pain | Dry mouth, drowsiness, dizziness, headache, nausea, vomiting, diarrhea, hepatotoxicity, nephrotoxicity, hyponatremia and Stevens–Johnson syndrome |
| | Valproate sodium | Parenteral (intravenous) | | |
| Other medication types: | Duloxetine, venlafaxine | Oral (tablet, capsule) | Neuropathic pain Duloxetine and clonazepam work well against burning mouth syndrome type painful conditions. | Headache, nausea, vomiting, dizziness, somnolence, dry mouth, depression exacerbation, nervousness |
| | Clonazepam | Oral (tablet, lozenges, liquid) | | Drowsiness, dizziness, impaired coordination, fatigue, confusion, lightheadedness, dependency |

Skeletal muscle relaxants are a diverse group of centrally acting medications (see **Table 1**). They effectively manage pain associated with muscular disorders, such as myofascial orofacial pain or muscle spasms. The medications vary in the exact mechanism of action, dosing, and strengths. Common side effects include somnolence, dry mouth, nausea, and dizziness.[25] Furthermore, a potential limitation of muscle relaxants in HNC-related pain management is the lack of availability of these medications in liquid or intravenous formulations.

Tricyclic antidepressants (TCAs) are a group of versatile medications that are effective in managing HNC-pain conditions with characteristics of neuropathic pain disorders or in the management of conditions that may originate from muscles (see **Table 1**).[26,27] Furthermore, they have been shown to potentiate the analgesic response of nerve blocks in the management of neuropathic-type HNC-related pain.[5] TCAs inhibit serotonin and noradrenergic reuptake, block sodium, potassium, and calcium channels, and are NMDA receptor antagonists.[28,29] The analgesic response of TCAs is independent of their antidepressant effects. TCAs are associated with nausea, urinary retention, somnolence, dry mouth, constipation, and confusion.[17,28]

Gabapentinoids (gabapentin and pregabalin) are voltage-gated calcium channels that are considered to be effective in the management of HNC-related pain with features of neuropathic pain disorders, such as trigeminal neuralgia or persistent pain disorder.[26,30,31] Likewise, they have been shown to improve the outcome of chemical neurolysis in patients with HNC-related pain.[32] Common side effects include nausea, somnolence, and dizziness.[30] Other anticonvulsants, such as carbamazepine, oxcarbazepine, sodium valproate, divalproex sodium, and valproic acid, effectively manage neuropathic-type HNC-related pain. However, their use is associated with nausea, somnolence, and dizziness (see **Table 1**).[33]

Other medications may be used to manage HNC-related pain conditions. In those resembling burning mouth syndrome, clonazepam, a benzodiazepine, and serotonin-norepinephrine reuptake inhibitor (SNRI) medications, such as duloxetine and venlafaxine may be used (see **Table 1**).[8,19,20,28,34]

## NONPHARMACOLOGICAL INTERVENTIONS

Nonpharmacological interventions include physical (eg, cutaneous stimulation, transcutaneous electrical nerve stimulation, acupuncture), occupational, or behavioral (eg, cognitive behavioral therapy, relaxation, psychotherapy, hypnosis) therapies. In combination with pharmacotherapy, nonpharmacological interventions have been shown to help control cancer-related pain and improve quality of life.[35]

## INTERVENTIONS

Noninvasive modalities help improve pain control and reduce pain-associated disability and distress. However, in up to 20% of the cases, the pain may become refractory and nonresponsive. Such patients may benefit from interventional approaches, such as nerve conduction blocks, local nerve infiltration, trigger point injections, and neurolysis procedures.[5,6,19] Interventions help provide relief from refractory pain, can act as a bridging therapy, improve pain control, reduce reliance on medications, and increase the effectiveness of pharmacotherapy.

Trigger point injections, or tender point injections, are a technique in which a local anesthetic, with or without corticosteroid, is injected into the area of maximum tenderness or a trigger point in the muscle. Furthermore, the injection may include fanning or needling into the injection site. Trigger point injections can be used for the management of muscular-origin HNC-related pain. The procedure is safe and often well tolerated.

Nerve infiltration or blocks are procedures in which a local anesthetic, with or without corticosteroid, is injected along the nerve tract to block sensory nerves preferentially. Local anesthetics reversibility inhibit voltage-gated sodium channel, thereby impairing the conduction of nerve impulses.[36] The extent and duration of the block depend on various factors, such as the dose and pharmacokinetic properties of the anesthetic, nerve characteristics such as thickness and myelination, and the physiologic and anatomic properties of the injection site.[36–38] Nerve blocks or infiltrations may result in 75% or more pain relief for at least a month in nearly 60% of patients with neuropathic-type HNC-related pain. This relief was associated with the concurrent use of amitriptyline.[5]

Neurolysis is a technique that uses physical or chemical neurolytic agents to degenerate a targeted nerve temporarily.[39] Commonly used chemical neurolytic agents include phenol, glycerol, and alcohol. The type, concentration, and volume of agent used for the procedure are dictated by pain location and characteristics, armamentarium availability, and experience of the clinician.[6,39,40] The data on the effectiveness of chemical neurolysis in managing HNC-related pain are limited, and only a handful of studies are available.[6,32] Data suggest that chemical neurolysis is an effective modality in controlling refractory HNC-related pain when used as an adjunct to pharmacologic interventions in up to 86% of cases.[6] Furthermore, the patients may report nearly $89.26\% \pm 10.49\%$ reduction in characteristic pain intensity for a mean period of $8.79 \pm 5.11$ weeks. The positive outcome was associated with concurrent use of gabapentinoids and negatively with the chronicity of pain and the presence of pain in the auricular region.[32] Adverse effects from chemical neurolysis may occur in up to 10% of the patients, and effects include burning pain or ulceration at the site of injection, motor weakness, and sensory changes.[6]

## SUMMARY

Head and neck cancers (HNC) are aggressive tumors with a high prevalence of pain. There are no universally accepted diagnostic criteria or classification available for HNC-related pain. Furthermore, the understanding of various clinical phenotypes of HNC-related pain is limited, and due to this, there are no clinical-based guidelines available for the management of this type of pain, which may explain the poor outcomes. The current practices are based on expert opinion, retrospective, and open-labeled trials. Using robust investigation standards, more research is needed to classify and subsequently manage HNC-related pain.

## DISCLOSURE

The authors have nothing to disclose.

## REFERENCES

1. Gupta B, Johnson NW, Kumar N. Global Epidemiology of Head and Neck Cancers: A Continuing Challenge. Oncology 2016;91(1):13–23.

2. Epstein JB, Elad S, Eliav E, et al. Orofacial Pain in Cancer: Part II—Clinical Perspectives and Management. J Dent Res 2007;86(6):506–18.

3. Khawaja SN, Jamshed A, Hussain RT. Prevalence of pain in oral cancer: A retrospective study. Oral Dis 2021;27(7):1806–12.

4. van den Beuken-van Everdingen MHJ, de Rijke JM, Kessels AG, et al. Prevalence of pain in patients with cancer: a systematic review of the past 40 years. Ann Oncol 2007;18(9):1437–49.
5. Nasir KS, Hafeez H, Jamshed A, et al. Effectiveness of Nerve Blocks for Management of Head and Neck Cancer Associated Neuropathic Pain Disorders; a Retrospective Study. J Cancer Allied Spec 2020;6(2).
6. Khawaja SN, Scrivani SJ. Utilization of neurolysis in management of refractory head and neck cancer-related pain in palliative patients: A retrospective review. J Oral Pathol Med 2020;49(6):484–9.
7. Blasco MA, Cordero J, Dundar Y. Chronic Pain Management in Head and Neck Oncology. Otolaryngol Clin North Am 2020;53(5):865–75.
8. Ing JW. Head and Neck Cancer Pain. Otolaryngol Clin North Am 2017;50(4): 793–806.
9. International Classification of Orofacial Pain, 1st edition (ICOP). Cephalalgia 2020;40(2):129–221.
10. Olesen J. International Classification of Headache Disorders. Lancet Neurol 2018;17(5):396–7.
11. Epstein JB, Wilkie DJ, Fischer DJ, et al. Neuropathic and nociceptive pain in head and neck cancer patients receiving radiation therapy. Head Neck Oncol 2009; 1:26.
12. Cheng TMW, Cascino TL, Onofrio BM. Comprehensive study of diagnosis and treatment of trigeminal neuralgia secondary to tumors. Neurology 1993;43(11): 2298.
13. Puca A, Meglio M. Typical trigeminal neuralgia associated with posterior cranial fossa tumors. Ital J Neuro Sci 1993;14(7):549–52.
14. Schmidt BL. The Neurobiology of Cancer Pain. J Oral Maxillofac Surg 2015; 73(12):S132–5.
15. Yarom N, Sroussi H, Elad S. Orofacial pain in patients with cancer and mucosal diseases. In: Farah CS, Balasubramaniam R, McCullough MJ, editors. Contemporary oral medicine. Cham, Switzerland: Springer International Publishing; 2019. p. 2187–212.
16. Benoliel R, Epstein J, Eliav E, et al. Orofacial pain in cancer: part I--mechanisms. J Dent Res 2007;86(6):491–505.
17. Epstein JB, Miaskowski C. Oral Pain in the Cancer Patient. JNCI Monogr 2019; 2019(53):lgz003.
18. Woolf CJ. Central sensitization: uncovering the relation between pain and plasticity. Anesthesiology 2007;106(4):864–7.
19. Portenoy RK. Treatment of cancer pain. Lancet 2011;377(9784):2236–47.
20. Ripamonti CI, Bandieri E, Roila F. Management of cancer pain: ESMO Clinical Practice Guidelines. Ann Oncol 2011;22:vi69–77.
21. Trescot AM, Datta S, Lee M, et al. Opioid pharmacology. Pain Physician 2008; 11(2 Suppl):S133–53.
22. Moses VS, Bertone AL. Nonsteroidal anti-inflammatory drugs. Vet Clin North Am Equine Pract 2002;18(1):21–37.
23. Saba NF, Choi M, Muller S, et al. Role of cyclooxygenase-2 in tumor progression and survival of head and neck squamous cell carcinoma. Cancer Prev Res (Phila) 2009;2(9):823–9.
24. Jackson CH, MacDonald NC, Cornett JW. Acetaminophen: a practical pharmacologic overview. Can Med Assoc J 1984;131(1):25–32, 37.
25. See S, Ginzburg R. Skeletal Muscle Relaxants. Pharmacotherapy 2008;28(2): 207–13.

26. Mishra S, Bhatnagar S, Goyal GN, et al. A comparative efficacy of amitriptyline, gabapentin, and pregabalin in neuropathic cancer pain: a prospective random-ized double-blind placebo-controlled study. Am J Hosp Palliat Care 2012;29(3): 177–82.
27. Gillman PK. Tricyclic antidepressant pharmacology and therapeutic drug interac-tions updated. Br J Pharmacol 2007;151(6):737–48.
28. Trindade E, Menon D, Topfer LA, et al. Adverse effects associated with selective serotonin reuptake inhibitors and tricyclic antidepressants: a meta-analysis. CMAJ 1998;159(10):1245–52.
29. Hillhouse TM, Porter JH. A brief history of the development of antidepressant drugs: from monoamines to glutamate. Exp Clin Psychopharmacol 2015; 23(1):1–21.
30. Jordan RI, Mulvey MR, Bennett MI. A critical appraisal of gabapentinoids for pain in cancer patients. Curr Opin Support Palliat Care 2018;12(2):108–17.
31. Caraceni A, Zecca E, Bonezzi C, et al. Gabapentin for neuropathic cancer pain: a randomized controlled trial from the Gabapentin Cancer Pain Study Group. J Clin Oncol 2004;22(14):2909–17.
32. Nasir KS, Hafeez H, Hussain R, et al. P20-10 Chemical neurolysis for refractory head and neck cancer-related pain. Ann Oncol 2021;32:S340.
33. Tremont-Lukats IW, Megeff C, Backonja MM. Anticonvulsants for neuropathic pain syndromes: mechanisms of action and place in therapy. Drugs 2000; 60(5):1029–52.
34. Khawaja SN, Bavia PF, Keith DA. Clinical Characteristics, Treatment Effective-ness, and Predictors of Response to Pharmacotherapeutic Interventions in Burning Mouth Syndrome: A Retrospective Analysis. J Oral Facial Pain Headache 2020;34(2):157–66.
35. Singh P, Chaturvedi A. Complementary and alternative medicine in cancer pain management: a systematic review. Indian J Palliat Care 2015;21(1):105–15.
36. Malamed SF. Handbook of local Anesthesia. 5th edition. Cham, Switzerland: Elsevier/Mosby; 2004.
37. Yagiela JA. Local anesthetics. Anesth Prog 1991;38(4–5):128–41.
38. Levin M. Nerve blocks in the treatment of headache. Neurotherapeutics 2010; 7(2):197–203.
39. Sist T. Head and neck nerve blocks for cancer pain management. Tech Reg Anesth Pain Management 1997;1(1):3–10.
40. Varghese BT, Koshy RC, Sebastian P, et al. Combined sphenopalatine ganglion and mandibular nerve, neurolytic block for pain due to advanced head and neck cancer. Palliat Med 2002;16(5):447–8.

# Posttraumatic Stress Disorder and the Role of Psychosocial Comorbidities in Chronic Orofacial Pain

Roxanne Bavarian, DMD, DMSc[a,b,*], Michael E. Schatman, PhD[c,d,e],
Ronald J. Kulich, PhD[f,g,h]

## KEYWORDS

- TMJ • TMD • Orofacial pain • Facial pain • Chronic pain • PTSD • Trauma
- Behavioral care

## KEY POINTS

- Up to 59% of patients with chronic pain present with a comorbid psychiatric condition, with common conditions including depression, substance use, and anxiety.
- Chronic pain and posttraumatic stress disorder share common symptoms of hyperarousal, anxiety, and fear-based avoidance of activities that could exacerbate pain or trigger trauma, which can allow the 2 conditions to mutually maintain each other.
- Patients with chronic pain and psychiatric conditions such as PTSD have overall worse functional status, greater distress, and less favorable responses to medical intervention.
- Management of patient with both orofacial pain and PTSD is best performed with integration of behavioral therapy and biomedical care early in the course of treatment.

## CASE PRESENTATION

A 55-year-old woman presented to the Oral and Maxillofacial Surgery Clinic at Massachusetts General Hospital with the chief complaint of right-sided jaw pain as well as

[a] Department of Oral and Maxillofacial Surgery, Massachusetts General Hospital, 55 Fruit Street, #230, Boston, MA 02114, USA; [b] Department of Oral and Maxillofacial Surgery, Harvard School of Dental Medicine, 188 Longwood Ave, Boston, MA 02115, USA; [c] Department of Anesthesiology, Perioperative Care, & Pain Medicine, NYU Grossman School of Medicine, 550 1st Avenue, New York, NY 10016, USA; [d] Department of Population Health – Division of Medical Ethics, NYU Grossman School of Medicine, 550 1st Avenue, New York, NY 10016, USA; [e] School of Social Work, North Carolina State University, 10 Current Dr, Raleigh, NC 27607, USA; [f] Department of Anesthesia, Critical Care and Pain Medicine, Massachusetts General Hospital, 55 Fruit St, Boston, MA 02114, USA; [g] Department of Psychiatry, Massachusetts General Hospital, 55 Fruit St, Boston, MA 02114, USA; [h] Department of Diagnostic Sciences, Tufts University School of Dental Medicine, 1 Kneeland Street, Boston, MA 02111, USA
* Corresponding author. Department of Oral and Maxillofacial Surgery, Harvard School of Dental Medicine, 188 Longwood Ave, Boston, MA, 02115, USA
*E-mail addresses:* rbavarian@partners.org; roxanne_bavarian@hsdm.harvard.edu

Dent Clin N Am 67 (2023) 141–155
https://doi.org/10.1016/j.cden.2022.07.011
0011-8532/23/© 2022 Elsevier Inc. All rights reserved.

difficulty opening and closing her jaw. She reported having experienced jaw pain for as long as she could remember and had undergone several surgeries on her temporomandibular joint (TMJ) beginning in her early 20s. She reported receiving bilateral Proplast-Teflon interpositional implants (Vitek Inc.; Houston, TX, USA) in the 1980s, followed by a bilateral total joint replacement, and most recently removal of the right total joint prosthesis. Her primary concern at her initial visit was that she could neither open nor fully close her mouth to bring her teeth together. Her pain score at the initial visit was scored as 7 of 10 intensity, felt bilaterally but predominantly in her right jaw.

Her medical history was relevant for fibromyalgia; osteoarthritis with prosthetic joints in the knee, hip, in addition to her jaw; depression; and anxiety. For fibromyalgia and osteoarthritis, she reported taking gabapentin 300 mg twice daily over the past 3 years. For depression, she was taking bupropion 150 mg once daily and duloxetine 60 mg once daily both for approximately 5 years. She also reported a range of anxiety symptoms, for which she was prescribed alprazolam 0.5 mg as needed, which she took on average "10 tablets a week."

The patient's initial examination showed an extremely limited range of motion, with 14-mm maximum mouth opening. She was unable to get her teeth closer than 2 mm. She also had swelling of her bilateral preauricular areas, with pain worst in the right preauricular area. A panoramic radiograph revealed partial edentulism in the maxilla and mandible as well as a mass of hypertrophic bone in the right TMJ (**Fig. 1**). In her left TMJ, she had a left total joint prosthesis with the condylar component displaced out of the socket. She also had impingement of her right maxillary tuberosity on the right mandible, preventing her from fully closing her jaw.

The patient was diagnosed as having right TMJ ankylosis due to the hypertrophic mass of bone in the right TMJ, which was impinging on the right external auditory canal and causing chronic otitis media. She also had impingement of her right maxilla on the mandible, preventing normal mouth closing, as well as a failed prosthetic joint of her left TMJ. The cause of these failed prostheses was thought to be potentially related to her history of Proplast-Teflon interpositional implants, which were the first medical device that was recalled by the US Food and Drug Administration (FDA) due to high rates of adverse events due to breakdown of the implant and chronic foreign body reactions in the surrounding tissues.[1]

She was ultimately planned for a series of surgeries to (1) embolize the right maxillary artery to control vascular structures before surgery, (2) remove the heterotopic

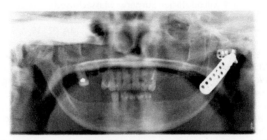

**Fig. 1.** Preoperative panoramic radiograph taken at the initial visit. The patient has a partially edentulous maxilla and mandible. On the right mandible, there is a large mass of heterotopic bone at the site of the right mandibular condyle fusing the mandible to the base of the skull. There is also impingement of the right maxillary tuberosity on the right mandible, accounting for the patient's inability to fully occlude. On the left mandible, a prosthetic implant of the TMJ appears dislocated from the glenoid fossa component.

bone as well as the left failed prosthesis, (3) reconstruct the TMJ and place temporary condylar implants, and (4) remove the temporary implants and place custom-made total TMJ implants.

The patient understandably had significant anxiety in anticipation of the surgeries. Her family was supportive, and her husband accompanied her to these visits. The surgeries proceeded uneventfully, and she was able to obtain a postoperative range of motion of 34 mm as well as the ability to fully occlude. Postoperative radiographs were unremarkable (**Fig. 2**), and upon clinical examination she demonstrated improved range of motion, although her pain persisted as a 7 of 10 intensity. She also developed synkinesis of her facial muscles, which improved with tizanidine 2 mg twice daily.

Psychosocial factors were not formally assessed before or following her surgery, and she was lost to follow-up after her initial postoperative visit. Although her prior records were reviewed, there was no documentation of contact with the patient's mental health or primary care providers—an important component of assessment given the patient's complex presentation.

The patient returned to the clinic 3 years later, with the chief complaint of persistent right-sided jaw pain of 8 of 10 intensity. She informed us that she had begun taking oxycodone 5 mg twice daily as prescribed by her primary care physician for her facial pain as well as her more diffuse fibromyalgia pain, although this did not reduce her pain below an 8 of 10 intensity. There were no aberrancies in her Prescription Drug Monitoring Program (PDMP) data. Clinical examination indicated that her range of motion was maintained at 34-mm mouth opening, with no changes in her occlusion. She had pain on palpation of her right preauricular area that duplicated her chief complaint. Her radiographic examination was within normal limits with no evidence of failure of the prosthetic hardware. Serology to rule out inflammatory arthritis was negative, as was metal allergy testing to rule out an allergy to the nickel contained in TMJ prostheses.

The patient then underwent a series of diagnostic nerve blocks and trigger point injections to identify the source of the pain. Although right-sided inferior alveolar and occipital nerve blocks reportedly reduced her pain from a 7 to 8 of 10 to a 4 to 5 of 10 pain for several hours, no treatment fully resolved her pain, nor did any treatment provide lasting relief. Additional medication trials with pregabalin, amitriptyline, baclofen, oxcarbazepine, and lamotrigine did not alleviate her pain, nor did botulinum toxin injections to her masticatory muscles. Throughout this year-long process, the character

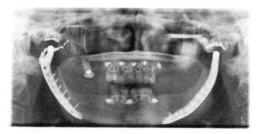

**Fig. 2.** Postoperative panoramic radiograph taken at 1 month following the patient's final surgery. The heterotopic bone has been removed, and the patient's TMJs have been replaced bilaterally with custom-made total TMJ prosthetic implants. On the right, there is a coil seen where the right maxillary artery was embolized before surgical intervention. The teeth are occluded, with temporary intermaxillary fixation in place with wires and screws.

of her pain progressed from a constant ache in the right preauricular area to a constant burning sensation over the posterior scalp as well as a paroxysmal electric shocklike sensation in the right side of her face, triggered by touch or cold air, in the distribution of the second and third branch of the trigeminal nerve.

Given continued refractory pain as well as her increasing distress and anger regarding her lack of progress, she was referred to a pain psychologist. She described to the psychologist her different sources of pain throughout her head, neck, and body, consistent with her previous diagnosis of fibromyalgia. The patient also revealed that her experience with TMJ surgeries beginning at age 29 years was a traumatic experience for her, and that she continued to find herself becoming upset when she was reminded of this experience and experienced flashbacks of the past surgical experience. She confirmed having periods of greater than 2 weeks during which she felt little interest or pleasure in engaging in normally enjoyable activities and feeling depressed without suicidal ideation. The patient reported panic attacks occurring once or twice a month. She acknowledged positive support from her husband but lamented that she spent much of her time in bed due to the pain. The patient also had reduced her daily activities, with walking limited to 10 minutes, and was fearful of driving because she felt her "balance was off due to the pain and medications." She also reported restless sleep, napping regularly, and having "no energy." The psychologist diagnosed the patient with a posttraumatic stress disorder (PTSD) and recurrent major depression. Although the patient was somatically focused and sought a "cure" to her problem, she was not thought to have symptoms suggestive of a somatoform disorder, and she also did not display any indication of malingering or a substance use disorder despite taking multiple concurrent medications with potential for abuse. The PDMP continued to indicate no aberrancies associated with acquiring her medications, and the standard Tobacco, Alcohol, Prescription medications, and other Substance Use (TAPS) screening tool revealed no major substance use risks.[2] A discussion with her primary care physician confirmed that she had been suffering from chronic diffuse pain for the more than 20 years that he had known her, although her depression and anxiety had increased over the previous 5 years. She continued to seek multiple concurrent providers for a resolution of her symptoms.

During the period in which she was lost to follow-up, she also sought additional consultations regarding her facial pain. The patient reported that she was diagnosed with trigeminal neuralgia, and ultimately underwent a balloon compression rhizotomy of the right trigeminal nerve performed by a neurosurgeon. Although she stated that this did resolve the lancinating, electric shock-like pain, she was left with a severe "excruciating" ache of 8 to 9 of 10 in her right TMJ that she described "like a bad ear infection," with the pain radiating to her right cheek, sinus, eye, and forehead. The patient continued on tizanidine 2 mg twice daily as well as baclofen 10 mg 3 times daily. No further surgical intervention was indicated due to her otherwise normal clinical and radiographic examination. Consultation with pain medicine specialists resulted in a recommendation of hydromorphone 2 mg every 4 hours, with this prescription being contingent on receiving concomitant psychological care to help her cope with this pain.

## THE ASSOCIATION OF PSYCHOSOCIAL COMORBIDITIES IN CHRONIC OROFACIAL PAIN

The case of a patient with persistent right-sided jaw pain with a history of multiple TMJ surgeries in the setting of persistent widespread body pain is presented, the causes of which were fibromyalgia, osteoarthritis with multiple joint replacements, as well as a PTSD, depression, and anxiety. The patient originally presented with clear signs of prosthetic joint failure, with heterotopic bone formation on her right joint as well as a displaced prosthetic hardware on the left joint. However, despite addressing these potential sources of pain and improving her TMJ from a functional perspective, her pain persisted and her distress increased, leading her to seek additional providers in search of a cure.

In patients suffering from chronic pain, which is generally defined as pain lasting longer than 3 months, there are generally known changes that can allow pain to persist beyond normal healing.[3] Patients experiencing chronic pain often experience emotional distress due to their pain and will often avoid any activity that perpetuates it, which can lead to further disability due to muscle atrophy and decreased flexibility that maintains a cycle of pain.[4] A systematic review of patients with temporomandibular disorders identified high rates of chronic pain comorbidities, including chronic back pain (66%), myofascial syndrome (50%), chronic stomach pain (50%), chronic migraines (40%), irritable bowel syndrome (19%), and fibromyalgia (14%).[5] Similarly, this patient had both fibromyalgia and osteoarthritis, with a history of prosthetic joint replacement in the knee and hip in addition to her longstanding TMJ disorder. Given the high rates of overlapping chronic pain conditions, such as fibromyalgia, temporomandibular disorder, headaches, and migraines, it has been proposed that these conditions are part of a spectrum indicating a central sensitivity syndrome that predisposes a person to multifocal and chronic pain as well as psychological symptoms, such as depression, anxiety, and PTSD.[6]

The relationship between chronic pain and mood disorders has been well established, with one study on patients with chronic lower back pain showing that 59% of patients exhibited symptoms of one or more psychiatric disorders, including depression (45%), substance abuse (19%), and anxiety disorder (16%).[7] Data regarding the rates of psychiatric disorders in patients with TMJ disorders are sparse, although psychosocial comorbidities increase as the patient's pain persists over time.[8,9]

In the case presented earlier, the patient reported symptoms of PTSD thought to relate to her history of past TMJ surgeries, including flashbacks as well as anxiety and avoidance of activities that remind her of her jaw pain and surgical history. The diagnostic criteria for PTSD are featured in **Box 1**, with the *Diagnostic and Statistical Manual of Mental Disorders* (Fifth Edition) defining trauma as "actual or threatened violent death, serious injury or accident, or sexual violence," whether this is directly witnessed by the patient or indirectly experienced via eyewitness accounts, exposure to a close family member, or with extreme or repeated exposure to the consequences of trauma.[10] For our patient, her PTSD was reportedly secondary to the life-altering effects and powerlessness experienced following TMJ surgery with a prosthetic implant, the Proplast-Teflon interpositional implant, that later was recalled by the FDA due to harmful adverse events related to the breakdown of the product causing a foreign body reaction in the surrounding tissues.[1] The possibility of other earlier trauma unrelated to her multiple surgeries also requires further investigation, because it has been established that histories of abuse and domestic violence are predictors of treatment-resistant facial pain.[11]

It is estimated that 10% to 50% of patients with chronic pain present with symptoms satisfying the criteria for PTSD, with studies on patients with orofacial pain showing rates of PTSD ranging from 15% to 23%.[12–14] In addition, the 2 conditions share a number of overlapping symptoms, including hyperarousal, fear avoidance, anxiety, and emotional lability, all of which can lead to a synergistic relationship in which each condition potentiates the other.[15,16] Specifically, chronic pain may serve as a constant reminder of the traumatic event and trigger an arousal response as well as

---

**Box 1**
**Diagnostic criteria for posttraumatic stress disorder[10]**

A. Exposure to actual or threatened death, serious injury, or sexual violence, whether directly experienced by the patient or indirectly experienced via eyewitness account, learning of an event occurring to a close family member or friend, or through repeated or extreme exposure to the consequences of trauma

B. Presence of recurrent, involuntary, and intrusive distressing memories associated with the traumatic event, which can present as recurrent distressing dreams or dissociative reactions (flashbacks)

C. Persistent avoidance of memories, thoughts, or feelings associated with the traumatic event, which can include external reminders of the trauma, such as people, places, objects, or situations

D. Negative changes in cognition and mood associated with the traumatic event, which can include dissociative amnesia; feelings of fear, horror, anger, guilt, or shame; feeling detached from others; and inability to experience positive emotions

E. Notable changes in arousal and reactivity associated with the traumatic event, such as hypervigilance, an exaggerated startle response, difficulty concentrating, insomnia, irritable mood, and reckless or self-destructive behavior

F. Symptoms present for more than 1 month

G. Symptoms leading to significant distress or impairment in personal or work life

H. Symptoms are unrelated to another medical condition or the effects of a substance (medication or alcohol)

---

anxiety. The patient may catastrophize, which refers to an irrational thought pattern that leads the patient to believe that his or her pain is much worse than is actually the case.[17] The patient may also avoid activities that have the potential to exacerbate pain or cause reinjury (fear avoidance), which leads to reduced activity levels and perpetuated or exacerbated physical disability. This physical disability can also lead to lethargy, fatigue, and depression. In fact, approximately 80% of patients with PTSD present with symptoms of at least one other psychiatric disorder, with studies most commonly demonstrating comorbidities of depression, anxiety, and substance use disorders.[18] In addition, these patients often have exacerbated pain due to insomnia and other sleeping disorders, which not only increases pain but also reduces energy and activity levels even further.[19] Demonstrating this, the patient presented in this case reported symptoms of PTSD as well as more generalized anxiety, avoidance of activities that exacerbate pain, depression, as well as insomnia, as comorbidities with her diffuse chronic pain.

The comorbidities of chronic pain, such as temporomandibular disorder in conjunction with psychiatric pain conditions such as PTSD is clinically meaningful. Patients with chronic pain and history of trauma have been determined to have overall worse functional status, greater distress, and less favorable responses to medical intervention.[20]

## PSYCHOLOGICAL ASSESSMENT OF THE PATIENT WITH OROFACIAL PAIN

Given the prevalence of comorbid psychiatric conditions in patients with chronic pain, as well as the impact of untreated psychiatric conditions that influence treatment outcomes, it is important to incorporate an early psychological assessment when evaluating a patient with orofacial pain. For example, in the case presented, the presence of chronic multifocal pain comorbidities and psychiatric conditions likely played a major role in the patient's persistent pain despite improvement in her range of motion following TMJ surgery. In hindsight, the psychological assessment was initially neglected due to the noteworthy pathology associated with prosthetic joint failure that was seen at her first visit. Clinicians need to recognize that the presence of pathophysiology does not necessarily preclude comorbid psychopathology, because such a "binary" approach to patients with complex chronic pain fails to capture the gestalt of these individuals' conditions.

The psychological assessment of the patient should be initiated at the initial visit and continue to be performed periodically throughout the duration of care. It is important to consider the patient's behavioral and emotional health throughout his or her treatment, whether the orofacial pain is improving, remaining stable, or worsening.

A thorough pain history is at the crux of the orofacial pain examination to make the most accurate diagnosis and tailor treatment accordingly. Although the patient's chief complaint should be reviewed, the clinician should enquire whether the patient has pain in other parts of the body, as well. For example, in our case, the patient presented with the chief complaint of jaw pain and limited mouth opening, but additionally suffered from fibromyalgia as well as osteoarthritis, with a history of multiple invasive surgeries. This information is clinically relevant not only in determining whether there is a systemic disease contributing to the patient's chief complaint but also because the presence of multifocal pain may be a sign of central sensitivity and a predictor of poor outcome. Similarly, in review of the patient's medical history, the clinician should consider other chronic pain diagnoses, such as fibromyalgia, chronic fatigue syndrome, irritable bowel syndrome, headache, migraines, chronic joint pain, or chronic back pain. Although this can be time consuming, it can be helpful to know what treatments the patient received for these conditions, whether they be pharmacologic, restorative, interventional, or surgical, and the degree to which each of these treatments helped.

In a patient presenting with jaw pain, it is standard practice to ascertain whether the patient has a parafunctional jaw grinding or clenching habit, whether it be unconsciously while sleeping or subconsciously during the day.[21] Doing so provides an opportunity for the provider to assess the contribution of stress and anxiety to the patient's pain as well as sleep quality. There are several brief screening questionnaires that can alert the clinician to the presence and intensity of anxiety, depression, and trauma, as well as substance use risk. Indeed, many of these are already considered the standard of care in primary care practices and patients are becoming increasingly comfortable with being asked about sensitive content as this becomes the standard.[22] **Table 1** provides examples of validated screening tools that are of relevance to the patient with chronic pain, and a subset of these can be incorporated into the assessment of all patients presenting to an orofacial practice.

Last, the clinician should also try to gain insight into patients' daily lives, including their energy levels, ability to perform the activities that they enjoy, and whether the patient reports social support from family and friends. Substance use should also be reviewed, including alcohol, tobacco, and prescription or recreational drugs. **Table 1** reviews screening tools for substance use, including the National Institute on Drug Abuse's TAPS questionnaire.[2] In cases in which chronic opioid therapy is being initiated or continued, the Screener and Opioid Assessment for Patients with Pain (SOAPP-R) and the Current Opioid Misuse Measure (COMM) Screener should be considered, and abbreviated versions of these measures are now available.[23,24] Most importantly, the PDMP database should also be reviewed consistently as a means of precluding doctor shopping and concomitant use of other controlled substances that may not be in the patient's best interest.[25]

**Table 1**
**Screening tools in the psychological assessment of the patient with chronic orofacial pain**

| Name | Purpose | Description |
|------|---------|-------------|
| PHQ-9[43] | Depression | 9-item questionnaire for symptoms of depression |
| GAD-7[44] | Anxiety | 7-item questionnaire for symptoms of anxiety |
| PHQ-15[45] | Somatization | 15-item questionnaire assessing somatization (eg, back pain, headaches, fatigue, insomnia) |
| MSPQ | Somatization | 13-item questionnaire assessing somatic symptoms (eg, stomach pain, neck ache, dry mouth, neck ache) |
| PROMIS-PF-4 | Disability/functionality | 4-item questionnaire assessing functionality (eg, walking 15 minutes, doing chores, running errands) |
| TAPS tools[2] | Substance use | 4-item questionnaire regarding use of tobacco, alcohol, illicit drugs, and nonmedical use of prescription drugs |
| SOAPP-R[23] | Substance use | 24-item questionnaire intended to screen for risk for opioid abuse in patients being considered for initiating or currently on opioid treatment |
| COMM[24] | Substance misuse for patients on long-term opioid therapy | 17-item questionnaire to identify risk factors for substance misuse or abuse in patients receiving long-term opioid therapy |

*Abbreviations:* COMM, Current Opioid Misuse Measure; GAD-7, General Anxiety Disorder-7; MSPQ, Modified Somatic Perception Questionnaire; PHQ, Patient Health Questionnaire; PROMIS-PF-4, Patient-Reported Outcomes Measurement Information System – Physical Function; SOAPP-R, Screener and Opioid Assessment for Patients with Pain-Revised.

Regarding PTSD, it is common practice in orofacial pain to enquire whether the patient has a history of trauma to the jaw, whether direct trauma (eg, fall, injury, altercation) or indirect trauma (eg, whiplash). Given the high rates of comorbidity between chronic pain and PTSD, the clinician should consider integrating a screener for a history of any trauma in their examination. There are self-report questionnaires, such as the PTSD Checklist (PCL), or alternatively a clinician can learn to ask direct questions regarding PTSD symptoms.[26] Various scripts have been developed that can help clinicians become more comfortable with asking a patient about a history of trauma.[16]

Ultimately, the onus is not on the orofacial pain clinician to provide a psychiatric diagnosis, but rather to introduce the concept of chronic pain as a disorder that can be impacted by stress, anxiety, depression, or PTSD. Following this discussion, the clinician may perform a screening to assess for risk of psychosocial comorbidities. In patients in whom there is concern for an undiagnosed psychiatric or substance use disorder, the clinician should underscore the importance of referral and collaboration with a mental health provider, preferably a clinician who has some familiarity with chronic pain. When the role of psychosocial health is introduced to the patient as a normal component of interdisciplinary pain management, the suggestion of collaboration with a mental health provider rarely meets with resistance from the patient. Unfortunately, collaboration with a mental health provider is often initiated after the patient "fails" treatment, and an adversarial relationship with the clinician has evolved.[17]

## MANAGEMENT OF PATIENTS WITH OROFACIAL PAIN WITH POSTTRAUMATIC STRESS DISORDER

Chronic pain is caused by a complex biopsychosocial interplay of factors, which acknowledges the role of biological, psychological, and social factors in perpetuating pain.[7] Management of chronic orofacial pain thus is most effectively addressed through a multidisciplinary approach that considers each of these factors, and includes specialists in orofacial pain, pain medicine, physical therapy, psychology, and, if necessary, psychiatry. The role of the primary care provider (PCP) should not be neglected, either, and regularly scheduled visits between the patient and PCP can help both streamline care and minimize anxiety and the risk of a crisis.

When the patient in this case presented with persistent pain despite improved range of motion after surgical treatment to correct her failed TMJ prostheses, it became clear to her providers that her pain was multifactorial, with elements of central sensitization and neuropathic pain as well as PTSD, anxiety, depression, and disability. Thus, her orofacial pain team included a pain psychologist, a neurologist, and a neurosurgeon, all in coordination with her primary care provider. Holding a multidisciplinary conference composed of specialists in facial pain can be helpful to coordinate and streamline care. For example, in our practice, a bimonthly conference is held, including representatives from pain medicine, neurology, neurosurgery, orofacial pain, oral and maxillofacial surgery, facial plastic surgery, and psychology, in which patients' cases are presented and discussed to review appropriate treatment options and referrals.

## BEHAVIORAL THERAPY

Given the central role of symptoms such as catastrophizing and avoidance in both chronic pain and PTSD, cognitive behavioral therapy (CBT) is a psychological treatment that has been demonstrated to be effective for treating both conditions by teaching patients to identify these negative feelings and behaviors and replace them with better adaptive skills and strategies.[27] For example, CBT could help to identify pain-catastrophizing and fear-avoidant behaviors in the patient and then introduce better coping strategies to replace these behaviors, such as relaxation training, distraction techniques, and reintroducing activities on a time-based quota.[28] CBT has been well studied, with studies demonstrating long-term relief in symptoms of chronic pain and depression and helping patients increase activity levels and return to work.[29] Other studies, however, emphasize that although CBT has a strong track record for helping alleviate the emotional and behavioral sequelae of chronic pain, its efficacy for reducing pain severity, per se, is not particularly impressive.[30,31]

Acceptance-based therapies, such as acceptance and commitment therapy (ACT), have also been demonstrated as helpful for patients living with chronic pain. The premise of ACT is to accept chronic pain without judgment and recognize that chronic pain may not ever fully resolve or "be cured." By accepting pain, the goal is for the patient to be able to focus on their other goals in life and avoid overengaging in symptoms and treatment of their pain. In a systematic review, patients who underwent ACT displayed increased acceptance of their pain, reduced symptoms of anxiety and depression, as well as increased functioning when compared with control groups who received treatment as usual.[32]

## INTERDISCIPLINARY PAIN REHABILITATION PROGRAMS

Interdisciplinary pain rehabilitation refers to intensive programs that address the physical, behavioral, and emotional aspects of chronic pain, typically through outpatient programs that combine aspects of pain medicine, physical therapy, occupational therapy, and behavioral health services. The goal of interdisciplinary rehabilitation is to provide physical reconditioning and teach activity pacing as well as relaxation training and health education to help patients cope more effectively with their chronic pain and eliminate pain behaviors, with an overarching goal of "functional restoration."[33]

With traditional operant or "functional restoration" programs, a focus is placed on encouraging activity and exercise in spite of pain; this is in contrast with passive approaches that focus on pain relief or efforts to "fix" the patients' underlying presumed tissue pathology. With a functional restoration approach, the patient is taught that there is a difference between "hurt" and "harm," and engagement in activity rarely causes harm. If a patient's choice of activity depends on the risk of pain, he or she may unintentionally become phobic about engaging in any functional pursuits. Consequently, deconditioning and isolation from enjoyable activities often follow suit, and are likely to result in exacerbated depression and anxiety.

This integrated model of pain rehabilitation also serves in contrast to the typical journey that patients with pain often follow, which often involves being referred from specialist to specialist without an integrated, holistic approach to their treatment. Sequential treatment such as this places patients at risk for unnecessary diagnostic or treatment procedures that can further exacerbate pain and emotional distress as well as distrust of the medical system.[7] In one larger study of patients with chronic pain and PTSD by Gilliam and colleagues,[33] participation in an interdisciplinary pain rehabilitation pain program resulted in 86.7% of patients experiencing improved functioning and 50.6% of patients reporting a reduction in PTSD symptoms.

## PSYCHOPHARMACOLOGY

For the pain specialist, there are several medications that have been demonstrated to be dually effective for treatment of both pain and mental health disorders, such as serotonin-norepinephrine reuptake inhibitors (SNRIs), tricyclic antidepressants (TCAs), and anticonvulsant medications.[28]

SNRIs selectively inhibit the reuptake and increase the period during which serotonin and norepinephrine remain in the synaptic cleft, thereby improving neurotransmission. These are 2 neurotransmitters important in the regulation of mood as well as decreasing pain by activating the descending inhibitory pain pathways. Commonly used SNRIs include venlafaxine, desvenlafaxine, and duloxetine. Although originally indicated for the treatment of depression, randomized controlled trials have also demonstrated duloxetine to be effective in reducing pain and depression in conditions such fibromyalgia,[34,35] neuropathic pain,[36] and musculoskeletal pain.[37,38] TCAs represent an older class of antidepressants that are thought to have a similar mechanism of modulating serotonin and norepinephrine to modulate pain. Although they are no longer widely used in the treatment of depression due to side effects at higher doses, low doses of TCAs such as amitriptyline and nortriptyline have been demonstrated as efficacious in the treatment of fibromyalgia[34,35] and chronic neuropathic pain.[36] Of note, TCAs should be prescribed with caution in patients with concomitant depression due to a significant risk of overdose coupled with the potential cardiotoxicity of this class of medications.

Anticonvulsants such as gabapentin and pregabalin have been used to treat a wide variety of chronic pain conditions, including fibromyalgia and neuropathic pain.[35,36]

Although not approved by the FDA for the treatment of anxiety, pregabalin has been demonstrated to be efficacious in the treatment of general anxiety disorder.[39]

With any of the aforementioned considerations, side effects also must be considered. Nonadherence is common, especially with agents that impact cognition, weight, or sexual function.

## LONG-TERM OPIOID THERAPY

In the case presented, the patient returned 3 years after her TMJ surgeries to replace her failed prostheses with the chief complaint of persistent pain. She reported that she had been taking oxycodone 5 mg 3 times daily as prescribed by her PCP for her facial pain as well as more diffuse pain related to fibromyalgia and osteoarthritis. Although opioids may be effective in reducing the patient's pain in the short term, studies have suggested that nonopioid medications and nonpharmacologic treatments are superior and have less risk of adverse events.[40] An important caveat is that common nonopioid analgesics such as acetaminophen and nonsteroidal anti-inflammatory drugs are approved by the FDA for mild to moderate pain, although not for severe pain, for which opioids are approved. Accordingly, sound practice involves careful assessment of each patient as an individual, and avoidance of attempts to "fit a square peg into a round hole" by prescribing weak analgesics as monotherapies for severe pain.

It should be considered that many patients with chronic pain and concomitant psychiatric conditions are at risk for suicide and overdose.[41] Thus, for patients on long-term opioid therapy (and, perhaps for other medications that may be used for vehicles for suicide), regular assessments such as TAPS and SOAPP-R and use of the PDMP should be performed to analyze risk factors for substance misuse.[25] The 2016 Centers of Disease Control and Prevention Guideline for Prescribing Opioids for Chronic Pain provides some structure for assessing risk, and it was noted that in the case presented, the patient's dosing of oxycodone was 5 mg 3 times daily, which is considered a low dosage.[25] If tapering is considered for a patient on higher dosages, the US Department of Health and Human Services offers an outline for patient care.[42]

## SUMMARY AND CLINICS CARE POINTS

In summary, chronic pain is a complex condition influenced by biological, psychological, and social factors. In reviewing the biopsychosocial model of pain within the context of the case provided here, the patient presented with clear evidence of underlying peripheral tissue damage within the TMJ. Her symptoms of chronic TMJ pain began following the placement of a Proplast-Teflon interpositional implant, which ultimately was recalled by the FDA due to the breakdown of the Proplast material in the surrounding tissues and chronic foreign body reactions that led to pain, arthritis, and heterotopic bone formation. In addition, the patient was diagnosed with fibromyalgia as well as osteoarthritis, with a history of multiple joint replacements. Given her widespread chronic pain, the patient aligns with the concept of a central sensitization potentially making her prone to chronic pain conditions. From a psychological standpoint, the patient revealed to her psychologist that she experienced symptoms of PTSD related to her history of surgeries, with flashbacks and anxiety regarding her medical visits, as well as symptoms of insomnia and depression. The combination of her chronic pain and PTSD had social consequences, because she described avoiding activities she had previously enjoyed and withdrew into social isolation. Given the role of psychological and social factors in perpetuating pain, it is imperative that psychological assessment and screening for mood disorders is performed with every patient presenting with chronic pain, with referral to psychology when indicated.

Chronic pain and PTSD, in particular, are 2 conditions that share a common mechanism that can "mutually maintain" each other, which is thought to be due to common symptoms of catastrophizing, anxiety, and avoidance. Although management of patients with chronic pain and PTSD is best performed through interdisciplinary care with a pain specialist and a psychologist, the case presented here was complicated by the patient's history of medical trauma and her consequent mistrust of the medical system. Her medical team discussed her case within a multidisciplinary group as well as with her PCP, although the patient ultimately declined further psychological care and continued to seek a cure for her pain. Most recently, the decision was made that she could not obtain further treatment at our center unless she participated in a longitudinal psychologic program integrated with her overall pain care. With longitudinal psychological care, time could be spent discussing the contribution of psychological and social factors in the maintenance of her chronic pain and introducing coping skills training as a cornerstone to her treatment.

## CLINICS CARE POINTS

- A thorough patient intake including psychological assessment and screening for conditions such as depression, anxiety, and substance use should be performed with all patients presenting with chronic orofacial pain.
- Management of patients with chronic pain and psychological comorbidities is best performed with interdisciplinary care, including orofacial pain, behavioral treatment, and physical therapy, as well as the primary care medical management.
- Behavioral therapy should be integrated into the patient's course of treatment at the start of care, rather than as a last resort after other treatment modalities have failed.

## DISCLOSURE

The authors have nothing to disclose.

## REFERENCES

1. Bavarian R, Schatman ME, Keith DA. Persistent pain following proplast-teflon implants of the temporomandibular joint: a case report and 35-year management perspective. J Pain Res 2021;14:3033–46.
2. McNeely J, Wu LT, Subramaniam G, et al. Performance of the tobacco, alcohol, prescription medication, and other substance use (TAPS) tool for substance use screening in primary care patients. Ann Intern Med 2016;165(10):690–9.
3. Treede RD, Rief W, Barke A, et al. Chronic pain as a symptom or a disease: the IASP classification of chronic pain for the international classification of diseases (ICD-11). Pain 2019;160(1):19–27.
4. Morgan L, Aldington D. Comorbid chronic pain and post-traumatic stress disorder in UK veterans: a lot of theory but not enough evidence. Br J Pain 2020; 14(4):256–62.
5. Kleykamp BA, Ferguson MC, McNicol E, et al. The prevalence of comorbid chronic pain conditions among patients with temporomandibular disorders: a systematic review. J Am Dent Assoc 2022;153(3):241–250 e10.
6. Ablin K, Clauw DJ. From fibrositis to functional somatic syndromes to a bell-shaped curve of pain and sensory sensitivity: evolution of a clinical construct. Rheum Dis Clin North Am 2009;35(2):233–51.

7. Cheatle MD, Gallagher RM. Chronic pain and comorbid mood and substance use disorders: a biopsychosocial treatment approach. Curr Psychiatry Rep 2006;8(5):371–6.
8. Velly AM, Look JO, Carlson C, et al. The effect of catastrophizing and depression on chronic pain–a prospective cohort study of temporomandibular muscle and joint pain disorders. Pain 2011;152(10):2377–83.
9. Fillingim RB, Ohrbach R, Greenspan JD, et al. Associations of psychologic factors with multiple chronic overlapping pain conditions. J Oral Facial Pain Headache 2020;34:s85–100.
10. American Psychiatric Association. *Diagnostic and Statistical Manual of Mental Disorders*. 5th ed. Washington, DC: American Psychiatric Association; 2013.
11. Curran SL, Sherman JJ, Cunningham LL, et al. Physical and sexual abuse among orofacial pain patients: linkages with pain and psychologic distress. J Orofac Pain Fall 1995;9(4):340–6.
12. Sharp TJ. The prevalence of post-traumatic stress disorder in chronic pain patients. Curr Pain Headache Rep 2004;8(2):111–5. https://doi.org/10.1007/s11916-004-0024-x.
13. Sherman JJ, Carlson CR, Wilson JF, et al. Post-traumatic stress disorder among patients with orofacial pain. J Orofac Pain. Fall 2005;19(4):309–17.
14. De Leeuw R, Bertoli E, Schmidt JE, et al. Prevalence of post-traumatic stress disorder symptoms in orofacial pain patients. Oral Surg Oral Med Oral Pathol Oral Radiol Endod 2005;99(5):558–68. https://doi.org/10.1016/j.tripleo.2004.05.016.
15. Gasperi M, Afari N, Goldberg J, et al. Pain and trauma: the role of criterion a trauma and stressful life events in the pain and PTSD relationship. J Pain 2021;22(11):1506–17.
16. Kind S, Otis JD. The interaction between chronic pain and PTSD. Curr Pain Headache Rep 2019;23(12):91.
17. Patterson EKR, Hernandez-Nuno de la Rosa MF, Roselli M, et al. Psychological Assessment of Pain and Headache. In: Brenner GJ, Rathmell JP, editors. The Massachusetts General Hospital Handbook of Pain Management. 4th edition. Philadelphia, PA: Lippincott Williams & Wilkins; 2020. p. 60–75.
18. Brady KT. Posttraumatic stress disorder and comorbidity: recognizing the many faces of PTSD. J Clin Psychiatry 1997;58(Suppl 9):12–5.
19. Finan PH, Goodin BR, Smith MT. The association of sleep and pain: an update and a path forward. J Pain 2013;14(12):1539–52.
20. Otis JD, Keane TM, Kerns RD. An examination of the relationship between chronic pain and post-traumatic stress disorder. J Rehabil Res Dev 2003;40(5):397–405.
21. Schiffman E, Ohrbach R, Truelove E, et al. Diagnostic criteria for temporomandibular disorders (DC/TMD) for clinical and research applications: recommendations of the international RDC/TMD Consortium Network* and Orofacial Pain Special Interest Groupdagger. J Oral Facial Pain Headache Winter 2014;28(1):6–27.
22. Mulvaney-Day N, Marshall T, Downey Piscopo K, et al. Screening for behavioral health conditions in primary care settings: a systematic review of the literature. J Gen Intern Med 2018;33(3):335–46.
23. Black RA, McCaffrey SA, Villapiano AJ, et al. Development and validation of an eight-item brief form of the SOAPP-R (SOAPP-8). Pain Med 2018;19(10):1982–7.
24. Butler SF, Budman SH, Fanciullo GJ, et al. Cross validation of the current opioid misuse measure to monitor chronic pain patients on opioid therapy. Clin J Pain 2010;26(9):770–6.

25. Dowell D, Haegerich TM, Chou R. CDC guideline for prescribing opioids for chronic pain - united states, 2016. MMWR Recomm Rep 2016;65(1):1–49.
26. Blevins CA, Weathers FW, Davis MT, et al. The posttraumatic stress disorder checklist for DSM-5 (PCL-5): development and initial psychometric evaluation. J Trauma Stress 2015;28(6):489–98.
27. Butler AC, Chapman JE, Forman EM, et al. The empirical status of cognitive-behavioral therapy: a review of meta-analyses. Clin Psychol Rev 2006;26(1):17–31.
28. Hooten WM. Chronic pain and mental health disorders: shared neural mechanisms, epidemiology, and treatment. Mayo Clin Proc 2016;91(7):955–70. https://doi.org/10.1016/j.mayocp.2016.04.029.
29. Richmond H, Hall AM, Copsey B, et al. The effectiveness of cognitive behavioural treatment for non-specific low back pain: a systematic review and meta-analysis. PLoS One 2015;10(8):e0134192.
30. Bernardy K, Fuber N, Kollner V, et al. Efficacy of cognitive-behavioral therapies in fibromyalgia syndrome - a systematic review and metaanalysis of randomized controlled trials. J Rheumatol 2010;37(10):1991–2005.
31. Velleman S, Stallard P, Richardson T. A review and meta-analysis of computerized cognitive behaviour therapy for the treatment of pain in children and adolescents. Child Care Health Dev 2010;36(4):465–72.
32. Hughes LS, Clark J, Colclough JA, et al. Acceptance and commitment therapy (ACT) for chronic pain: a systematic review and meta-analyses. Clin J Pain 2017;33(6):552–68.
33. Gilliam WP, Schumann ME, Craner JR, et al. Examining the effectiveness of pain rehabilitation on chronic pain and post-traumatic symptoms. J Behav Med 2020;43(6):956–67.
34. Hauser W, Petzke F, Uceyler N, et al. Comparative efficacy and acceptability of amitriptyline, duloxetine and milnacipran in fibromyalgia syndrome: a systematic review with meta-analysis. Rheumatology (Oxford) 2011;50(3):532–43.
35. Hauser W, Bernardy K, Uceyler N, et al. Treatment of fibromyalgia syndrome with antidepressants: a meta-analysis. JAMA 2009;301(2):198–209.
36. Finnerup NB, Attal N, Haroutounian S, et al. Pharmacotherapy for neuropathic pain in adults: a systematic review and meta-analysis. Lancet Neurol 2015;14(2):162–73.
37. Wang ZY, Shi SY, Li SJ, et al. Efficacy and safety of duloxetine on osteoarthritis knee pain: a meta-analysis of randomized controlled trials. Pain Med 2015;16(7):1373–85.
38. Hochberg MC, Wohlreich M, Gaynor P, et al. Clinically relevant outcomes based on analysis of pooled data from 2 trials of duloxetine in patients with knee osteoarthritis. J Rheumatol 2012;39(2):352–8.
39. Perna G, Alciati A, Riva A, et al. Long-term pharmacological treatments of anxiety disorders: an updated systematic review. Curr Psychiatry Rep 2016;18(3):23.
40. Dowell D, Haegerich TM, Chou R. CDC guideline for prescribing opioids for chronic pain–united states, 2016. JAMA 2016;315(15):1624–45.
41. Chou R. Five things to know when a psychiatric patient is prescribed opioids for pain. JAMA Psychiatry 2021;78(2):220–1.
42. Dowell D, Compton WM, Giroir BP. Patient-centered reduction or discontinuation of long-term opioid analgesics: the HHS guide for clinicians. JAMA 2019;322(19):1855–6.
43. Kroenke K, Spitzer RL, Williams JB. The PHQ-9: validity of a brief depression severity measure. J Gen Intern Med 2001;16(9):606–13.

44. Lowe B, Decker O, Muller S, et al. Validation and standardization of the General-ized Anxiety Disorder Screener (GAD-7) in the general population. Med Care 2008;46(3):266–74.
45. Kroenke K, Spitzer RL, Williams JB. The PHQ-15: validity of a new measure for evaluating the severity of somatic symptoms. Psychosom Med 2002;64(2): 258–66.

# Management of Episodic Migraine with Neuromodulation: A Case Report

Thiago D. Nascimento, DDS, MMedSc, MS[a,b], Dajung J. Kim, PhD[a,b],
Conrad Chrabol, MD[a,b], Manyoel Lim, PhD[a,b], Xiao-Su Hu, PhD[a,b],
Alexandre F. DaSilva, DDS, DMedSc[a,b,*]

## KEYWORDS

- Migraine • Neuromodulation • Transcranial direct current stimulation
- Primary motor cortex (M1)

## KEY POINTS

- Migraine is a prevalent neurologic disorder in orofacial pain practice.
- Clinicians should be able to identify the essential diagnostic characteristics of migraine defined by The International Classification of Headache Disorders.
- Experimental noninvasive neuromodulation of the primary motor cortex (M1) by high-definition transcranial direct current stimulation (HD-tDCS) is a research tool with potential therapeutic effect for managing episodic migraine.
- tDCS is an experimental device. Currently, tDCS is not a US Food and Drug Administration-approved treatment.

## INTRODUCTION

Despite recent pharmacologic advances in the acute and preventive management of migraine patients,[1,2] there is still a need for safe and well-tolerated non-pharmacological treatment strategies[3] to minimize the risks of medication side effects and avoid poorly managed ictal episodes that can lead to the transformation of episodic to chronic migraine.[4] Non-pharmacological interventions can provide pain relief for migraineurs that (1) are unresponsive to medications[5]; (2) have a contraindication to a particular drug (eg, triptans in those with cardiovascular disease[6]; (3) have low adherence to their medication regimen[7]; or (4) simply prefer nondrug interventions.[8]

[a] Department of Biologic and Materials Sciences & Prosthodontics, University of Michigan School of Dentistry, Ann Arbor, MI, USA; [b] Michigan Neuroscience Institute (MNI), Headache & Orofacial Pain Effort (H.O.P.E.) Laboratory, 205 Zina Pitcher Pl, Room 1027, Ann Arbor, MI 48109, USA
* Corresponding author. Michigan Neuroscience Institute (MNI), Headache & Orofacial Pain Effort (H.O.P.E.) Laboratory, 205 Zina Pitcher Pl, Room 1027, Ann Arbor, MI 48109.
*E-mail address:* adasilva@umich.edu

Dent Clin N Am 67 (2023) 157–171
https://doi.org/10.1016/j.cden.2022.07.012
0011-8532/23/© 2022 Elsevier Inc. All rights reserved.

Transcranial direct current stimulation (tDCS) is a practical and affordable investigational device that has been shown to be effective in the management of migraine.[9]

This case report is part of a clinical trial funded by the National Institutes of Health – National Institute of Neurological Disorders to investigate the endogenous μ-opioid pain system (arguably the principal pain modulatory system in the brain) and its modulatory effects through high-definition transcranial direct current stimulation (HD-tDCS) over the primary motor cortex area (M1).

The clinical trial was a randomized, double-blind, sham-controlled, HD-tDCS intervention in episodic migraineurs. It involved [$^{11}$C] carfentanil, a selective μ-opioid receptor (μOR) radioligand, PET before and after 10-daily active or sham sessions of contralateral (to the predominant side of migraine pain) M1 HD-tDCS.

The outcome measures included moderate/severe (M/S) headache days, headache attack intensity, and abortive medication use over 1 month after the HD-tDCS trial. As a molecular imaging outcome, we tracked changes in μOR availability.

This case report describes a single patient from the 25 participants that completed the trial, selected because of her clinical history and improved clinical outcomes in the 30-day follow-up period.

### Case Presentation

A 36-year-old Hispanic woman with a chief complaint of "severe headaches" was enrolled in our clinical trial in 2019. Her main goals in participating in the clinical trial were to potentially obtain "pain relief" from the HD-tDCS sessions and, through research, to help other patients suffering from migraine.

### HISTORY OF PRESENT ILLNESS
### Onset and Treatment History

The pain started spontaneously in 2014 when the patient was 31 year old. She experienced a single, sharp, left-sided, severe headache attack for 24 h. It was not associated with any other symptoms. She described a possible relationship between the attacks and the stress from her graduate studies and upcoming thesis defense. Otherwise, she reported no physically or emotionally traumatic events or precipitating factors that could have been related to the episode.

As this was her first headache of that type, she was concerned that it possibly was a brain lesion. After the pain subsided, she consulted with a neurologist for a medical evaluation. Based on the presentation history and a normal clinical examination, the neurologist diagnosed it as a migraine and recommended that she manages future attacks with non-opioid analgesics and avoid common migraine triggers such as red wine and dark chocolate. Routine physical exercise was also recommended. No brain imaging was ordered.

She reported being headache-free until 2018, when the headache attacks reoccurred unexpectedly. She recalled experiencing approximately four similar headache attacks that year, which were also not associated with any other symptoms. She experienced some mild pain relief by taking naratriptan 2.5 mg during the attacks; however, the medication was associated with mild to severe somnolence. Owing to the limited efficacy and troublesome side effects, she discontinued the medication.

The attacks became frequent approximately a year later with her move to the United States to continue her doctoral degree. After seeing an advertisement for our study, she contacted our research laboratory, wishing to enroll.

During her screening session for the study in August of 2019, she reported a falling accident onto her back a few weeks prior resulting in a sacral fracture. After a comprehensive emergency room evaluation, the treatment plan consisted of a 7-day course of hydrocodone 5 mg/acetaminophen 325 mg (an analgesic combination containing an opioid) for the acute management of her back pain, followed by physical therapy for 3 months.

Her participation in our study was delayed for 6 months because of her opiate intake (exclusionary for the clinical trial). She returned after the wash-out period, and her clinical presentation at that time is described below. She reported a full and uneventful recovery, no low back pain, and no changes in headache symptoms after the injury.

### Location

The pain was localized (described and pointed) to the left parietal and temporal regions. She denied having any pain on the right side, or any referred or radiating pain.

As an aid for pain intensity and area localization, we used a three-dimensional (3D)-pain tracking mobile application developed in-house (PainTrek, University of Michigan, MI, USA). As shown in **Fig. 1**, the patient was able to precisely identify the location in the head in which the headache attacks occurred. She was also able to rate her pain level for each area within the same region. The image also confirmed her history of not having any referred or radiating pain.

During the screening visit, the migraine headache area and intensity were recorded. The pain area with matching intensity was hand-drawn on the 3D representation of the head and neck area (consisting of 220 cells) using the PainTrek application (University of Michigan, MI, USA). The Pain Area and Intensity Number Summation (PAINS) value was calculated with the calculation: 12 (averaged pain intensity * the number of cells representing pain) divided by 660 cells in the region (maximum pain intensity × total number of cells). The pain intensity rating is defined as follows: mild (1—light red), moderate (2—red), and severe (3—dark red).

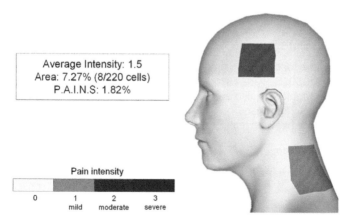

Average Intensity: 1.5
Area: 7.27% (8/220 cells)
P.A.I.N.S: 1.82%

Pain intensity

0    1    2    3
   mild  moderate  severe

**Fig. 1.** Baseline migraine severity measured by PainTrek. During the screening visit, the migraine headache area and intensity were recorded. The pain area with matching intensity was hand-drawn on the 3D representation of the head and neck area (consisting of 220 cells) using the PainTrek application (University of Michigan, MI, USA). The Pain Area and Intensity Number Summation (PAINS) value was calculated with the calculation: 12 (averaged pain intensity * the number of cells representing pain) divided by 660 cells in the region (maximum pain intensity × total number of cells). The pain intensity rating is defined as follows: mild (1—light red), moderate (2—red), and severe (3—dark red).

### Intensity and Quality

The pain intensity was rated as a 7 on a 0 to 10 numerical rating scale (NRS), 0 representing no pain and 10 being the worst pain imaginable. This pain persisted at the same intensity throughout the headache attacks. It was described as pulsating, like a "heartbeat."

### Pain Impact and Disability

To evaluate the impact of the headache attacks on her function and daily life, we used the Migraine Disability Assessment (MIDAS) questionnaire.[10] Her score of 31 indicated severe disability attributed to her migraine, based on the number of days of reduced productivity and days of missed work and activities.

### Temporal Pattern

The pain had been chronic and recurrent since 2019. She did not identify any pattern with respect to the morning, afternoon, or evening onset of attacks.

### Frequency and Duration

The average number of attacks per month was 6, and each episode lasted approximately 48 h (either if untreated or unsuccessfully treated). Thus, her number of headache days was 12 per month at the time of enrollment in the clinical trial.

### Aggravating Factors and Triggers

Physical activity and head movements increased her headache pain.
    Triggers included emotional stress (mainly associated with her doctoral studies), fatigue, and food such as dark chocolate and red wine.

### Alleviating Factors

In addition to avoiding triggers and aggravating factors, she noted that a warm shower, massage (neck, shoulder, periorbital, and frontal), sleep, relaxation, and rest in a dark environment were successful pain-relieving tools.

### Associated Signs and Symptoms

She denied the presence of visual aura, sensory loss, or weakness. Some of the attacks (fewer than 50%) were associated with a left-sided "tightness" in her neck. Each headache attack was also associated with nausea, occasional vomiting, photophobia (sensitivity to light), and phonophobia (sensitivity to sound). The attacks were not associated with her menses.

### Relationship with Sleep

No pain episodes were reported upon awakening, nor did she report pain that would awaken her.

### Current Medications

Since 2019, for her abortive treatment, she had been taking a non-opioid analgesic combination containing acetaminophen 250 mg/aspirin 250 mg/caffeine 65 mg, up to two tablets, in half of the attacks (usually those with severe accompanying nausea and fatigue). This medication provided moderate relief of her symptoms in approximately half of her attacks.

    The patient was not taking any preventive medications. She reported no known drug allergies or adverse drug reactions.

## Medical History

At the time of presentation, her general health status was good, and her past medical history was noncontributory. Other than the sacral fracture, no other history of trauma or concussion was reported. She was not pregnant nor planning to become pregnant during her participation in the study. A negative pregnancy test was also required before initiating the clinical trial.

A comprehensive review of systems was conducted, and no abnormalities were found other than the patient's chief complaint (neurologic system).

Her habit history was negative for any oral parafunctional habits, awake bruxism, and sleep bruxism. She reported good overall posture at work.

The patient's family history was also noncontributory, apart from a positive history of migraine in her brother.

## Psychosocial History

At the time of the study, the patient was single, with one healthy school-age son, and reported having a good social support system. Her perceived emotional stress was mild overall, with occasional stress related to her dissertation that she felt were associated with the onset of some headache attacks. She reported suitable coping mechanisms and no catastrophizing. Her Beck Depression Inventory-2 yielded a score of 0, which indicated a lack of depressive symptoms (higher scores indicate more severe depressive symptoms).

The patient was a dentist-scientist by profession, working on her doctoral degree. She routinely engaged in physical exercise as it also helped prevent headache attacks. She was a nonsmoker, denied any substance use, drank minimal alcohol, and consumed low amounts of caffeine daily. She reportedly ate a balanced diet with adequate daily water intake.

She described her sleep quality as restorative, feeling refreshed in the morning, without daytime sleepiness, fatigue, or impairment. The patient reported a regular sleep schedule, averaging seven to 8 h per night. Her self-reported sleep latency was, on average, 20 min. She slept alone on her left side and was unaware of nighttime symptoms, such as snoring or apnea. The patient had no difficulties falling asleep or maintaining sleep and did not report frequent awakenings. Mallampati classification and neck circumference were not measured due to the scope of the clinical trial. However, her total Pittsburgh Sleep Quality Index (PSQI) score[11] was calculated to be a 2, which is suggestive of good sleep quality.

## Physical Examination

During her voluntary screening for the clinical trial, the patient was calm, in no acute distress, alert and well-oriented. She was well-developed and well-nourished, appearing to her stated age. She was 5' 4", 116 pounds, with a body mass index of 19.9. She displayed coherent speech and well-organized thought processes. The patient was ambulatory and showed good balance and coordination. She denied any pain at the time of her visit.

During the head and neck inspection, there was no apparent facial asymmetry, good facial coloration and contour, and no involuntary movements of the head and neck. The patient displayed no autonomic symptoms and had no skin lesions. Palpation was negative for pain in both temporal arteries, sinuses (including percussion), and salivary glands (parotid/submandibular glands). There were no signs of masseter hypertrophy and no abnormalities upon visual inspection of the eyes, nose, and ears.

Palpation of the neck was normal at the carotid arteries, and there was no detectable lymphadenopathy.

Her postural evaluation was satisfactory, noting no forward head posture or rolled shoulders.

Cervical range of motion was within normal limits, including rotation, extension, flexion, and lateral side bend.

Mandibular range of motion (including opening and excursive movements) was pain-free, symmetric, without restriction, and within normal limits. Her left temporomandibular joint (TMJ) displayed an opening click (also noticed by the patient) without pain or crepitation. No significant deflection/deviations of the mandible were present. No TMJ locking was reported. TMJ palpation was negative.

Masticatory muscle palpation was positive solely for the bilateral bodies of the masseter, showing non-familiar tenderness to palpation without referred pain. Cervical palpation was positive for the suboccipital muscles, also without referred pain.

Intraoral examination revealed no dental pain or sensitivity. Her occlusion was stable. Oral cancer screening was negative for signs of malignancy. She denied any bite changes.

Cranial nerve II–XII examination revealed no gross abnormalities.

## DISCUSSION

This case report describes a classical clinical presentation of episodic migraine. The patient's medical history and physical examination were unremarkable. She did not present with any red flags or somatosensory abnormalities. Owing to the classic presentation and normal history, no additional testing was performed. Still, the impact of pain on her quality of life was significant. Although she was stable with abortive medication, she sought further pain relief that would not involve additional medications.

### Headache Classification and Differential Diagnosis

According to the International Classification of Headache Disorders (ICHD-3),[12] there are two main types of headaches: primary and secondary. In primary headaches, the headache itself is the disease. In secondary headaches, the headache is produced by another disease process because of its pathophysiology. The three main types of primary headaches are migraine, tension-type headache (TTH), and trigeminal autonomic cephalalgias (TAC). A relevant secondary headache associated with orofacial pain is headache attributed to temporomandibular disorder (TMD). It is discussed later in this section.

As migraine is a clinical diagnosis, a comprehensive patient history is paramount. First, the clinical presentation of our patient lacked autonomic symptoms. Hence, TAC was not considered in the differential diagnosis. The pain was described as unilateral, severe, with a pulsating quality, aggravated by regular physical activity, and associated with nausea, photophobia, and phonophobia. All of these descriptors match the ICHD-3 classification of migraine, as shown in **Tables 1** and **2**, comparing features of migraine (without aura) versus frequent TTH (Yes/No indicates the presence or absence of each feature in our patient).

An important observation accounted for in the ICHD-3 is that if the clinical presentation fulfills all criteria A through D (**Table 1**) other than one (in addition to not fulfilling any other criteria for another headache disorder, and not better accounted for by another ICHD-3 diagnosis), the migraine should be classified as a probable migraine without aura. For instance, when the patient first visited a neurologist in 2014 after experiencing

**Table 1**
**Migraine (without Aura) Diagnostic Criteria**

| Migraine (without Aura) Diagnostic Criteria | | Yes | No |
|---|---|---|---|
| A. At least five attacks fulfilling criteria B-D | | X | |
| B. Headache attacks lasting 4–72 h (untreated or unsuccessfully treated) | | X | |
| C. Headache has *at least two* of the following: | Unilateral location | X | |
| | Pulsating quality | X | |
| | Moderate or severe pain intensity | X | |
| | Aggravation by or causing avoidance of routine physical activity | X | |
| D. During headache *at least one* of the following: | Nausea and/or vomiting | X | |
| | Photophobia and phonophobia | X | |
| E. Not better accounted for by another ICHD-3 diagnosis. | | X | |

only a single headache attack, her diagnosis of migraine did not meet Criteria A and would have been more accurately classified as a probable migraine.

It is crucial to consider the two major subtypes of migraine during the clinical examination: migraine with and without aura. Aura are recurrent and fully reversible focal neurologic disturbances, including sensory, visual, or motor symptoms, that can occur before or during a migraine attack, and occasionally without an accompanying headache. They occur in approximately 30% of migraineurs.[13] Our case did not involve a present or past history of aura, so the diagnosis was directed toward migraine without aura. However, for completeness, the diagnostic criteria for migraine with aura are presented in **Table 3**.

Another aspect of the classification refers to the frequency of attacks. The ICHD-3[12] recommends that a "headache occurring on 15 or more d/mo for more than 3 months, which, on at least 8 d/mo, has the features of migraine headache" should be classified as chronic migraine. However, the International Headache Society guidelines for controlled clinical trials in chronic migraine also recommend that "Subjects having at least 14 headache days within 28 calendar days, with at least 8 days with migrainous features during the 28-day period, should qualify for a diagnosis of chronic migraine."[14] Our patient had less than 14 headache days; therefore, she was included in the study as having episodic migraine.

**Table 2**
**Frequent Episodic TTH Diagnostic Criteria**

| Frequent Episodic TTH Diagnostic Criteria | | Yes | No |
|---|---|---|---|
| A. At least 10 episodes of headache occurring on 1–14 d/mo on average for >3 mo ($\geq$12 and < 180 d/y) and fulfilling criteria B–D | | | X |
| B. Lasting from 30 min to 7 d | | X | |
| C. *At least two* of the following: | Bilateral location | | X |
| | Pressing or tightening (non-pulsating) quality | | X |
| | Mild or moderate intensity | | X |
| | Not aggravated by routine physical activity such as walking or climbing stairs | | X |
| D. *Both* of the following: | No nausea or vomiting | | X |
| | No more than one of photophobia or phonophobia | | X |
| E. Not better accounted for by another ICHD-3 diagnosis. | | | X |

**Table 3**
**Migraine (with Aura) Diagnostic Criteria**

| Migraine (with Aura) Diagnostic Criteria | | Yes | No |
|---|---|:---:|:---:|
| A. At Least two Attacks Fulfilling Criteria B and C | | X | |
| B. Aura consists of *at least one* of the following fully reversible symptoms: | Visual | | X |
| | Sensory | | X |
| | Speech and/or language | | X |
| | Motor | | X |
| | Brainstem | | X |
| | Retinal | | X |
| C. *At least three* of the following: | At least one aura symptom spreads gradually $\geq$5 min | | X |
| | Two or more aura symptoms occur in succession | | X |
| | Each individual aura symptom lasts 5–60 min | X | X |
| | At least one aura symptom is unilateral | | X |
| | At least one aura symptom is positive | | X |
| | The aura is accompanied, or followed within 60 min, by headache | | X |
| D. Not better accounted for by another ICHD-3 diagnosis. | | | X |

Migraine is a highly prevalent and debilitating neurovascular disorder.[15] On the basis of the data collected through the MIDAS questionnaire, approximately 3% of episodic migraineurs and close to 25% of chronic migraineurs reported a high level of disability relating to severe headaches.[16] Although episodic migraines do not cause the same high frequency of disability as chronic migraines, chronification can occur if risk factors such as ineffective acute treatment and stressful life events are not addressed.[17] Our patient presented both as contributing factors in her migraine attacks. Therefore, it is essential to recognize these risk factors and implement adequate treatment to manage migraine symptoms.

The first-line treatment of episodic migraines is pharmacologic, with triptans usually recommended as the initial choice. Unfortunately, triptans frequently cause adverse effects, one of which is somnolence (reported by our patient). It is also the most troublesome adverse event.[18] Non-pharmacological treatment modalities, such as neuromodulation through transcranial direct current stimulation (tDCS) over the primary motor cortex (M1), are a safe and well-tolerated treatment approach to migraine.[9,19,20] We report her clinical trial results that include PET with [$^{11}$C] carfentanil (a selective $\mu$OR radioligand) before and after ten-daily active or sham sessions of contralateral M1 HD-tDCS (the manuscript detailing the complete clinical trial results is under review elsewhere).

As mentioned at the beginning of this section, headache attributed to TMD is a common and relevant secondary headache caused by a disorder involving structures in the temporomandibular region.[12] It is imperative to consider this type of secondary headache disorder as a differential diagnosis, for instance, in cases where the headache has a temporal relationship to the onset of TMD and/or the headache is aggravated by the motion, function, or parafunction of the jaw. The complete ICHD-3 diagnostic criteria for Headache attributed to TMD are shown in **Table 4**.

Considering non-pharmacological treatment options for chronic TMD patients, our laboratory has investigated the neuromodulatory effects of repetitive M1 HD-tDCS in patients with chronic TMD,[21] with some patients also having pain in the temporalis region as part of their masticatory dysfunction. The study was a randomized controlled

| Table 4 | | |
|---|---|---|
| **Headache attributed to TMD Diagnostic Criteria** | | |
| Headache Attributed to TMD Diagnostic Criteria | Yes | No |
| A. Any headache fulfilling criterion C | | X |
| B. Clinical evidence of a painful pathological process affecting elements of the temporomandibular joint(s), muscles of mastication and/or associated structures on one or both sides | | X |
| C. Evidence of causation shown by *at least two* of the following:     The headache has developed in temporal relation to the onset of the temporomandibular disorder, or led to its discovery | | X |
|     The headache is aggravated by jaw motion, jaw function (eg, chewing) and/or jaw parafunction (eg, bruxism) | | X |
|     The headache is provoked on physical examination by temporalis muscle palpation and/or passive movement of the jaw | | X |
| D. Not better accounted for by another ICHD-3 diagnosis. | | X |

trial consisting of five daily applications of 20 min of sham or active two milliamps (mA) HD-tDCS. At 1-month follow-up, among some of the outcome measures collected, the active HD-tDCS group had more patients with TMD who responded to treatment with higher than 50% pain relief in the visual analog scale (VAS). Overall, our study adds to the body of evidence reported in the literature supporting the use of HD-tDCS for the management of TMD and migraines.

### Neuroimaging Analyses, Results, and Interpretation of Outcome Measures

The patient's M/S headache days over 1-month after M1 HD-tDCS decreased by 50%, from 12 days to 6 days per month. Her pain intensity was reduced from 7 to 5 on an NRS, indicating that HD-tDCS may efficiently reduce M/S headache days and symptom severity. Also, as her headaches became less frequent and severe, she required less medication to manage her migraines compared with before the treatment.

We acquired longitudinal PET with [$^{11}$C] carfentanil 6 and 7 days before and after M1 HD-tDCS, respectively, expecting that it would help explain the clinical improvement with the underlying mechanism. μOR binds to endogenous peptides (eg, β-endorphin) and various opiate drugs (eg, morphine, fentanyl), exerting strong analgesic effects and motivational and rewarding properties.[22–24]

After 1 week of tDCS, we observed an increased μOR availability in the limbic-descending pain modulatory regions, measured during a sustained thermal pain threshold (STPT) challenge in the PET scanner (**Fig. 2**). Based on our visual examination, change in μOR availability was notable in the parahippocampal gyrus and temporal pole ipsilateral to the stimulation and rostral Anterior Cingulate Cortex (ACC) contralateral to the stimulation. The STPT paradigm was developed in-house to measure the pain threshold of the trigeminal mandibular region (V3) ipsilateral to the worst headache side by using a 16 mm$^2$ thermal probe system (MEDOC Pathway Model, Ramat Yishai, Israel). Experimental details have been described previously.[25]

Two PET acquisitions were performed 1 week before and after HD-tDCS over M1. Increased μOR availability, measured through [$^{11}$C] carfentanil non-displaceable

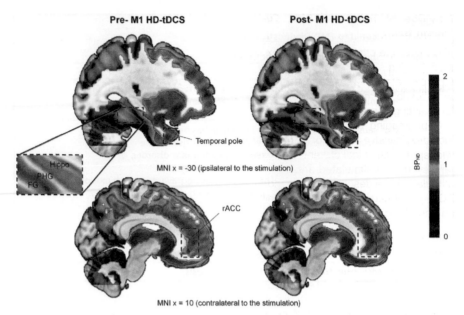

Fig. 2. PET studies of μ-opioid receptor availability. Two PET acquisitions were performed 1 week before and after HD-tDCS over M1. Increased μOR availability, measured through [$^{11}$C] carfentanil non-displaceable binding potential (BP$_{ND}$), during thermal pain threshold stimulation (late phase: 45–90 min after radioligand injection) in this patient is indicated by the dashed rectangle.

binding potential (BP$_{ND}$), during thermal pain threshold stimulation (late phase: 45–90 min after radioligand injection) in this patient is indicated by the dashed rectangle.

### Is there a relationship between these increases in μOR availability and clinical improvement?

Our previous [$^{11}$C] carfentanil PET and voxel-wise analyses showed that relative to episodic migraineurs, patients with chronic migraine showed lower μOR availability, indicating either lower receptor concentration or greater release, in the parahippocampal gyrus and amygdala.[26] Importantly, the lower μOR availability in the amygdala was related to higher migraine attack severity.

Having experienced moderate pain and accompanying emotional distress for more than 6 years, this patient is likely to show downregulated μOR concentration. Research suggests that the chronic pain experience itself (neuropathic injury model) reduces endogenous central nervous system μOR expression, as shown in an animal model.[27] Thus, an increase in receptor expression with treatment might be beneficial in modulating pain symptoms and impeding the progression from episodic to chronic migraine.

The parahippocampal gyrus and temporal pole, both of which are part of the limbic system, are implicated in migraine pathophysiology.[28] Moulton and colleagues[29] showed that hyperactivity of these regions in response to sensory stimuli underpins migraineurs' hypersensitivity to pain. Their role in migraine can additionally be through altered functional connectivity with the hypothalamus,[30,31] contributing to failure in autonomic regulation linked to migraine attacks. These results align with the view that dysautonomia is suggested in the pathogenesis of migraine.[32]

### How Does M1 Transcranial Direct Current Stimulation Change Endogenous Opioid Transmission?

tDCS over the primary motor cortex (M1) has been extensively investigated over the past 20 years as a target for chronic pain management. A weak electric current (approximately 1–2 mA) applied to the scalp induces changes in neuronal firing via modification of resting-membrane potential at a subthreshold level, which can induce long-lasting neural plasticity.[33,34]

Neuroimaging and computational modeling studies show that M1 stimulation, including invasive motor cortex stimulation (MCS) and noninvasive modalities, induces widespread electrical current changes in cortical, subcortical, and brainstem regions far beyond the stimulated areas.[9,35] Among the regions showing changes following stimulation, the descending pain modulatory pathway, including the prefrontal cortex, ACC, periaqueductal gray (PAG), and rostral ventral medulla, has been suggested as an underlying neural correlate for ameliorating chronic pain symptoms.[36,37]

### Translational Neuroscience: The endogenous opioid system and the clinical implication for migraine pathophysiology

An MCS study to treat refractory neuropathic pain with pre- and postoperative [$^{11}$C] diprenorphine PET identified endogenous opioid release in pain control regions (including the anterior and middle cingulate cortex, and PAG) to be associated with pain relief.[38] Our previous tDCS study involving healthy subjects and [$^{11}$C] carfentanil PET showed a reduction in μOR availability in the PAG, precuneus, and prefrontal cortex, and an increase in pain threshold immediately after active M1 tDCS.[39] Although there is limited knowledge of the neurobiological factors that underlie changes in μOR, these pieces of evidence suggest that M1 stimulation works, at least in part, through opioid-mediated top–down modulation of pain processing.

It should be noted that this is the result for a single subject; thus, the current imaging representation cannot rule out expectation-induced placebo (as we have done using sham tDCS). It is widely known that the expectation of pain relief induces μ-opioid transmission in the limbic and prefrontal regions.[40–43] Another possibility is that changes in endogenous opioid signaling partly reflect relief from pain, as shown in an animal[44] and human study.[45] This explanation is relevant given that the μOR is closely implicated in hedonic homeostasis.[46]

As in this patient's case, stress is one of the most well-known triggers for migraine attacks.[47] μOR can act as a modulator of emotional and physical stress.[48] Knowing that repeated stressors and attacks can induce maladaptive brain neuroplasticity in migraineurs, hampering adaptation and promoting chronification,[49,50] future migraine research will benefit from an improved understanding and remodeling of the μOR system involved in stress and pain regulation.

### Limitations

- The tDCS method we used is currently labeled by the Food and Drug Administration (FDA) as an investigational device for investigational use only. Its use in clinics is restricted to research or under strict Institutional Review Board (IRB)-approved protocols for "expanded access."
- The neuroimaging results presented here are part of a group of analyses of several migraineurs included in the clinical trial. It is not intended to be a prescription for tDCS use.
- We only reported clinical outcomes up to 30 days associated with pain reduction. However, longitudinal studies are needed to evaluate the long-term effect of tDCS on migraine.

## CLINICS CARE POINTS

- Migraine may be effectively treated with neuromodulation in those who are unresponsive to medications, complicated by medication side effects, contraindicated to drug treatment, or simply prefer non-pharmacologic management.
- Patients presenting with classical primary headache symptoms are common in orofacial pain practice. Clinicians should be able to identify these patients and provide adequate treatment or referral.
- The International Classification of Headache Disorders criteria are useful to navigate difficult headache diagnoses and prevent the harms of delayed or improper treatment.

## ACKNOWLEDGMENTS

This study was supported by the Grant "Investigation and Modulation of the Mu-Opioid Mechanisms in Migraine (In Vivo)", National Institutes of Health – National Institute of Neurological Disorders and Stroke (NIH-NINDS) R01-NS094413 (Principal Investigator: Dr A.F. DaSilva). The Institutional Review Board (IRB) number of the study is HUM00107286.

## DISCLOSURE

The content described in this study has been developed at the University of Michigan (UM) and disclosed to the UM Office of Tech Transfer. All intellectual property rights, including but not limited to patents/patent applications, trademark, and copyright of software, algorithms, reports, displays, and visualizations, are owned by the Regents of UM. Dr A. F. DaSilva isthe major creator of PainTrek, a technology that tracks and analyzes pain data used in **Fig. 1**. The remaining authors have no conflicts of interest to disclose.

## REFERENCES

1. Vos T, Flaxman AD, Naghavi M, et al. Years lived with disability (YLDs) for 1160 sequelae of 289 diseases and injuries 1990-2010: a systematic analysis for the Global Burden of Disease Study 2010. Lancet Lond Engl 2012;380(9859):2163–96.
2. Steiner TJ, Stovner LJ, Vos T. GBD 2015: migraine is the third cause of disability in under 50s. J Headache Pain 2016;17(1):104.
3. Cai G, Xia Z, Charvet L, et al. A Systematic Review and Meta-Analysis on the Efficacy of Repeated Transcranial Direct Current Stimulation for Migraine. J Pain Res 2021;14:1171–83.
4. Thorlund K, Toor K, Wu P, et al. Comparative tolerability of treatments for acute migraine: A network meta-analysis. Cephalalgia Int J Headache 2017;37(10): 965–78.
5. D'Antona L, Matharu M. Identifying and managing refractory migraine: barriers and opportunities? J Headache Pain 2019;20(1):89.
6. Dodick D, Lipton RB, Martin V, et al. Consensus statement: cardiovascular safety profile of triptans (5-HT agonists) in the acute treatment of migraine. Headache 2004;44(5):414–25.
7. Hepp Z, Dodick DW, Varon SF, et al. Adherence to oral migraine-preventive medications among patients with chronic migraine. Cephalalgia Int J Headache 2015; 35(6):478–88.

8. Ailani J, Burch RC, Robbins MS, et al. The American Headache Society Consensus Statement: Update on integrating new migraine treatments into clinical practice. Headache 2021;61(7):1021–39.

9. Dasilva AF, Mendonca ME, Zaghi S, et al. tDCS-induced analgesia and electrical fields in pain-related neural networks in chronic migraine. Headache 2012;52(8): 1283–95.

10. Stewart WF, Lipton RB, Whyte J, et al. An international study to assess reliability of the Migraine Disability Assessment (MIDAS) score. Neurology 1999;53(5): 988–94.

11. Buysse DJ, Reynolds CF, Monk TH, et al. The Pittsburgh Sleep Quality Index: a new instrument for psychiatric practice and research. Psychiatry Res 1989; 28(2):193–213.

12. Headache Classification Committee of the International Headache Society (IHS). The International Classification of Headache Disorders, 3rd edition. Cephalalgia Int J Headache 2018;38(1):1–211.

13. Viana M, Sances G, Linde M, et al. Prolonged migraine aura: new insights from a prospective diary-aided study. J Headache Pain 2018;19(1):77.

14. Tassorelli C, Diener HC, Dodick DW, et al. Guidelines of the International Headache Society for controlled trials of preventive treatment of chronic migraine in adults. Cephalalgia Int J Headache 2018;38(5):815–32.

15. Ashina M, Katsarava Z, Do TP, et al. Migraine: epidemiology and systems of care. Lancet Lond Engl 2021;397(10283):1485–95.

16. Buse DC, Manack AN, Fanning KM, et al. Chronic migraine prevalence, disability, and sociodemographic factors: results from the American Migraine Prevalence and Prevention Study. Headache 2012;52(10):1456–70.

17. May A, Schulte LH. Chronic migraine: risk factors, mechanisms and treatment. Nat Rev Neurol 2016;12(8):455–64.

18. Dodick DW, Martin V. Triptans and CNS side-effects: pharmacokinetic and metabolic mechanisms. Cephalalgia Int J Headache 2004;24(6):417–24.

19. Przeklasa-Muszyńska A, Kocot-Kępska M, Dobrogowski J, et al. Transcranial direct current stimulation (tDCS) and its influence on analgesics effectiveness in patients suffering from migraine headache. Pharmacol Rep PR 2017;69(4): 714–21.

20. Bikson M, Grossman P, Thomas C, et al. Safety of Transcranial Direct Current Stimulation: Evidence Based Update 2016. Brain Stimulat 2016;9(5):641–61.

21. Donnell A, Nascimento T D, Lawrence M, et al. High-Definition and Non-invasive Brain Modulation of Pain and Motor Dysfunction in Chronic TMD. Brain Stimulat 2015;8(6):1085–92.

22. Schoffelmeer AN, Warden G, Hogenboom F, et al. Beta-endorphin: a highly selective endogenous opioid agonist for presynaptic mu opioid receptors. J Pharmacol Exp Ther 1991;258(1):237–42.

23. Bodnar RJ. Endogenous opiates and behavior: 2014. Peptides 2016;75:18–70.

24. Gibula-Tarlowska E, Kotlinska JH. Crosstalk between Opioid and Anti-Opioid Systems: An Overview and Its Possible Therapeutic Significance. Biomolecules 2020;10(10):E1376.

25. Nascimento TD, DosSantos MF, Lucas S, et al. μ-Opioid activation in the midbrain during migraine allodynia - brief report II. Ann Clin Transl Neurol 2014;1(6): 445–50.

26. Jassar H, Nascimento TD, Kaciroti N, et al. Impact of chronic migraine attacks and their severity on the endogenous μ-opioid neurotransmission in the limbic system. Neuroimage Clin 2019;23:101905.

27. Thompson SJ, Pitcher MH, Stone LS, et al. Chronic neuropathic pain reduces opioid receptor availability with associated anhedonia in rat. Pain 2018;159(9): 1856–66.

28. Chong CD, Schwedt TJ, Dodick DW. Migraine: What Imaging Reveals. Curr Neurol Neurosci Rep 2016;16(7):64.

29. Moulton EA, Becerra L, Maleki N, et al. Painful heat reveals hyperexcitability of the temporal pole in interictal and ictal migraine States. Cereb Cortex N Y N 1991 2011;21(2):435–48.

30. Moulton EA, Becerra L, Johnson A, et al. Altered hypothalamic functional connectivity with autonomic circuits and the locus coeruleus in migraine. PLoS One 2014; 9(4):e95508.

31. Messina R, Rocca MA, Valsasina P, et al. Clinical correlates of hypothalamic functional changes in migraine patients. Cephalalgia Int J Headache 2022;42(4–5): 279–90.

32. Gazerani P, Cairns BE. Dysautonomia in the pathogenesis of migraine. Expert Rev Neurother 2018;18(2):153–65.

33. Nitsche MA, Paulus W. Excitability changes induced in the human motor cortex by weak transcranial direct current stimulation. J Physiol 2000;(527 Pt 3):633–9.

34. Yavari F, Jamil A, Mosayebi Samani M, et al. Basic and functional effects of transcranial Electrical Stimulation (tES)-An introduction. Neurosci Biobehav Rev 2018; 85:81–92.

35. DaSilva AF, Truong DQ, DosSantos MF, et al. State-of-art neuroanatomical target analysis of high-definition and conventional tDCS montages used for migraine and pain control. Front Neuroanat 2015;9:89.

36. Mercer Lindsay N, Chen C, Gilam G, et al. Brain circuits for pain and its treatment. Sci Transl Med 2021;13(619):eabj7360.

37. DosSantos MF, Ferreira N, Toback RL, et al. Potential Mechanisms Supporting the Value of Motor Cortex Stimulation to Treat Chronic Pain Syndromes. Front Neurosci 2016;10:18.

38. Maarrawi J, Peyron R, Mertens P, et al. Motor cortex stimulation for pain control induces changes in the endogenous opioid system. Neurology 2007;69(9): 827–34.

39.. DosSantos MF, Martikainen IK, Nascimento TD, et al. Building up Analgesia in Humans via the Endogenous μ-Opioid System by Combining Placebo and Active tDCS: A Preliminary Report. PLoS ONE 2014;9(7):1–9. Available at: https://www.ncbi.nlm.nih.gov/pmc/articles/PMC4100885/ [cited 2020 Nov 23].

40. Wager TD, Scott DJ, Zubieta JK. Placebo effects on human mu-opioid activity during pain. Proc Natl Acad Sci U S A 2007;104(26):11056–61.

41. Scott DJ, Stohler CS, Egnatuk CM, et al. Placebo and nocebo effects are defined by opposite opioid and dopaminergic responses. Arch Gen Psychiatry 2008; 65(2):220–31.

42. Prossin A, Koch A, Campbell P, et al. Effects of placebo administration on immune mechanisms and relationships with central endogenous opioid neurotransmission. Mol Psychiatry 2022;27(2):831–9.

43. Zubieta JK, Bueller JA, Jackson LR, et al. Placebo Effects Mediated by Endogenous Opioid Activity on μ-Opioid Receptors. J Neurosci 2005;25(34):7754–62.

44. Navratilova E, Xie JY, Meske D, et al. Endogenous opioid activity in the anterior cingulate cortex is required for relief of pain. J Neurosci Off J Soc Neurosci 2015;35(18):7264–71.

45. Sirucek L, Price RC, Gandhi W, et al. Endogenous opioids contribute to the feeling of pain relief in humans. Pain 2021;162(12):2821–31.

46. Darcq E, Kieffer BL. Opioid receptors: drivers to addiction? Nat Rev Neurosci 2018;19(8):499–514.
47. Sauro KM, Becker WJ. The stress and migraine interaction. Headache 2009; 49(9):1378–86.
48. Ribeiro SC, Kennedy SE, Smith YR, et al. Interface of physical and emotional stress regulation through the endogenous opioid system and mu-opioid receptors. Prog Neuropsychopharmacol Biol Psychiatry 2005;29(8):1264–80.
49. Maleki N, Becerra L, Borsook D. Migraine: maladaptive brain responses to stress. Headache 2012;52(Suppl 2):102–6.
50. Borsook D, Youssef AM, Simons L, et al. When pain gets stuck: the evolution of pain chronification and treatment resistance. Pain 2018;159(12):2421–36.

# Challenges for the Dentist in Managing Orofacial Pain

Reny de Leeuw, DDS, PhD, MPH*, Diego Fernandez-Vial, DDS

## KEYWORDS

- Endodontist • Orthodontist • Prosthodontist • Temporomandibular joint
- Orofacial pain • Dentist • Root canal treatment • Extraction

## KEY POINTS

- Lack of understanding of orofacial pain conditions may lead to multiple irreversible treatments by dentists and specialists in other disciplines.
- Lack of pain relief may result in doctor shopping and puts the patient at risk for unnecessary and potentially damaging treatments.
- Providers should be warned that repeating procedures (ie, multiple root canal treatments, oral appliances, and other treatments by different providers) that fail to reduce pain and expecting different results is usually not beneficial and usually costly to the patient.

## IDENTIFICATION INFORMATION

- Age: 67 years old.
- Sex: Female.

## CHIEF COMPLAINT

- *Chief complaint:* "Continued discomfort at tooth extraction sites and jaw pain."
- *Patient goals:* She stated that she did not have any expectations from this appointment, and that she came only because her current dentist insisted.

## HISTORY OF PRESENT ILLNESS/PROBLEM

The patient reported that 7 years before consulting our clinic, she started experiencing episodes of intense sharp pain in the upper left molar area, sometimes waking her up in the middle of the night. After clinical examination and imaging, her primary dentist (Provider #1) found neither evident pathologic condition nor any explanation for the pain and recommended doing a root canal treatment in the maxillary left second molar (tooth #15) based only on the location of the pain. Because the pain did not resolve in

Division Orofacial Pain, University of Kentucky College of Dentistry, Kentucky Clinic, Second Floor, Wing C, Room E214, 740 South Limestone, Lexington, KY 40536-0284, USA
* Corresponding author.
*E-mail address:* renydeleeuw@uky.edu

Dent Clin N Am 67 (2023) 173–185
https://doi.org/10.1016/j.cden.2022.07.013
0011-8532/23/© 2022 Elsevier Inc. All rights reserved.

the following weeks, the same dentist repeated the root canal treatment. After this did not result in pain relief, an endodontist (Provider #2) repeated the procedure 2 more times. The endodontist decided not to repeat the procedure a third time because he decided that her pain was *"clearly a bite issue"* and she was referred her to an orthodontist (Provider #3).

After a "meticulous and thorough examination," which included radiographs and a 2-night home sleep apnea test (pulse oximetry only that revealed some episodes of oxygen desaturation that reached a minimum of 90%), the orthodontist explained to her that her pain was caused by an *"alignment problem."* The dentist warned her that the problem was something more serious than just dental pain because it was also correlated with a significant narrowing of her airway, and the dentist *"was afraid that this would shorten her life unless she had orthodontic and surgical treatment to correct the problem."* She was evaluated by an oral and maxillofacial surgeon (Provider #4), who agreed with the plan of surgically facilitated orthodontic treatment (SFOT). She underwent this surgical intervention and started orthodontic treatment with clear aligners. Almost 8 months later, still undergoing orthodontic treatment, she reported that she started experiencing intense sharp pain in the area of the mandibular left molars that was described with the same characteristics as the pain in the maxillary area but more intense and frequent. Because it was not possible to get the necessary tooth movements with the aligners and the new pain, the providers decided to change the treatment plan. They recommended a full-mouth reconstruction with crowns on all her teeth (28 teeth without previous restorative treatments other than composites) to achieve occlusal stability, to alleviate her pain and to improve the "life-threatening airway narrowing." She consulted the endodontist (Provider #2) again because of the pain who decided not to proceed with any further treatment at that time because the cause and origin of the pain was not clear. One week later, because there was no resolution of the new pain, she was evaluated by a different endodontist (Provider #5), who decided to do a root canal treatment in the mandibular left second molar (tooth #18). She stated that the pain slightly reduced in frequency and intensity, reaching the same characteristics as the pain in the maxillary area.

Next, she was evaluated by the prosthodontist (Provider #6) who was affiliated with the orthodontist and the oral surgeon. The prosthodontist planned to start with the preparation of the crowns of the premolars and molars and their temporary crowns, and then to prepare the anterior teeth to cement all the final crowns at the same time. The patient reported that during the period that she had the provisional crowns on the posterior teeth, she started experiencing a new type of pain in addition to the previously described maxillary and mandibular and still unresolved pain. She mentioned that the new pain was located bilaterally in the masseter areas and angle of the mandible (more intense on the left side), and described it as deep aching, with variable intensity between 2/10 and 6/10 (worse at the end of the day), aggravated by weather changes and chewing hard and chewy food. She stated she started taking high doses of ibuprofen (3200 mg/d) and acetaminophen (total 3250 mg/d). Even though the patient was experiencing intense pain, the prosthodontist recommended that she proceed with the restorative treatment, and they prepared the anterior teeth and placed the temporary crowns. Motivated by the pain and no signs of improvement, she decided to obtain a "second opinion" and consulted another orthodontist (Provider #7), who agreed with the treatment plan and explained that the *"bite issues would be resolved in the provisional stage."* After she completed the full-mouth reconstruction and her "bite misalignment was corrected" the pain remained unchanged. The prosthodontist recommended soft-diet and fabricated upper and lower appliances to be used 24/7 to help with the pain. After multiple adjustments of the appliances, the prosthodontist notified the patient that the appliance adjustments "*would no longer be considered part of the post-operative care.*"

The patient's primary dentist (Provider #1) referred her to be evaluated by a different orthodontist to get another "second opinion." The patient reported that the new orthodontist (Provider #8) told her: "*I have seen too many cases like this,*" and he delivered a new set of appliances. Due to no improvement, the primary dentist (Provider #1) and the initial endodontist (Provider #2) decided to order a computerized tomography (CT) scan. The CT scan showed an abscess of tooth #15. Additionally, the endodontist mentioned that tooth #18 was "*depressible,*" and recommended extraction of both teeth. An oral surgeon (Provider #9) extracted the teeth and performed a bone graft to prepare the area for implants to be placed in the future. The extractions did not improve the pain.

Subsequently, the patient consulted a new dentist (Provider #10), who after evaluating her (including panoramic radiograph) mentioned that "*the oral cavity enlargement surgery and other treatments were unnecessary. I am sorry that someone in my profession did this to you.*" She was referred to a "TMJ specialist" (Provider #11), who ordered a bilateral temporomandibular joint (TMJ) MRI that showed the disc of the right TMJ to be in an anterior position in closed and open mouth positions and decided to fabricate a new set of appliances and recommended home exercises. Shortly after she started using the new appliances, she had a follow-up appointment with her endodontist (Provider #2), who questioned that the pain could originate in a muscle or the joint. The patient decided to visit her original dentist (Provider #1), who recommended a trial of cyclobenzaprine 15 mg at bedtime. The patient stated that for the first time she started noticing improvement of her overall pain, reaching 60% to 70% improvement after 1 month. After that, the "TMJ specialist" (Provider #11) gave her a diagnosis of "phantom pain" and decided to try injecting a mix of local anesthetic, Sarapin (an aqueous solution containing select soluble salts from the Pitcher plant in benzyl alcohol) and D5W (dextrose 5% in water) solution around the area of tooth #18. She noticed some improvement that lasted for a couple of weeks. The specialist was in transition to retirement and recommended returning to the original treating dentist to be referred to a new provider, stating that "*it was better not to see a surgeon, as they do not know what they are doing.*" She was evaluated by a new dentist (Provider #12), who referred her to another "TMJ specialist" and provided the name of a neurosurgeon in case of wanting a different perspective from outside of the dental field. The new specialist (Provider #13) recommended continuing using a previously fabricated maxillary appliance during day and nighttime, taking cyclobenzaprine 5 mg at bedtime and starting physical therapy. Additionally, this specialist referred the patient to our clinic for further evaluation and to explore other treatment modalities.

At the time the patient presented to our clinic (Provider #14), 7 years after she started experiencing the initial pain, she reported 2 types of pain. She described the first type as episodic, intense "*hot needles,*" with an average frequency of 3 episodes per week with a duration from seconds up to a couple of minutes, and with an intensity that could reach 9/10, located in the area of the extracted left maxillary and mandibular second molars. Touching the areas (intraorally), cold food and drinks, and weather changes were reported as triggering and aggravating factors and applying pressure over the painful areas and taking cyclobenzaprine at bedtime were reported as alleviating factor. The patient denied associated symptoms or motor alterations during the episodes. She described the second type of pain as a constant deep aching, located bilaterally in the masseter and angle of the mandible, with an intensity varying between 2/10 and 6/10 (worse at the end of the day), aggravated by weather changes and chewing hard and chewy food. She mentioned that physical therapy, the use of cyclobenzaprine, and ibuprofen alleviated this type of pain. She stated that her bite had been progressively changing, with the current occlusal contact being only between the right mandibular canine and the maxillary appliance. Additionally, she reported a history of occasional asymptomatic right preauricular clicking noises that started when she was in her twenties, and denied locking episodes.

The patient stated being frustrated because of the multiple providers that she had visited since her pain started, all with different and sometimes contradictory treatment recommendations that resulted in a long history of failed irreversible treatment attempts.

## MEDICAL HISTORY

- Endocrine: Parathyroid adenoma.
- Hospitalizations: For surgical procedures.
- Pulmonary: Obstructive sleep apnea (using continuous positive airway pressure [CPAP] machine).
- Surgical history:
  - Bilateral cataract surgery.
  - Tooth extractions.
  - SFOT.
  - Parathyroidectomy.
- Allergies/adverse drug reactions:
  - Codeine.
  - Latex.
  - Macrodantin.
  - Morphine.
  - Ofloxacin.
- Medications:
  - Cholecalciferol (Vitamin D-3) 50 mcg: 1 capsule per day.
  - Cyclobenzaprine 5 mg at bedtime.
  - Multiple vitamins/minerals over the counter.
  - Ibuprofen 400 mg as needed (infrequent use).

*Review of Prior Records/Communication with other Providers*: The patient provided extensive documentation, including the notes of the previous providers, imaging studies with their reports, and a timeline with a self-report including the evolution of her pain and treatments since her pain started. All the documents supported the history provided by the patient and were described in the "history of the present illness" section. A brain MRI taken recently by her primary care physician was unremarkable.

## PSYCHOSOCIAL ASSESSMENT

- Habit history: The patient denied parafunctional habits.
- Patient reported that currently the pain produced moderate interference of her day-to-day activities and reduction of satisfaction in social and recreational activities.
- History of substance use/current: She denied use of tobacco, alcohol, or recreational drugs.
- History of psychological/psychiatric treatments: Negative.

## CURRENT AFFECTIVE SYMPTOMS/SUICIDAL IDEATION

- Sleep disorder symptoms: She reported restful sleep, with a total duration of 8 hours, and a sleep latency of 30 minutes and occasional awakenings.

- Anxiety symptoms: Patient reported mild anxiety and denied symptoms of depression or current/past suicidal ideation.
- Psychosocial history: She mentioned that her husband is supportive, and that he is always attentive and worried about her suffering.
- Overt pain behavior: Negative.

*Diagnostic studies/imaging*: None at this time.

## PHYSICAL EXAMINATION

1. Pulse rate: 121 bpm.
2. Blood pressure: 164/106 mm Hg.
3. Oxygen saturation: 95%.
4. Temperature: 97.4 °F.
5. Height: 5′ 3″.
6. Weight: 156 lb.
7. Body mass index: 27.67 kg/m$^2$.
8. Pain level: 3/10.

## REVIEW OF SYSTEMS

- Skin: Unremarkable.
- Head, eyes, ears, nose, throat: Tinnitus.
- Neck: Unremarkable.
- Cardiac: Unremarkable.
- Respiratory: Snoring.
- Abdomen: Unremarkable.
- Musculoskeletal: Jaw pain.
- Neurologic: Unremarkable.

## MAXILLOFACIAL EXAMINATION

- General appearance: Unremarkable.
- Mental status: The patient was alert, oriented and was able to answer all the questions and did not exhibit any signs of confusion or memory loss.
- Facial symmetry: Unremarkable.
- Head and neck examination: Head and neck movements were not painful or restricted. No lymphadenopathy observed.
- Oral cavity examination:
  - Hyperalgesia elicited on applying light touch and pressure stimulus over periodontal tissues behind tooth #14. After a couple of minutes, the patient reported she started feeling familiar pain in the area.
  - Palatal tori.
  - No swelling, masses, or lesions noted.
- Masticatory muscle examination: Tenderness elicited on palpation of bilateral temporalis muscles and temporalis tendons (left temporal tendon familiar to jaw pain). No evidence of functional disability or pain to provocation.
- Mandibular function examination: Maximal comfortable opening 34 mm, maximal assisted opening 42 mm (discomfort reported in the left masseter area; no deviation), left excursive 12 mm, right excursive 11 mm, protrusive 8 mm, vertical overlap 2 mm, horizontal overlap 2 mm.
- Occlusal examination: Occlusal contacts identified in the right molar and canine area only (with shim stock). No gross occlusal interferences.

- TMJs: No sounds or interferences noted.
- Cervical muscle examination: Nonfamiliar tenderness elicited on palpation of bilateral sternocleidomastoid (left side radiating to scapular area), occipital, trapezius, and paracervical muscles.
- Description of dentition:
  ○ Absence of teeth #1, 15, 16, 17, 18, and 32.
  ○ All remaining teeth with monolithic ceramic crowns (adequately restored).
- Attrition status: Unremarkable.
- Oral appliances: When wearing only the maxillary appliance (hard flexible retainer), occlusal contacts were observed on teeth #2 and 6. When using both the maxillary and mandibular appliances, contacts were observed on the right molar and canine areas and left first molar.
- Neurologic examination (cranial nerves): Cranial nerves II–XII were grossly intact with no gross observed deficiencies.

*Contributing factors:* Trauma after dental procedures (?), multiple procedures.
*Alternative/differential diagnoses:* Based on International Classification of Orofacial Pain, first edition.[1]

- Differential diagnoses for the pain located in the areas of extraction of teeth #15 and 18:
  ○ Trigeminal neuralgia.
    ▪ Classic trigeminal neuralgia, purely paroxysmal.
    ▪ Secondary trigeminal neuralgia.
    ▪ Idiopathic trigeminal neuralgia, purely paroxysmal.
  ○ Posttraumatic trigeminal neuropathic pain.
  ○ Idiopathic trigeminal neuropathic pain.
  ○ Trigeminal autonomic orofacial pain.
  ○ Neurovascular orofacial pain.
  ○ Referred pain from other structures (heterotopic pain).
- Differential diagnoses for the pain located bilaterally in the masseter and angle of the mandible areas:
- Chronic, highly frequent primary myofascial orofacial pain without pain referral.
- Myofascial orofacial pain attributed to tendonitis of the temporalis muscle.

## IMPRESSIONS
### Problem-Oriented Workup

- Problem list pain in certain areas unresolved after multiple interventions:
  ○ Pain in the area of extraction of tooth #15.
  ○ Pain in the area of extraction of tooth #18.
  ○ Pain located bilaterally in the masseter area and angle of the mandible.
- Problem additional evaluation—diagnostic tests:
  ○ A topical medication in Orabase (amitriptyline 2%, carbamazepine 5%, and benzocaine 6%) was placed over the extraction site of tooth #15. The medication was applied after the patient stated that she started feeling the "*hot needles*" pain in that area during the intraoral examination. Patient reported complete relief after less than 1 minute.
  ○ Left temporalis tendon diagnostic block: A total of 1 mL of 3% mepivacaine (without vasoconstrictor) was injected in the area. Preoperative jaw pain: 4/10. After 10 minutes, the patient reported significant improvement, being able to open wider without pain. No pain elicited on palpation of left temporalis muscle.

- Rule out reasoning for the different pain complaints:
- For the pain located in the areas of extraction of teeth #15 and 18:
  - Trigeminal neuralgia.
    - Classic or secondary trigeminal neuralgia, purely paroxysmal. Ruled out because there was no evidence of neurovascular compression of the trigeminal nerve or any disease in brain MRI.
    - Idiopathic trigeminal neuralgia, purely paroxysmal. Ruled out because of the presence of positive somatosensory symptoms (hyperalgesia) associated with the pain.
  - Posttraumatic trigeminal neuropathic pain. *Potential diagnosis* because the pain was located in the distribution of the trigeminal nerve, recurring for more than 3 months, with a history of injury to the trigeminal nerve. Additionally, positive somatosensory symptoms (hyperalgesia) were observed during examination.
  - Idiopathic trigeminal neuropathic pain. Ruled out because of traumatic factor (infection, root canal treatment, and other treatments) associated with the current pain.
  - Trigeminal autonomic orofacial pain. Ruled out because of absence of autonomic signs and symptoms.
  - Neurovascular orofacial pain. Ruled out because of absence of autonomic signs and symptoms or migrainous features.
  - Referred pain from other structures (heterotopic pain). Ruled out because local stimulation of the site of pain elicited familiar pain, and resolution of the pain was obtained after topical anesthetic block of the site of pain. In addition, the pain was not reproduced by palpation of any other structures.
- For the pain located bilaterally in the masseter muscles and angle of the mandible:
  - Chronic highly frequent primary myofascial orofacial pain without pain referral of the bilateral temporalis muscles. Ruled out because the location of the pain reported by the patient did not match the pain elicited when palpating the temporalis muscles and was not familiar to her complaint.
  - Myofascial orofacial pain attributed to tendonitis of the temporalis muscle. *Potential diagnosis* because familiar pain was elicited on palpation of the area, and the anesthetic block of the left temporalis tendon area resulted in a significant decrease of the pain.

## DIAGNOSES

- Posttraumatic trigeminal neuropathic pain—second and third branch of the left trigeminal nerve.
- Myofascial orofacial pain attributed to tendonitis of the temporalis muscles—bilateral.

## TREATMENT PLAN

- Reassurance and education of the patient's conditions.
- Self-care therapy recommendations including soft diet, muscle relaxation, habit control, sleep hygiene, and functioning within pain free limits.
- Temporalis tendon anesthetic block to be repeated in the future if proven beneficial.
- Use of topical medication tried in clinic along with cyclobenzaprine.
- Continue with physical therapy.

- Discontinue the daytime use of the current appliance. Fabrication of a maxillary hard acrylic stabilization appliance (full coverage providing simultaneous bilateral symmetric contacts) by referring dentist for use at nighttime only.
- The above recommendations were provided to the referring dentist.
- No follow-up was scheduled due to long travel distance; patient was assured we are available for follow-up.

## COURSE OF CARE AND OUTCOMES

One month after the appointment, the patient was contacted; the patient reported an average pain intensity of 1/10 to 2/10, aggravated by cold weather and rainy days. Patient reported taking cyclobenzaprine every night and using the topical medication for flare-ups. She stated to be satisfied with the results of our treatment, and that the current pain was *"something she can live with."*

## CLINICS CARE POINTS
### *Problems Identified in the Case that Are Common Pitfalls*

In the case presentation, multiple problems were identified that led to inappropriate care to which both the providers and the patient contributed. From the provider's perspective, there was a lack of agreement in diagnosis and subsequent treatment needs escalating to multiple incorrect invasive and irreversible interventions. From the patient's perspective, there was a pursuit for an explanation and resolution of the pain, resulting in visiting multiple different dental care providers and acceptance of multiple expensive and invasive treatments. In the following, these and additional items that may lead to challenges for the general dentist in the management of orofacial pain (OFP), and the authors' recommendations to approach them, will be discussed.

*Lack of educational resources in OFP.* In the United States, there are not enough OFP referral centers and specialists available to treat patients, which results in some dentists with insufficient training, attempting to treat conditions that they are not sufficiently trained to do. Additionally, there are several organizations with different philosophies providing conflicting continuing education programs, further confusing the field. OFP not being recognized as a specialty for a long time may have played a significant role in that as well. In 2020, the National Commission on Recognition of Dental Specialties and Certifying Boards (NCRDSCB) announced the recognition of OFP as the 12th dental specialty, with the American Academy of Orofacial Pain (AAOP) as the official dental specialty sponsoring organization. OFP was officially defined as "the specialty of dentistry that encompasses the diagnosis, management and treatment of pain disorders of the jaw, mouth, face, head and neck. The specialty of OFP is dedicated to the evidenced-based understanding of the underlying pathophysiology, etiology, prevention, and treatment of these disorders and improving access to interdisciplinary patient care."[2] OFP-associated disorders include but are not limited to temporomandibular disorders, jaw movement disorders, neuropathic and neurovascular pain disorders, headache, and sleep disorders.[3] In March of 2022, the American Board of Orofacial Pain (ABOP) was recognized by the NCRDSCB as the official specialty certifying board. These 2 important milestones will help unify the promotion of education and research in this area and provide higher standards of patient care. It is important for the general dentist and other dental specialists to establish a referral-network that includes recognized OFP specialists. The AAOP standard for a specialist in OFP "is a licensed dentist (DDS, DMD or equivalent degree) who has demonstrated an exceptional understanding of the diagnosis, management and treatment of orofacial pain through graduate or post graduate training, research or clinical experience and meets one or more of the following standards: (1) is a Fellow of the AAOP; (2) has successfully completed a formal advanced education program in orofacial pain of at least two years that is now accredited by the Commission on Dental Accreditation (CODA); and/or (3) has passed the ABOP certification examination. Additionally, the specialist adheres to the all legal requirements in accordance with the laws and regulations of their competent licensing and jurisdictional authority (state licensing administration/state dental board/commission, etc.)."[3]

*Noncompliance with essential principles of ethics and practicing beyond the scope of practice of dentistry.* The principles of patient autonomy, nonmaleficence, beneficence, justice and veracity, that form the foundation of the American Dental Association code of ethics,[4] were clearly not respected on multiple occasions in the case presented above. The intention of this article is not to provide a lecture about ethics, instead, to serve as a reminder that we, dentists, must always keep as the main goal to promote patient's welfare. Consequently, to achieve that, it is imperative to keep knowledge and skills current, to know the limitations of practice and when to refer to a specialist or other professional. It was also observed that the patient was diagnosed by one of the providers with an obstructive sleep breathing disorder based on a low-quality home sleep apnea test, without proper referral to a qualified medical provider for further evaluation and adequate management. Consequently, she underwent an invasive and irreversible treatment (failed SFOT, leading to full mouth rehabilitation) that was not founded by scientific evidence, and may have led to an inadequate management of a life-threatening condition. It is important to recognize the limits of dental practice and to recognize when other medical or dental providers need to be involved.

*Deficiency in clinical and diagnostic reasoning.* It is not necessary for a general dentist to know all the pain-related diagnoses that may affect the stomatognathic system and how to treat them. However, it is fundamental to be able to recognize when a painful condition does not fit the characteristics of classic dental and periodontal pain. This is important to avoid irreversible treatments that may aggravate a condition, especially in the absence of clinical evidence to support a decision to perform the treatment. Unquestionably, in the case history described there were clear characteristics of nonodontogenic pain that were not recognized by multiple providers, leading to a repetition of the endodontic treatment 4 times with the same failed outcome.

When talking about pain, several different types of pain can be distinguished.[5] First, in normal conditions, after exposure to a noxious stimulus such as something too hot or cold, *nociceptive pain* will help activate an early-warning protective system in order to avoid tissue damage. Second, also in physiologic conditions, *inflammatory pain* will usually start after tissue injury or infection in order to help avoid further risk of damage and to promote recovery. Some stimuli that were innocuous before (ie, light touch), will now elicit pain. In some cases, instead of being protective, pain can become *pathologic* because of maladaptation and abnormal functioning of the central nervous system after damage or disease (*neuropathic pain*) but also in circumstances in which there is no such damage (*dysfunctional pain*).[5] It is important to differentiate these different types of pain in order to direct treatment in the appropriate direction. **Table 1** summarizes pain quality descriptors and secondary symptoms associated with different pain categories that can affect the orofacial region. Additional validated questionnaires may be used to help identify specific types of pain, such as neuropathic pain (Leeds Assessment of Neuropathic Symptoms and Signs,[6] Douleur Neuropatique [DN4],[7] NPQ,[8] painDETECT,[9] ID Pain,[10] Neuropathic Pain Symptom Inventory).[11]

**Table 1**
**Pain quality descriptors and secondary symptoms associated with different pain categories that can affect the orofacial region**

| Type of Pain | Quality | Secondary Symptoms |
|---|---|---|
| Tooth pulp (acute/chronic) | Sharp, shooting, throbbing, dull | • Pain may refer and/or radiate to other ipsilateral orofacial locations<br>• Usually evoked by thermal or mechanical stimulus |
| Periodontium and gingivae | Dull, aching, throbbing | • Pain is exacerbated by physical stimuli applied to the tissue overlying the root<br>• Pain may also refer and/or radiate to other ipsilateral orofacial locations |
| Musculoskeletal | Dull, aching, pressure, depressing, tight, stiff, occasionally sharp | • Flushing, hyperalgesia, allodynia<br>• Can refer or be referred from distant sites<br>• Worse with function |
| Neurovascular | Throbbing, pulsating, stabbing, pounding, rhythmic | • Worsened by increasing intracranial pressure (eg, Valsalva bending over, physical activity), sensitivity to light and/or sounds, nausea, vomiting |
| Neuropathic | Shooting, bright, stimulating, burning, itchy, electric shock-like, cutting | • Numbness, hyperalgesia, paresthesia, allodynia, dysesthesia |
| Psychogenic | Descriptive | • Complaint patterns often do not match anatomic sensory supply |

*Adapted from* de Leeuw R, Klasser GD. Orofacial Pain: Guidelines for Assessment, Diagnosis, and Management. Vol 2018. 6th ed: Quintessence; 2018; with permission.

It is also important to be aware that, in some cases, the site of the pain (where the pain is felt) does not coincide with the source or origin of the pain (where the tissue injury is located), and this has been named *secondary* or *heterotopic pain*. In those cases, the pain can be emanating from structures of the central nervous system (*central pain*), in another area innervated by the same nerve (*projected pain*), or in an area innervated by a different nerve than the one that mediates the primary nociceptive input (*referred pain*).[12] **Table 2** summarizes identified structures that can produce secondary pain in the orofacial region.

**Fig. 1** contains the clinical and diagnostic reasoning algorithm proposed by the authors that may be helpful in identifying the source of painful conditions. This algorithm also addresses nonpainful conditions affecting the orofacial region. It may not be complete but it may help guide the user in the direction to provide appropriate care and to void unnecessary interventions.

*Open access health information and misinformation sources.* The World Health Organization defined the term *infodemic* as an "overabundance of information, both online and offline."[13] They also pointed out that misinformation and disinformation can result in physical and mental harm, stigmatization, and inappropriate use of recourses. Even though that definition was provided in 2020 in relation to the massive "outbreak" of information associated to the COVID-19 pandemic, it certainly also represents what has been happening at a lesser extent in the past decades in relation to health-related

**Table 2**
**Structures and diseases that can produce secondary pain felt in the orofacial region**

| Site of Pain (Secondary Pain) | Origin of Pain/Underlying Disease |
|---|---|
| Toothaches:<br>• Mandibular molars<br>• Maxillary incisors<br>• Maxillary premolars<br>• Maxillary molars<br>• Maxillary canines, premolars, and molars<br>• Mandibular incisors<br>• Left mandibular molars | • Superficial masseter<br>• Anterior temporalis<br>• Middle temporalis<br>• Posterior temporalis<br>• Maxillary sinus<br>• Anterior digastric<br>• Cardiovascular |
| Left angle and body of the mandible | Cardiovascular |
| Jaws, ears, headaches | Cervicogenic |
| Vascular headaches | Elevated blood pressure |
| Throat, ear, headaches, mandible | Thyroid disease |
| First, second, and third branches of the trigeminal nerve | Central or peripheral nervous system secondary to trauma, multiple sclerosis, vascular compression, or space-occupying lesions |
| TMJs, masticatory muscles | Systemic lupus erythematous |

data. As clinicians, we will see multiple patients that have already consulted "Dr Google" before coming to us, and that may predispose them to expect certain specific diagnoses and treatments, which may or may not coincide with the provider's approach. A large prospective study (n = 723) found that 24.5% of patients searched the Internet

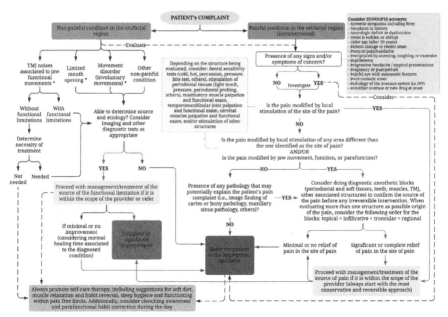

**Fig. 1.** Proposed clinical and diagnostic reasoning algorithm that may be helpful to identify the source of painful conditions. This algorithm also addresses nonpainful conditions affecting the orofacial region.

for their symptoms before going to the emergency department but only a minority of those (29%) searched for the diagnosis they eventually received after the visit.[14] These discrepancies may represent a barrier to establishing a patient–provider relationship, which is fundamental in providing adequate care. Therefore, it is important to always ask patients if they have any idea of what the cause of their pain/problem may be, if they have previously consulted other providers or the Internet, and what their expectations from the present consultation are. In the opinion of the authors, the World Wide Web represents an opportunity more than a threat because it can be used to provide evidence-based education to the general population but for that, it is also important to educate the patients to assume a critical attitude when looking for information online.

The case history exposed the fact that a lack of understanding of orofacial pain conditions may lead to multiple irreversible treatments without solving the real problem of the patient. Conversely, lack of pain relief may result in doctor shopping and puts the patient at risk for unnecessary and potentially damaging treatments. Providers should be warned that repeating failed procedures and expecting different results is usually not beneficial but can be costly to the patient. It is important to always respect the essential principles of ethics and to work within the scope of practice of each specialty, to strengthen the clinical and diagnostic reasoning skills, and to keep knowledge and skills current, to know our limitations and when to refer to a specialist or other professional.

## DISCLOSURE

The authors have nothing to disclose.

## REFERENCES

1. International Classification of Orofacial Pain, 1st edition (ICOP). Cephalalgia 2020;40(2):129–221.
2. National Commission on Recognition of Dental Specialties and Certifying Boards. Specialty Definitions. 2020. Available at: https://ncrdscb.ada.org/en/dental-specialties/specialty-definitions#. Accessed April 24, 2022.
3. American Academy of Orofacial Pain. Press Release: Orofacial Pain is Now the 12th ADA-Recognized Dental Specialty. 2020. Available at: https://aaop.org/wp-content/uploads/2021/01/AAOP-OFP-Specialty-Press-Release-Updated.pdf. Accessed April 24, 2022.
4. American Dental Association Principles of Ethics and Code of Professional Conduct: with official advisory opinions revised to November 2020. 2020. Available at: https://www.ada.org/en/about-the-ada/principles-of-ethics-code-of-professional-conduct. Accessed April 24, 2022.
5. Woolf CJ. What is this thing called pain? J Clin Invest 2010;120(11):3742–4.
6. Bennett M. The LANSS Pain Scale: the Leeds assessment of neuropathic symptoms and signs. Pain 2001;92(1–2):147–57.
7. Bouhassira D, Attal N, Alchaar H, et al. Comparison of pain syndromes associated with nervous or somatic lesions and development of a new neuropathic pain diagnostic questionnaire (DN4). Pain 2005;114(1–2):29–36.
8. Krause SJ, Backonja MM. Development of a neuropathic pain questionnaire. Clin J Pain 2003;19(5):306–14.
9. Freynhagen R, Baron R, Gockel U, et al. painDETECT: a new screening questionnaire to identify neuropathic components in patients with back pain. Curr Med Res Opin 2006;22(10):1911–20.

10. Portenoy R. Development and testing of a neuropathic pain screening question-naire: ID Pain. Curr Med Res Opin 2006;22(8):1555–65.

11. Bouhassira D, Attal N, Fermanian J, et al. Development and validation of the Neuropathic Pain Symptom Inventory. Pain 2004;108(3):248–57.

12. Okeson JP. Bell's oral and facial pain. 7th edition. Quintessence Publishing; 2014.

13. WHO U, UNICEF, UNDP, UNESCO, UNAIDS, ITU, UN Global Pulse, & IFRC. Man-aging the COVID-19 infodemic: Promoting healthy behaviours and mitigating the harm from misinformation and disinformation. World Health Organization. 2020. Available at: https://www.who.int/news/item/23-09-2020-managing-the-covid-19-infodemic-promoting-healthy-behaviours-andmitigating-the-harm-from-misinformation-and-disinformation. Accessed April 24, 2022.

14. McCarthy DM, Scott GN, Courtney DM, et al. What Did You Google? Describing Online Health Information Search Patterns of ED patients and Their Relationship with Final Diagnoses. West J Emerg Med 2017;18(5):928–36.

# Language Access and Orofacial Pain

Roxanne Bavarian, DMD, DMSc[a,b], Rachel Harris, DMD[b], Nicole Holland, DDS, MS[c],*

## KEYWORDS

- Orofacial pain • Health literacy • Access to care • Language access
- Limited English proficiency • Interpreter services

## KEY POINTS

- Language access is integral to attaining health literacy and achieving health equity. Individuals with limited English proficiency are subject to greater communication challenges and obstacles when navigating the healthcare system.
- Clear communication is essential to obtain an accurate history and establish a proper diagnosis for successful pain management.
- Providing culturally and linguistically appropriate, patient-centered care in the orofacial pain practice setting is of utmost importance to care quality and treatment outcomes.
- Future research on language access, particularly in the field of orofacial pain, is warranted.

| Abbreviations | |
| --- | --- |
| LEP | Limited English Proficiency |
| OFP | Orofacial pain |

## CASE REPORT

An 84-year-old woman presented to the Massachusetts General Hospital (MGH) Orofacial Pain (OFP) Clinic on referral from her oral surgeon for the evaluation of right-sided, intraoral pain. Her medical record showed Vietnamese as her preferred language, so telephonic interpretation was provided by the hospital. She was accompanied by her adult daughter. Briefly after initiating the visit, the patient's daughter stated that the interpreter was not interpreting her mother's symptoms correctly so she preferred to interpret for her mother.

[a] Department of Oral and Maxillofacial Surgery, Massachusetts General Hospital, 55 Fruit Street, Boston, MA 02114, USA; [b] Harvard School of Dental Medicine, 188 Longwood Avenue, Boston, MA 02115, USA; [c] Tufts University School of Dental Medicine, 1 Kneeland Street, Boston, MA 02111, USA
* Corresponding author.
E-mail address: Nicole.Holland@tufts.edu

Dent Clin N Am 67 (2023) 187–198
https://doi.org/10.1016/j.cden.2022.07.014
0011-8532/23/© 2022 Elsevier Inc. All rights reserved.

dental.theclinics.com

The patient's daughter stated her mother had been having pain for at least 3 months in her right upper jaw. Her mother pointed to her right anterior maxilla, which was completely edentulous. Her pain began 3 months prior following multiple extractions in the maxilla by her local dentist, in preparation for a complete denture. Her daughter confirmed that the remaining maxillary teeth were nonrestorable and not painful before the extractions, although notes from other providers stated the pain was present *before* the extractions. The patient described the pain as constant in nature, with an "aching," "squeezing," and "pulling" sensation, per interpretation through her daughter. She also experienced paroxysms of sharp, shooting pain, which would occur sporadically without any inciting event and last for 2 seconds at a time.

The pain would wake her at night. The pain could also spread throughout the entire maxilla and face, with the patient pointing to her anterior and left maxilla as well to her bilateral temporal and frontal areas. No numbness, tingling, fever, chills, nor symptoms of swelling of the face or mouth were reported.

Following dental extractions, she returned to her local dentist due to persistent pain but no further treatment was recommended. She was not able to wear her dentures and unintentionally lost 10 pounds due to pain and difficulty eating. Approximately 1 month following the extractions, she presented to the MGH Emergency Department where the Oral and Maxillofacial Surgery service was consulted. The consulting oral surgeon documented no signs of acute infection on clinical or radiographic examination but noted the presence of sharp, buccal bony edges underlying the thin gingival tissue of the maxilla. An alveoloplasty was recommended and performed, when a residual root tip of tooth #6 was identified and extracted. Two weeks following the alveoloplasty, the patient reported persistent severe pain and was referred to the OFP clinic. She reported no pain relief with analgesics, including ibuprofen, acetaminophen, and oxycodone 5 mg. The oral surgeon had prescribed oxcarbazepine 150 mg nightly, which she reported taking 300 mg nightly for about a week with no relief. **Fig. 1** depicts a timeline of the case.

Review of her medical history revealed a history of papillary thyroid carcinoma treated with a total thyroidectomy, with hypothyroidism, for which she took levothyroxine 75 mcg. She also had diagnoses of hypertension, for which she took amlodipine 5 mg; stage 3 chronic kidney disease; bronchiectasis, using bronchodilator inhalers; and reflux gastritis, taking ranitidine as needed. She has drug allergies to amoxicillin, which causes a rash. The patient's daughter revealed that the patient lived with her husband, who is also an older adult with medical issues. The patient's daughter is

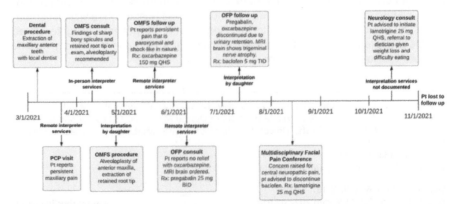

**Fig. 1.** Timeline of patient's history of present illness to date. BID, twice daily; QHS, nightly.

her health-care proxy and accompanies her mother to all appointments. The daughter expressed worry of her mother's ongoing pain and lack of definitive diagnosis.

She was concerned that her mother was not sleeping and waking due to pain. Her mother had been waking confused, scared, and disoriented, and her daughter confirmed that her mother never had any cognitive issues before the onset of facial pain. Review of notes from other providers show the patient has told her daughter that she thinks she may be dying. Of note, the daughter is married and has 2 children. Both she and her husband work full-time and coordinating care of her mother's ongoing health issues has been challenging.

On examination, the patient was seated in a wheelchair due to fatigue and weakness related to her pain and difficulty eating and sleeping. She did not make eye contact during the visit and let her daughter interpret for her. She spoke only with brief phrases in Vietnamese in response to questions. Extraoral examination showed cranial nerves V and VII were intact. Her mandibular range of motion was within normal limits, with 40 mm mouth opening without pain and lateral range of motion approximately 5 mm in both directions. She had tenderness on palpation of her right masseter and right temporalis muscles but this was not consistent with her chief complaint. Palpation of the right infraorbital notch and right anterior maxillary alveolar ridge best duplicated her pain. There was no evidence of erythema or edema of the maxillary alveolar ridge. The alveolar bone was smooth without evidence of sharp bony spicules.

Her differential diagnoses included posttraumatic trigeminal neuropathy of the right anterior maxilla, persistent idiopathic dentoalveolar pain of the anterior maxilla, and trigeminal neuralgia of the right V2 distribution. She also had a component of right-sided myofascial pain. Determining a definitive diagnosis for her neuropathic pain was difficult because it was unclear precisely when the patient's symptoms began (specifically, before or following the dental extractions), the quality of pain, and any exacerbating or relieving factors because the description and chronology of her symptoms seemed to be described differently from visit to visit. Review of her medical records showed inconsistent use of an interpreter, relying on the patient's daughter for interpretation. A brain MRI with trigeminal protocol was ordered to rule out central pathologic condition. For treatment, she was recommended to continue oxcarbazepine 300 mg nightly and initiate pregabalin 25 mg twice daily. Verbal and written instructions were provided to the patient and her daughter to help clarify the dosing.

At 1 month follow-up, the patient and her daughter returned to the OFP clinic. The patient continued to have no relief from her medications. She also developed abdominal pain, bloating, and difficulty urinating, prompting an urgent care visit. The urgent care physician recommended discontinuation of pregabalin. It was unclear for how long the patient had taken pregabalin before discontinuing. She was then advised to discontinue oxcarbazepine. Baclofen was prescribed for her ongoing neuropathic pain, with verbal and written instructions given to begin with 5 mg nightly and gradually increase to 3 times daily as tolerated. A nerve block to the right infraorbital nerve was performed with the patient's consent but led to no relief of pain, raising concern for central neuropathic pain.

The brain MRI revealed atrophy of the cisternal portion of the trigeminal nerve. The case was reviewed in an interdisciplinary meeting with facial pain specialists from neurology, neurosurgery, plastic surgery, and pain psychology. Concern for a central neuropathic pain condition (namely, a trigeminal ganglionopathy) was raised. The patient did not present for her follow-up appointment but a discussion with the patient's daughter through telephone led to recommendations to discontinue baclofen, which had not helped reduce her pain after 4 weeks of use, and initiate lamotrigine 25 mg nightly. Serology for an immune-mediated neuropathy was ordered, including SS-A,

SS-B, ANA, rheumatoid factor, and SPEP. A referral was placed to a neurologist specializing in facial pain, and the neurologist encouraged the patient to initiate lamotrigine 25 mg, which she had not yet started given her history of medication intolerance. The patient was also referred to a dietician for her weight loss since the dental extractions. The patient was subsequently lost to follow-up with no further visits with OFP, neurology, or her PCP.

## HEALTHCARE DISPARITIES, LITERACY, AND LIMITED ENGLISH PROFICIENCY

A quick review of this case may lead one to conclude that it is simply an unfortunate situation involving a noncompliant patient who does not speak English. After all, more than 66 million Americans (21.5%) speak a language other than English at home, with more than 25 million (8.2%) speaking English "less than very well."[1] However, individuals with limited English proficiency (LEP), which is defined as "individuals who do not speak English as their primary language and who have a limited ability to read, speak, write, or understand English,"[2] are subject to greater communication challenges and obstacles when navigating the healthcare system. Clear communication, regardless of language, enhances care quality, improves clinical outcomes, and helps to drive down health-care costs.[3–5] Despite research showing that clear, effective communication is vital to quality patient care, a national survey revealed that 88% of adults lack the health literacy skills required to successfully manage the demands of the US healthcare system.[6] Furthermore, as this case illustrates, language barriers further complicate many aspects of care.

Language, culture, and literacy are closely intertwined, and addressing language differences is integral to attaining health literacy and achieving health equity. As reflected in Healthy People 2030, health literacy (**Box 1**) is required to achieve health and well-being.[7] In fact, increasing the proportion of adults with LEP who say their providers explain things clearly is a national health objective[8] (along with 15 oral health-related objectives and many other high-priority public health issues).[9] Furthermore, the National CLAS (culturally and linguistically appropriate services) Standards also has language access (defined as "providing LEP people with reasonable access to the same services as English-speaking individuals"[10]) fully integrated into its mission—as stated in the Principal Standard: "Provide effective, equitable, understandable, and respectful quality care and services that are responsive to diverse cultural health beliefs and practices, preferred languages, health literacy, and other communication needs."[11] Standards 5 to 8 directly address communication and language assistance in healthcare settings.

---

**Box 1**
**Healthy People 2030 Health Literacy Definition**

*Personal health literacy* is the degree to which individuals have the ability to find, understand, and use information and services to inform health-related decisions and actions for themselves and others.

*Organizational health literacy* is the degree to which organizations equitably enable individuals to find, understand, and use information and services to inform health-related decisions and actions for themselves and others.

*From* Health Literacy in Healthy People 2030. US Department of Health and Human Services - Office of Disease Prevention and Health Promotion. Accessed April 30, 2022. https://health.gov/our-work/healthy-people/healthy-people-2030/health-literacy-healthy-people-2030

Moreover, federal and state laws have been enacted to protect individuals with LEP from discrimination across many societal sectors in this country, including health care. The legal foundation for language access was established with Title VI of the 1964 Civil Rights Act,[12] which has historically been interpreted as failure to provide language access having a discriminatory impact because of national origin.[13] Section 1557 of the Affordable Care Act further prohibits discrimination on the grounds of race, color, national origin, sex, age, or disability by dental practices and other health-care providers receiving federal funds through HHS. Furthermore, state laws provide additional specificity and protections.[14]

Research studies have shown language-related barriers to be associated with medical errors, decreased patient satisfaction, poorer self-management, and worsened clinical outcomes.[15–20] Contrarily, the use of professional interpreters and other quality language assistance services facilitate effective communication across languages, thereby enhancing language access and improving patient engagement and satisfaction, overall care quality, and clinical outcomes; however, language assistance services remain underutilized.[17,21–26]

Although the aforementioned research and policy point to the generalized need for language access in health care, there is a paucity of research on the effects of linguistic diversity on OFP outcomes. The relationships between language, health literacy, and chronic pain have been studied, albeit not robustly. Results of a 2019 study on health literacy, opioid misuse, and pain experience indicated that health literacy was negatively associated with pain severity and pain disability (as well as opioid misuse and severance of opioid dependency) among adults with chronic pain.[27] When examining the relationship between language spoken and pain outcomes, the most robust research focuses on the acculturation literature and yields inconsistent results. For example, greater use of the Spanish language has been associated with disparities in healthcare visits for OFP, not having a usual dentist, having greater pain, increased difficulty eating and sleeping, and more depression.[28] However, other studies have shown greater use of the Spanish language to be associated with less functional limitation due to pain even after adjusting for known risk factors.[29]

Although further research is warranted, the significance of effective communication cannot be understated. Given that (1) a proper diagnosis is foundational to successful pain management and (2) an accurate history is critical to pain diagnosis, we must carefully consider how language barriers influence pain care. Consider the multiple factors considered when eliciting a complete pain history: location, onset, characteristics of initial presentation, duration, clinical course, prior treatment outcomes, relevant physical and emotional background, and prior trauma, infection, or systemic illness. Given the subjective nature of one's pain experience, language concordance between patient and provider likely plays a large role in management. In cases such as this with neuropathic pain, the presence of normal-appearing structures renders the clinician reliant on the patient's description of their pain history for diagnosis and management. Asking appropriate questions to obtain specific, meaningful, patient-reported descriptors accurately describing the pain followed by adequate provider understanding that leads to a clear and useful explanation of findings and treatment plan can be difficult, even when language is concordant between patient and provider.

## LANGUAGE ACCESS AND WORKFORCE CONSIDERATIONS
### Orofacial Pain Practice Areas and Service Populations

Access to quality OFP care is a challenge, and language barriers further complicate many aspects of the care continuum. OFP is a relatively "young" specialty within dentistry, which began in 1975, and only became recognized by the American Dental Association in 2020.[30,31] Consequently, OFP specialists are not only few in number but primarily located in metropolitan cities. As of April 2022, the American Board of Orofacial Pain (ABOP) lists 264 board-certified OFP providers in the United States.[32] **Fig. 2** demonstrates the distribution of board-certified OFP specialists, showing a predominance of providers in major cities and along the coastlines. It is worth noting that this map only features board-certified OFP providers, whereas other dentists may still practice OFP. In addition, there are currently 13 OFP training programs located in 10 large, US metropolitan areas (see **Fig. 2**). It is estimated that 80.7% of the US population lives in urban areas,[33] a plausible explanation for the predominance of OFP specialists in major cities.

### Orofacial Pain Practice Models

In addition to the total number of specialists and their geographic distribution, the type of practice model also affects language access. OFP practice models include, but are not limited to, hospital-based practice (such as with this case), dental school-based practice, solo private practice, group practice with multiple OFP providers, group practice with other dentists and specialists, and group practice with nondental providers specializing in pain (eg, physicians, physical therapists, and psychologists). Minimal data exists on the types and frequency of OFP practice models; however, offering language assistance services in solo or small group practice settings can be difficult,[34] whereas larger hospital-based and dental school-based practices (often with training programs and greater resources) are generally better equipped to offer such services.[35]

### Equipping the Workforce: Orofacial Pain Training Programs

As noted previously, there are only 13 OFP training programs in the United States. (12 of which are currently accredited.) Although there are no accreditation requirements specific to managing patients with LEP in order to graduate from dental school, all dental students "must be competent in managing a diverse patient population and

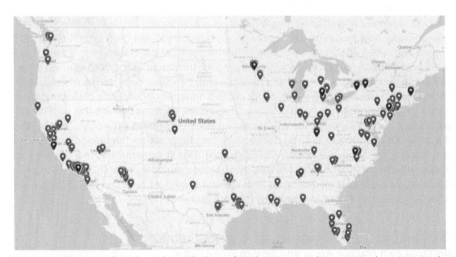

**Fig. 2.** Distribution of (A) board-certified, orofacial pain specialist practice locations in the United States according to the American Board of Orofacial Pain and (B) US-based orofacial pain training programs.

have the interpersonal and communications skills to function successfully in a multicultural work environment" (Standard 2–17).[36] The Accreditation Standards (Standards) for Advanced Dental Education Programs in Orofacial Pain clearly require all OFP residency programs to include training related to the basic mechanisms and the anatomic, physiologic, neurologic, vascular, behavioral, and psychosocial aspects of OFP.[37] However, unlike the standards for predoctoral dental curricula, issues of health literacy, effective patient-provider communication, and working with diverse patient populations are not explicitly written into the standards for OFP residency programs.[37] Although cultural competency is included as an example of evidence to demonstrate compliance with Standard 3-8 (The program must show evidence of an ongoing *faculty* development process.), there is no specific mention of OFP trainees.

Furthermore, the results of a 2016 survey of academic deans assessing interpreter services at US dental school clinics indicated that the proportion of patients with LEP treated at dental schools was perceived to be higher than that of the general population.[38] A subsequent 2017 survey of dental students found that a large proportion of dental students (46%) do not consider adequately prepared to manage LEP patients following graduation.[39] Given this curricular gap in predoctoral dental education, it is imperative that the OFP training programs intentionally set out to train residents to effectively treat patients with LEP.

### Other Considerations: the Current State of Language Access

The COVID-19 pandemic significantly influenced health care in a myriad of ways. Pandemics have historically had a disproportionate impact on vulnerable populations,[40] and this unfortunate pattern has persisted with the COVID-19 pandemic.[41–43] Specific to language access, the pandemic magnified the many challenges in providing equitable, culturally and linguistically appropriate care to patients with LEP. Although the use of an in-person interpreter is often considered ideal,[44] heightened safety precautions in healthcare settings coupled with hierarchical provisioning of personal protective equipment resulted in a rapid increase in demand for and use of remote interpreter services—impacting not only patients and their families but the interpreter services profession.[45]

In this case, remote interpreter services had been preferentially used for ambulatory care since March 2020 due to hospital social distancing policies. Telephonic interpreter services were attempted during the first visit; however, the patient's daughter, who also speaks Vietnamese and serves as the patient's health-care proxy, reported poor interpretation via the service and requested to personally interpret for her mother, to which her mother agreed. Although the use of qualified interpreters is recommended, an individual with LEP has a right to decline such services. Section 1557 Final Rule (revised in 2020) maintains that when interpreters are needed, interpretation must still be accurate, timely, and free of charge, and individuals with LEP cannot be required to bring their own interpreter or rely on a minor child or accompanying adult to interpret.[46] As noted in our case, language assistance services were offered and subsequently declined. Perceived competence of the interpreter by the patient and her daughter was lacking in this case. Interpretation in the interdisciplinary field of OFP requires a unique skillset that draws on many health disciplines. Future research on interpreter training and services in oral health settings, specifically OFP, is warranted.

### SUMMARY

In the case presented, significant communication challenges influenced the diagnosis and management of this patient with LEP who was suffering from neuropathic facial pain.

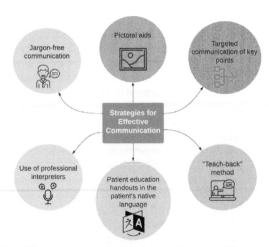

**Fig. 3.** Strategies for effective communication in health-care settings.

Before her initial visit to the OFP clinic, the need for language assistance was identified via preferred language (Vietnamese) documentation in her medical record. Qualified, remote (telephonic) interpreter services were procured, offered free of charge, and ready for use.

Unfortunately, inaccurate interpretation (per her daughter's report) by the interpreter services company resulted in reliance on a family member for all future communication. Consequently, obtaining a thorough pain history regarding the onset, quality, intensity, and frequency of pain was challenging. Her daughter reported difficulty understanding, and thus interpreting, the doses her mother tried and for how long she took each medication before discontinuing—further enhancing the difficulty in obtaining an accurate history.

Qualified healthcare interpreters (a) ought to have appropriate training to interpret with skill and accuracy (although this case brings into question the definition of "appropriate training"), (b) are assessed for professional skills, and (c) are required to adhere to an ethical code.[47] They are trained to be objective and neutral and speak directly on behalf of the patient.[48] Although the use of ad hoc interpreters, such as family members and friends, is generally discouraged due to the lack of confirmed: (a) neutrality, (b) confidentiality, and (c) knowledge of complex dental/medical terminology. Furthermore, general language fluency does not always equate to proficiency in interpreting complex health information. As noted in this case, ad hoc interpretation was preferred over "qualified" language assistance services offered by the hospital. Although professional interpreter services were ultimately declined in this case, it is still critically important for clinicians to (1) consistently use effective communication strategies (**Fig. 3**) across all language proficiency levels and (2) use recommended strategies for working with various types of interpretation (**Fig. 4**).

Language access protections existed before the COVID-19 pandemic.[35] Although language access policies exist to protect individuals with LEP from discrimination, implementation varies and oversight is limited—particularly within the dental profession.[35] Policy-driven motivation is limited, at best. Regardless of whether a specific policy is required of one's clinical practice, language and communication needs directly affect patient care, particularly pain care, thus solidifying the critical role language access plays in OFP. Providing patient-centered care that is culturally and

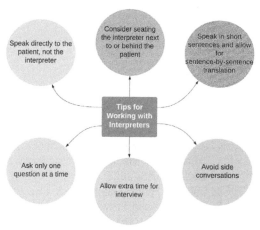

**Fig. 4.** Tips for working with interpreters in the clinical setting.

linguistically appropriate in the OFP practice setting is of utmost importance to care quality and treatment outcomes.

## CLINICAL CARE POINTS
### Conduct a Language Needs Assessment

Determine which languages your patients are most comfortable speaking and reading, and assess whether your current language assistance options meet those needs. Identify unmet needs by systematically asking the preferred language in which your patients would prefer to receive their OFP care on your intake form.

### Train all Members of Your OFP Team

Establish practice policies for working with LEP individuals, and train your team on effective communication practices, cultural competency, respectful assessment and documentation of preferred language and interpreter needs, and working with interpreters.

*Identify which language assistance options are most reasonable to offer in your practice.* Given language assistance services are required to be of no-cost to the patient, implementation can be challenging. Prioritize resources according to the languages most commonly used by your patients. Language assistance options might include: (a) hiring staff who reflect the linguistic and cultural diversity of your community, (b) designating time blocks in the schedule for when appropriate interpreter services are available, and (c) contracting with an interpreter services company to provide remote interpreter services.

### Working with Interpreters

Individuals with LEP cannot be required to bring their own interpreter or rely on a minor child or accompanying adult to interpret. Although multilingual providers and/or staff members can interpret if they have adequate skills and training, it is important to remember that general language fluency does not always equate to proficiency in interpreting complex health information.

**DISCLOSURE**

The authors have nothing to disclose.

**REFERENCES**

1. Table ID. S1601: Language Spoken at Home. American Community Survey 5-Year Estimates, 2016 – 2020. U.S. Census Bureau. Available at: https://data.census.gov/cedsci/table?q=S1601&tid=ACSST5Y2020.S1601. Accessed April 30, 2022.
2. Limited English Proficiency: Commonly Asked Questions. U.S. Department of Justice, Civil Rights Division. Available at: https://www.lep.gov/commonly-asked-questions. Accessed April 15, 2022.
3. National Action Plan to Improve Health Literacy. U.S. Department of Health and Human Services – Office of Disease Prevention and Health Promotion. 2010. Available at: https://health.gov/our-work/national-health-initiatives/health-literacy/national-action-plan- improve-health-literacy. Accessed April 30, 2022.
4. Improving Health Literacy Could Prevent Nearly 1 Million Hospital Visits and Save Over $25 Billion a Year. Available at: https://www.unitedhealthgroup.com/content/dam/UHG/PDF/About/Health-Literacy-Brief.pdf. Accessed April 30, 2022.
5. Berkman ND, Sheridan SL, Donahue KE, et al. Low health literacy and health outcomes: an updated systematic review. Ann Intern Med 2011;155(2):97–107.
6. Kutner M, Greenberg E, Jin Y, et al. The health literacy of America's adults: results from the 2003 national assessment of adult literacy (NCES 2006–483). Washington, DC: U.S. Department of Education - National Center for Education Statistics; 2006.
7. Healthy People 2030: Framework. U.S. Department of Health and Human Services, Office of Disease Prevention and Health Promotion. Available at: https://health.gov/healthypeople/about/healthy-people-2030-framework. Accessed April 30, 2022.
8. Increase the proportion of adults with limited English proficiency who say their providers explain things clearly — HC/HIT-D11. U.S. Department of Health and Human Services - Office of Disease Prevention and Health Promotion. Available at: https://health.gov/healthypeople/objectives-and-data/browse-objectives/health- communication/increase-proportion-adults-limited-english-proficiency-who-say-their-providers- explain-things-clearly-hchit-d11. Accessed April 30, 2022.
9. Oral Conditions. US Department of Health and Humans Services - Office of Disease Prevention and and Health Promotion. Available at: https://health.gov/healthypeople/objectives-and-data/browse-objectives/oral-conditions. Accessed April 30, 2022.
10. Frequently Asked Questions on Legal Requirements to Provide Language Access Services. Migration Policy Institute. https://www.migrationpolicy.org/programs/language%C2%A0access-translation-and-interpretation-policies-and-practices/frequently-asked. Accessed April 29, 2022.
11. CLAS Standards. U.S. Department of Health and Human Services. Available at: https://thinkculturalhealth.hhs.gov/clas/standards. Accessed April 30, 2022.
12. 42 U.S.C. 2000d.
13. Chen AH, Youdelman MK, Brooks J. The legal framework for language access in healthcare settings: Title VI and beyond. *J Gen Intern Med* Nov 2007;22(Suppl 2): 362–7.

14. Youdelman M. Summary of State Law Requirements Addressing Language Needs in Health Care. National Health Law Program. Available at: https://healthlaw.org/resource/summary-of-state-law-requirements-addressing-language-needs- in-health-care-2/. Accessed April 15, 2022.
15. Flores G, Abreu M, Barone CP, et al. Errors of medical interpretation and their potential clinical consequences: a comparison of professional versus ad hoc versus no interpreters. Ann Emerg Med 2012;60(5):545–53.
16. Wisnivesky JP, Krauskopf K, Wolf MS, et al. The association between language proficiency and outcomes of elderly patients with asthma. Ann Allergy Asthma Immunol 2012;109(3):179–84.
17. Gany F, Leng J, Shapiro E, et al. Patient satisfaction with different interpreting methods: a randomized controlled trial. J Gen Intern Med 2007;22(Suppl 2):312–8.
18. Khan A, Yin HS, Brach C, et al. Association Between Parent Comfort With English and Adverse Events Among Hospitalized Children. JAMA Pediatr 2020;174(12):e203215.
19. Wasserman M, Renfrew MR, Green AR, et al. Identifying and preventing medical errors in patients with limited English proficiency: key findings and tools for the field. J Healthc Qual 2014;36(3):5–16.
20. Tseng W, Pleasants E, Ivey SL, et al. Barriers and Facilitators to Promoting Oral Health Literacy and Patient Communication among Dental Providers in California. Int J Environ Res Public Health 2020;18(1).
21. Karliner LS, Jacobs EA, Chen AH, et al. Do professional interpreters improve clinical care for patients with limited English proficiency? A systematic review of the literature. Health Serv Res 2007;42(2):727–54.
22. Tang AS, Kruger JF, Quan J, et al. From admission to discharge: patterns of interpreter use among resident physicians caring for hospitalized patients with limited english proficiency. J Health Care Poor Underserved 2014;25(4):1784–98.
23. Schenker Y, Perez-Stable EJ, Nickleach D, et al. Patterns of interpreter use for hospitalized patients with limited English proficiency. J Gen Intern Med 2011;26(7):712–7.
24. Bagchi AD, Dale S, Verbitsky-Savitz N, et al. Examining effectiveness of medical interpreters in emergency departments for Spanish- speaking patients with limited English proficiency: results of a randomized controlled trial. Ann Emerg Med 2011;57(3):248–256 e1-4.
25. Karliner LS, Perez-Stable EJ, Gregorich SE. Convenient Access to Professional Interpreters in the Hospital Decreases Readmission Rates and Estimated Hospital Expenditures for Patients With Limited English Proficiency. Med Care 2017;55(3):199–206.
26. Ngo-Metzger Q, Sorkin DH, Phillips RS, et al. Providing high-quality care for limited English proficient patients: the importance of language concordance and interpreter use. J Gen Intern Med 2007;22(Suppl 2):324–30.
27. Rogers AH, Bakhshaie J, Orr MF, et al. Health Literacy, Opioid Misuse, and Pain Experience Among Adults with Chronic Pain. Pain Med 2020;21(4):670–6.
28. Riley JL 3rd, Gibson E, Zsembik BA, et al. Acculturation and orofacial pain among Hispanic adults. J Pain 2008;9(8):750–8.
29. Jimenez N, Dansie E, Buchwald D, et al. Pain among older Hispanics in the United States: is acculturation associated with pain? Pain Med 2013;14(8):1134–9.
30. Heir GM. Orofacial pain, the 12th specialty: The necessity. J Am Dent Assoc 2020;151(7):469–71.

31. AAOP History. American Academy of Orofacial Pain. Available at: https://aaop. org/history/. Accessed April 30, 2022.

32. ABOP Diplomate Search. https://www.abop.net/search/default.asp. Accessed April 20, 2022.

33. Urban Areas Facts. United States Census Bureau. https://www.census.gov/ programs-surveys/geography/guidance/geo-areas/urban-rural/ua-    facts.html. Accessed April 30, 2022.

34. 68 FR 47311.

35. Holland N. A Historical Overview of Language Access in Dentistry: The Impact of Language Access Protections on Oral Health Care. J Calif Dental Assoc 2021; 49(12):749–56.

36. Accreditation Standards For Dental Education Programs. Committee on Dental Accreditation. 2021. Available at: https://coda.ada.org/~/media/CODA/Files/ predoc_standards.pdf?la=en. Accessed April 30, 2022.

37. Commission on Dental Accreditation. Accreditation Standards for Advanced Dental Education Programs in Orofacial Pain. 2020. Available at: https://coda. ada.org/~/media/CODA/Files/Orofacial_Pain_Standards.pdf?la=en.    Accessed April 30, 2022.

38. Simon L, Hum L, Nalliah R. Access to Interpreter Services at U.S. Dental School Clinics.Educ, 2016. J Dent Educ 2016;80(1):51–7.

39. Simon L, Hum L, Nalliah R. Training to Care for Limited English Proficient Patients and Provision of Interpreter Services at U.S. Dental School Clinics. J Dent Educ 2017;81(2):169–77.

40. Wade L. From Black Death to fatal flu, past pandemics show why people on the margins suffer most. Science 2020. https://doi.org/10.1126/science.abc7832.

41. Woolf SH, Masters RK, Aron LY. Effect of the covid-19 pandemic in 2020 on life expectancy across populations in the USA and other high income countries: simulations of provisional mortality data. BMJ 2021;373:n1343.

42. L Hill SA. COVID-19 Cases and Deaths by Race/Ethnicity: Current Data and Changes Over Time. Kaiser Family Foundation. Available at: https://www.kff. org/coronavirus-    covid-19/issue-brief/covid-19-cases-and-deaths-by-race-ethnicity-current-data-and-changes- over-time. Accessed April 30, 2022.

43. Data from: COVID Data Tracker. Centers for Disease Control and Prevention. Available at: https://covid.cdc.gov/covid-data-tracker. Accessed April 30, 2022.

44. Betancourt JR, RM, Green AR, et al. Improving patient safety systems for patients with limited English proficiency: a guide for hospitals. Rockville, MD: Agency for Healthcare Research and Quality; 2012.

45. NCIHC Research Work Group. Remote Interpreting Challenges During the Covid-19 Pandemic. Access: the NCIHC Journal. National Council on Interpreting in Health Care. 2022. Available at: https://heyzine.com/flip-book/6b2a493290. html#page/14. Accessed April 19, 2022.

46. 85 FR 371602020

47. FAQ - Healthcare Professionals. National Council on Interpreting in Health Care. Available at: https://www.ncihc.org/faq-healthcare-professionals. Accessed April 30, 2022.

48. Rimmer A. Can patients use family members as non-professional interpreters in consultations? BMJ 2020;368:m447.

# *Moving?*

## Make sure your subscription moves with you!

To notify us of your new address, find your **Clinics Account Number** (located on your mailing label above your name), and contact customer service at:

**Email: journalscustomerservice-usa@elsevier.com**

**800-654-2452** (subscribers in the U.S. & Canada)
**314-447-8871** (subscribers outside of the U.S. & Canada)

**Fax number: 314-447-8029**

**Elsevier Health Sciences Division**
**Subscription Customer Service**
**3251 Riverport Lane**
**Maryland Heights, MO 63043**

Printed and bound by CPI Group (UK) Ltd, Croydon, CR0 4YY

03/10/2024

01040469-0002